SPORTS MEDICINE

(Curious Queries)

Dr. P.K. Pande

KHEL SAHITYA KENDRA
7/26, Ansari Road, Daryaganj
New Delhi-110002

Published by:
KHEL SAHITYA KENDRA
7/26, Ansari Road, Darya Ganj, New Delhi-110002
Ph.: (O) 011-65190343, 43551324, 42564726
(M) 9811088729, (Fax) 011-42564726
(Res.) 011-47091605
E-mail: khelsahitya1@rediffmail.com
Website: www.khelsahitya.com

ISBN : 978-81-7524-149-7

PRINTED IN INDIA 2026

Laser Typeset by:
ROYAL GRAPHICS
Delhi

Printed by:
ASIAN OFFSET PRINTERS,
Delhi

CONTENTS

CHAPTER 1
DO YOU KNOW

Q.1 Please, list the main items of Sports Medicine.

Ans. a) Medical treatment of Injuries and illnesses.

b) Medical advice on life style and athletic nutrition.

c) Scientifically-based control of training.

d) Medical check-up before starting a sport to detect any damage which could be worsened by the sport.

e) Performance investigation to assess the performance capacity and Heart, circulation, respiration, metabolism and the skeletal musculature.

f) Performance diagnosis specific to the type of sport.

g) Medical assistance in developing optional training method.

Q.2 What definition Council of Europe has given for Sports Medicine.

Ans. In 1973 the Definition given is as under :-
"The application of the art and science of medicine from a prenentive and therapeutic point of view to the practice of sports and physical activity in order to utilize the opportunities afforded by sports for maintaining or improving health and to avoid dangers."

Q.3. Is it possible to define the word 'Sports Medicine'?

Ans. The strict definition of this area of medical practice is made difficult by the fact that many designations are historically rather than logically developed. There is also considerable overlapping of research interests and clinical practices among the different fields. Since it has developed gradually, though sporadically, over a period of 2500 years, and draws upon many scientific and non-scientific areas of inquiry and practice, attempts to define it are considerably hampered by both the factors. Though sports medicine includes the word 'medicine', its practice is by no means restricted to physicians. At the field site, it is mostly practised by sports officer or coaches.

Q.4. What is the origin of term 'Sports Medicine'?

Ans. It appears to be in February, 1928, during the Second Olympic Winter Games at St. Moritz, Switzerland, where medical doctors W. Knoll of Switzerland and F. Laterjet of France called together 33 physicians who were attending the games with the teams of eleven nations. They established a committee to draw a plan for the First International Congress of Sports Medicine, to take place in Amsterdam during the games of the IX Olympiad in August the same year. It was also decided to propose and plan to set up an organization to work as a permanent International assembly on Sports Medicine.

Q.5. What are the three principal purposes in first constitution of Sports Medicine?

Ans. They are the following :

1. To inaugurate scientific research in biology, psychology and sociology in relation to sports.
2. To promote the study of medical problems encountered in physical exercises and sports in collaboration with various international sports federations.
3. To organise international congress on sports medicine.

Q.6. What can be the latest definition of Sports Medicine ?

Ans. In a nutshell, it can be said :

"To create a positive environment, an athlete converts his all genetic potentialities into the phenotypes realities." Dr. P.K. Pande.

In a very simple way Dr. Alok Ghosh has mentioned, "The application of medical science and arts i.e., theory, practice and research, for sports on healthy and handicapped human beings, to maintain positive health and to avoid any physical damage connected with hyper-activities, in order to devise ways and means for adequate, effective prevention, therapy and rehabilitation measures as well as, sensible and scientific improvements of performing capabilities in stages, in all age groups."

Q.7. In what proportions the various medical and other designations may be clubbed together for Sports Medicine ?

Ans. In India where limited resources are available, it may comparise of :

10% Orthopaedics;	Internal or general medicine, viz, first aid and resuscitation;
10% Psychology;	Nutrition and Hygiene;
10% Physiology	Individual and team medical care;
10% Physical Medicine	Fatigue factors;
10% Massage/physiotherapy and the rest, i.e., 50%	Gastro-Intestinal and environmental issues, e.g., heat, cold, underwater or encompasses altitude training or acclimatisation; drugs and dopes; sex problems etc.

Where experts are available, the most important aspect of athletic injury and preventive sports medicine makes 50% of total sports medicine coverage.

Q.8. What is the role of Sports Medicine ?

Ans. The very processes by which physical fitness is achieved may give rise to pathological conditions of the kind and another which remain outside the scope of 'normal' clinical practice. It is with these special problems that sports medicine is concerned in the same way as Geriatrics is concerned with the special problems of old age, or paediatrics with the peculiarities of diseases in the children.

A British doctor has commented, "We (doctors) are so concerned in our clinics with the grossly subnormal, that slightly disabled by usual standards, are apt to receive scanty attention, yet to the athlete himself as light disability a great deal." At this level role of sports medicine expert is important to solve the problems of athletes in practice.

Q.9. In the same way, what you mean by Sports Psysiology?

Ans. The use of Phychological knowledge to enhance the development, performance and the personal satisfaction of athletes and others associated with sports, such as coaches and sports officers. An idea and knowledge about basic assumption is that there is a model form of athletic preparation behaviour which should be followed in order to produce or help maximum performances.

Q.10. Can you define 'Sports Biomechanics' also ?

Ans. It is the study of human motion in Sports, in which the knowledge and methods of mechanics are applied to the structure and functions of the human system.

Q.11. What is Physical conditioning ?

Ans. Physical conditioning is the development of motor qualities to the desired level with acquired magnitude of emphasis on particular motor qualities in view of the requirements of the game concerned and also keeping in view the limitations of the sportsman concerned. It may be divided into 2 parts-general and specific.

Q.12. What is 'FIMS'?

Ans. It is the changed name of 'Federation International medico-Sportive et Scientifique', where 'Scientifique' word is dropped. It was done during second congress (1933)

Q.13. What is IASM ?

Ans. In the year 1970, Prof. G.La Cava desired that in India a branch should be formed under name of 'Indian Association of Sports Medicine'. Initially its headquarter was at Calcutta. Later on it was shifted to Patiala.

Q.14. What do you understand by word 'Athlete' ?

Ans. The Athlete is one who takes part in those activities of running, walking, jumping and throwing which for the programme of track and field events are collectively known as 'Athletics'. But the definition must be more universal, and embrace all who strive for victory in feats of strength, speed, endurance or agility, and who train their bodies to this end.

Q.15. What is the concept of Sports Medicine ?

Ans. Ryan has indicated that the concept of Sports Medicine consists of :

— medical supervision of the athlete;
— special (adapted) physical education;
— the rapeutic exercise;
— exercise in the prevention of chronic degenerative diseases.

Q.16. What is exercise Physiology or Sports Physiology ?

Ans. The study of how the body functions, adopts to changes during exercise, sports, games and other physical activity.

Q.17. What is the role of Subcommission on 'Sports Medicine and orthopaedics'?

Ans.
1. It takes part in the fight against doping.
2. Alongwith the Boxing Federations, it has carried out a study, which has brought out a study complete revision of the rules in order to provide greater protection to the boxers.
3. It has the task of studying and eliminating the dangers relating to certain sports.
4. It works closely with subcommission on coordination with the NOG.

Q.18. What is Athletic Trainer ?

Ans. A person with specific qualifications who, upon the advice and consent of his sports physician, carries out the practice of prevention and on physical rehabilitation of injuries incurred by athletes. To carry out these functions, the athletic trainer is authorised to use physical modalities such as heat, light, sound, cold, electricity or mechanical devices related to rehabilitation and treatment. For the time being, in our country this work may be taken from qualified Coach or Director Physical Education after giving him orientation in Sports Physiotherapy.

Q.19. What are the common functions that fall into the category of Athletic Trainer ?

Ans. In the true sense, an athletic trainer, who may also be a sports physiotherapist, is likely to carry on the following functions:

— prevention of athletic trauma or conditions that adversely affect the health or the performance of the athlete.

— management (first aid, evaluation, treatment and rehabilitation) of athletic trauma or other medical problems that affect the athlete.

— counselling of the athlete in various health related areas such as.

— nutrition.

— relaxation and tension control.
— personal health habits.

Q.20. Explain in details the meaning and role of team physician ?

Ans. Team Physician directly supervises the athletic trainer, and advises on the over all conditioning programme. He is responsible for performing or collecting and reviewing the pre-participation physical evaluation, and making the final determination of fitness for participation.

The team physician provides medical coverage for competitive events especially contact Sports, supplying emergency evaluation, treatment and triage of athletic injuries and illness. He also will provide primary call of athletic injuries or arrange referrals to the family physician or specialist consultants as indicated. Additionally, he oversees or establishes the guidelines and procedures for trainer personnal to respond to emergencies and can suggest emergency equipment needed.

Following injury or illness, the team physician is responsible for insuring that rehabilitation has been adequate. He should assess the athlete for readiness to return to activity.

Finally the team physician should educate coaches, trainees, administrators, athletes and parents regarding the medical aspects of sports.

Q.21. Mention the members of team approach ?

Ans.
1. Team physician.
2. Certified athletic trainer.
3. Coaches.
4. Student athletic trainers.
5. Resident physicians.
6. Athletic administrators.

Q.22. What is "Athletic Triangle" ?

Ans. It consists of athlete, coach and parents. The advantage of this triangle is to reduce the situational stress for the athlete and plan the stress management training programme for an athlete to help him in acquiring cognitive and physiological copying skills.

Q.23. What are the expected functions an Athletic Trainer in Schools ?

Ans. He or she interacts with school administrators, equipment supply staff, school physician, nurse, paramedical staff, teachers, parents and athletes. His/her primary responsibility may be considered in the following four areas :-

— Injury prevention among school children;
— First aid and emergency care;
— Treatment and rehabilitation;
— Programme Administration.

Q.24. How can Athletic Trainer provide treatment and rehabilitation for athletes ?

Ans. First aid measure is corner stone of rehabilitation control and prevention of haemorrhaged, effusion, oedema, inflammatory reaction, and spasm of skeletal muscles, reduce the damage to injured area. It also helps in earlier return to full safe participation.

Since he/she is skilled in using electro-and hydrotherapy equipments, so with the guidance of medical expert, injured area is treated. Trainer should also initiate a planned programme of reconditioning exercises to retain and restore range of motion, strength, power and endurance.

Since these people have thorough understanding of the special needs of the athlete, they can develop programmes to meet the athlete's unique demands, which usually are far greater than those of a non-athlete with similar type of injury. Such paramedical person will individualize the care to meet the needs of athletes in each sport, some of which may have specific physical requirements.

Q.25. What are the expected duties of Sports Health Centre ?

Ans. This concept is yet to develop in our country. It may have the following services of functions :

1. Preventive programmes for various types of athletic endeavours.
2. Athletic first aid and emergency care.
3. Evaluation and diagnostic services.

4. Non-surgical treatment.
5. Referral services when appropriate.
6. Rehabilitation to injured.
7. Teaching models for utilisation by various curricula in sports medicine field.

The sports centre could provide services to the programmes given below :

— Intercollegiate athletics.
— Intramural athletic club and recreational sports.
— Physical education departments.

Q.26. What is the basic concept of treatment ?

Ans. The following five A's of the treatment should be kept in mind :

1. Accept athletics : The physician should recognize the value of competitive athletics, otherwise, patient-doctor relationship suffers.
2. Avoid expediency : Outside influence must not be permitted to outweighs sound medical judgement. The boy's desire to compete, his fear of falling his team-mates, the parents desire to see their sons excel, the coach's hope that the player is not really hurt. All must be ignored if the proper conclusion is to be reached. The temporary convenience must be sacrificed for the ultimate goal.
3. Adopt the best method for treatment.
4. Act promptly : A definitive decision as to the proper method of treatment must be made at the earliest possible moment and then that method must be carried out according to the facilities available.
5. Achieve perfection : In most of the routine cases, the athlete is basically in a good condition and can well tolerate any reasonable measure if it serves to increase his chances of complete recovery.

Q.27. What is Unifying Principle ?

Ans. If there is one theme that unifies the whole concept of sports medicine, it is the study and observation of man in motion. "By moving express my being."

Q.28. What are the responsibilities of Scientific Commission of FIMS.

Ans. 1. Documentation and publication of position statements regarding specific problems in Sports Medicine.

2. The promotion of Scientific Research.
3. Cooperation with organisers of International sports medicine meetings and events regarding programme planning and the publication of proceedings.
4. Maintenance of contact with other international scientific organization institutions and individual professionals.
5. Cooperation with the editors of the official FIMS publication regarding scientific content of the Journal.

Q.29. How is the membership of FIMS made.

Ans. The membership is made up of honorary members, national associations, invited members, and representatives of the international sports federations. These member constitute the five bodies :

(i) the board of representatives;
(ii) the executive committee;
(iii) the plenary assembly;
(iv) the scientific commission;
(v) the inter-federal medical commission.

Q.30. How is the Plenary Assembly formed ?

Ans. On the occasion of Olympic Games, it meets every four years and consists of :

(i) the members of the executive committee;
(ii) the members of board of representatives;
(iii) the national delegates;
(iv) the four members of the scientific commission designated by executive committee;
(v) three delegates of the international college of sports physicians;
(vi) the delegates of the international groups of sports medicine recognized by FIMS and the delegates of the international institutions that have official dealings with FIMS.

The assembly is presided over by the President of FIMS. Its motion are submitted to the Board of Representatives.

Q.31. When does the Board of Representative meet and what are their exact duties ?

Ans. They meet every two years at the time and place of the International Congress. It is constituted of the delegates of the National Associations of Federations of Sports Medicine at the rate of one per country. The President FIMS presides. The exact duties and responsibilities of this board are not specified in the statutes.

Q.32. How is the Executive Committee formed ?

Ans. It is elected for a period of four years by the Board of Representatives except for the Honorary President who is appointed for the life time. The retiring president remains an ex-officio member. The committee is composed of :

(i) an Honorary President;
(ii) the President of FIMS;
(iii) two Vice-Presidents;
(iv) a Secretary General;
(v) a Treasurer; and
(vi) six members.

This committee meets at least twice annually to debate and decide the general outlines of the activities of FIMS in accordance with the deliberations of the Board Representatives.

Q.33. Explain, how the Scientific Commission is formed.

Ans. It is formed up of the invited members and is directed by the four members chosen by the executive committee, who represent :

(i) the sciences of physiology and biology as applied to sports;
(ii) the practice of sports medicine and sports medical examinations;
(iii) sports traumatology and the prevention of sports accidents; and
(iv) prevention and treatment of thorough physical activities.

Q.34. What can be the preventive functions of sports Medicine centres ?

Ans. They can be arranged like this.

A) Medical supervision and framing of people engage in games and physical activities, with special reference of several going children. It is also applicable to all levels as well as high performance sports. The intension should be enable them to attain the derived levels without endangering their health.

B) Assessment of the state of health and fitness of the individual with an intention to establishing the capacity and directing the concerned person to suitable activity/games/sports/jobs etc.
It should also include training for competition for gifted sportsman and women and courses of fitness or treatment for the others.

C) In relation to Bhartyam, mass participations, application of medical knowledge to Physical movements to gain, conserve and improve health at the level of "sports for All" and to guard against possible hazards example. Diabetic or cardiac rehabilitation care of people of high risk of developing such diseases etc.

D) Active participation in the planning and control of hygiene and safety precautions for all types of sports and facilities.

Q.35. What do you understand by word "Therapeutic Functions"?

Ans. Application of the techniques in the field of traumatology internal medicine, physical medicine as well as physiotherapy for treatment and functional rehabilitations of competitive and recreational athletes, to enable them to resume participation, training or competition as soon as desirable.

Q.36. What are the aims of Scientific Commission ?

Ans. Its aims are to promote research in sports medicine and to study the adaptation of scientific data and issue opinions on questions submitted by the Executive Committee.

Q.37. What is UNESCO ?

Ans. It includes an International Council of Sports and Physical Education. A research committee of this division was organized under the leadership of Professor Emst Joke in 1960 and has held many meetings in different countries since then. An international committee for the standardization of Physical Fitness Testing was organized in 1964 and has prepared a written set of standards to be used in scientific studies of the functional capacities and anthropometry of the world's population.

Q.38. What is CISM ?

Ans. It was founded in 1948 to promote healthful recreation and sports activities in international competition for the world armies. Its membership includes 37 nations. In the year 1970, it sponsored 21 international events, including 13 sports championships involving thousands of athletes. In 1961, an Academy was established which has undertaken research in diet, the medical control of athletes, physiology, philosophy and psychology of sports, coaching, training and physical conditioning. It holds regular conferences and publishes its findings in Sports International, the official CISM managing and leading research journals.

Q.39. Why do we need relationship of Sports Medicine with Exercise Physiology ?

Ans. Over the past 25 years, the members of exercise physiology laboratories have increased tremendously all over the world. As a result of that, much more knowledge dealing with how best to train the athletic team and develop fitness for health has appeared in the recent scientific literatures. More and more people are becoming directly involved in it. Example : American College of Sports Medicine, established in the year 1954, had membership of 2000 from 1954 to 1975, in 1978 it increased to 6000 and now it has crossed 15000. As has been mentioned Sports Medicine is a specialized area of science which deals with medical problems along with other inter-related specialities. For example :

— Athletic Injuries and Rehabilitation,

— Clinical medicine,

— Athletic nutrition,
— Bio-mechanics,
— Sports and Age, growth and development,
— Psycho-social aspects of sports,
— Exercise Physiology and Biochemistry.

This shows that a clear concept of Exercise Physiology is a must for a coach or player.

Q.40. Does the minute alteration in gravity affect the performance in certain athletic events ?

Ans. The influences of differences in gravity with variations in longitude, latitude and altitude, and the lessening of air density with higher altitude are important factors in altering the performance. Usually, intraindividual or biological variability is sufficiently large to obscure the small competitive advantage the athlete would have in the lessened air density and decreased gravitational force.

If we go into the details of theoretical aspect, shot put and long jump world records could be set at the highest possible terrestrial altitude where other competitive conditions are favourable.

The combined effects of decreased air density and resistance (increased take of speed) and lessened gravitational force combined could have made no more than about a 1% or a 4 inch contribution to the long jump record.

It shows that there may be at least theoretical possibility of affected performance due to mild change in gravitational force.

Q.41. Does noise have any effect on player's performance ?

Ans. In a game situation, noise has a complex factor. The cheering and applauses can stimulate the athlete to peak effort, but an inappropriate sound can ruin his concentration. In general, non-associated noise such as ground or air traffic and uncontrolled irrelevant crowd noise detracts the concentration on the event underway. It has been shown that sudden loud noise can facilitate a maximal muscular contraction or body effort. Karate and weight lifters frequently use a self-generated noise to this end.

Q.42. Does attitude affect performance ?

Ans. The force of gravity decreases slightly as one rises above the surface of earth. This tends to favour jumpers and weight-throwers at moderate altitudes. This advantage is very small as compared to the other effects which are produced on performance by the decreased barometric pressure.

Q.43. What do you understand by the word "Sports training" ?

Ans. It is a component of broader phenomenon - sports. In India it appeared, developed and is developing at the movement in unity with other aspects of sports activity. Before going for sports training one must have clear concept of sports.

Q.44. What do you mean by word "Sports" ?

Ans. It can be defined as "competitive activity proper, the specific form of which is a system of competitions, field of physical culture for a society as a special sphere of identifying and comparing human potential in a unified form. But if we go in a bit detail 'sports' does not only mean to achieve purely competitive goals. It is much broader. Sports is an activity which has many sided effects on man and as a sphere of diverse interhuman contacts. It has even a deeper meaning, conditioned in the final analysis by the aggregate of basic social relations of which the given activity is a part. The broader definition can be "the word sport encompasses the competitive activity proper, special preparation for it and specific relations in the sphere of this activity taken as a whole."

Q.45. Can the sports be explained as "Social Phenomenon" ?

Ans. As a many sided social phenomenon, sports is an active factor in physical education, one of the basic forms of preparing a person for labour and other socially necessary types of activity, and alongside this one of the important means of the ethic and aesthetic education, satisfaction of the moral requirements of society, consolidation and expansion of international ties.

Q.46. What is the basic difference between 'sports training' and 'training on athlete' ?

Ans. Though these two notions coincide in many aspects but are not similar. The second notion is broader both in scope and content and, therefore, can serve as one of the starting points in defining the notion 'sports' training. Athlete's training is a multi sided process of the expedient use of aggregate factors (means, methods and conditions) so as to influence the development of an athlete and ensure the necessary level of preparedness.

Q.47. Will you further explain the word 'training of an athlete' ?

Ans. It may include the following :

- — Sports training,
- — Competition (they serve as a means of training),
- — The use of extra training and extra competition factors supplementing and intensifying training and competition of speeding up the rehabilitation process after loads.

Q.48. Now explain the word sports training in the light of previous answer.

Ans. It is the basic form of an athlete's training. It is a systematic preparation organised with the help of exercises which in fact are pedagogically organised process of controlling an athlete's development, i.e. his sporting perfection. The course of fundamentals of sports training is an aggregate of the generalised knowledge concerning an athlete's preparation being realised in its main form-in the form of training. The course is aimed at identifying the most essential traits, the main contents and the requirements of planning and training-common for various sports.

Q.49. Will you highlight the importance and need of rest during training ?

Ans. During the training process rest is essential. Rest may be regarded as a truly organic component part of training only when it is organised in correspondence with its regularities. An excessive brief or on the contrary, excessively prolonged rest violates the training structure and turns in such cases into a factor of over-training or detraining. This is the reason that rest is to be given in optimum amount and duration. Rest, whether active or passive, has two main functions in training :

(a) It ensures the rehabilitation of work capacity after training loads and thus allows their repetition;
(b) It serves as one of the means of the optimisation of the load effect.

The more rationale use of both components is to be taken into consideration.

Q.50. How the rest is given as a rehabilitation during a training process ?

Ans. The rest in the training process is rationalised with the help of such means as the use of its various forms (including the shifting over to another form of activity from the one that caused fatigue); combining variants of active and passive rest introducing intervals between a series of exercises, elements of psycho-regulating training aimed at calming and toning up an athlete, rehabilitating massage, thermal treatment.

Example : A brief warning in sauna during the interval of swimming exercises.

The direct aim of training is not rest but the achievement of the optimal training effect. The dosage of rest is subordinated to it.

Q.51. What do you understand by continuity by the Training Process ?

Ans. Continuity, as the regularity of the training process in sports, is characterised by the following :

(a) The intervals between the training sessions are kept to the limits guaranteeing a steady development of the training level in the general tendency.
(b) Physical training is in fact a chain of year round and many year sessions, ensuring maximum effect of the sport specialization.
(c) The bond between the links of this process is ensured on the basis of continuity of the immediate, delayed and accumulative training effect.

Q.52. What do you understand by Cyclic Nature of Training Process ?

Ans. Full training process is built in the form of cycles, i.e. from childhood to adult. These can be divided in three broad categories:

— small or microcycles, i.e. weekly :

— middle or mesocycles, i.e. monthly ;

— large or macrocycles, i.e. yearly.

There may be another type of cycles of four years duration (Olympic) though so far their structure has not as yet been sufficiently studied. The cycles in this sense are a universal form of planning the training. This is exactly at what the principle of the cyclic nature of the training process is aimed at:

Q.53. Elaborate the principle of cyclic nature of training process ?

Ans. It can be explained under the following heads :

(a) As a rule it can be said that cyclic nature is expressed in these requirements. Its content is revealed more concretely in the detailed analysis of the structural foundations of the planning of the training process.

(b) To adjust the training loads as adopted to the regularities of the change of training phases, stages, and periods (micro, meso and macrocycles).

(c) While planning the training to proceed from the necessity to systematic, repeat the basic elements of its content and at the same time consecutively change the training assignments in correspondence with the logic of sequence of the phases, stages and periods of the training process.

(d) While solving the problems, the expedient use of the methods of training to find for them a corresponding place in the structure of the training cycle i.e. any training exercise, means and methods no matter how good in themselves, lose their effectiveness if not used timely, or used out of place without taking into account the specifics of training phases and periods.

(e) Any fragment of training process in its inter-relation with the bigger and lesser forms of the cyclic training structure taking into account that the structure of the microcycles, for instance, is greatly determined by their place in the structure of the average cycles, while the structure of the average cycles is conditioned, on the one hand, by the peculiarities of their microcycles and, on the other, by their place in the macrocycle's structure and so on.

Q.54. Give the list of common items expected to be in sports medical kit.

Ans.
— Soap and Sponage
— Wound cleansing solution, for example sterile physiological saline in single use containers, wound and eye douches.
— Disposable kidney dishes.
— First aid bandage.
— Sterile dressing.
— Gauze bandages.
— Cotton wool.
— Elastic bandages and elas top last adhesive bandages.
— Stretch and non-Stretch adhesive tape.
— Plasters and surgical tape.
— Foam rubber and felt.
— Disposable gloves.
— Scissors, forceps and safety pins.
— Oral thermometer.
— Pocket torch.
— Cold Pack or ice.
— Disposable cups.

Medications

— Analgesics such as acetylsalicy lic acid preparations and paracetamol preparation.
— Nasal drops in single dose pack
— Antiseptic/anaesthetic lozenges for sore throat, for eg-benzo-caine lozenges.
— Cough suppress-anls, for eg-1 dextro-methorphan
— Skin ointments to prevent friction sores, water repellent silicone ointments corticos-teroid ointments for the treatment of insects bites' and sun-screen lotins.
— Glucose.

Q.55. Enlist the requirement of sports physicians boys.

Ans.
- — Bandages as per above.
- — Chlorhexidine and surgical spirit.
- — Suturing material, single-luse suture sets.
- — Disposable syrings and needles.
- — Scalpel and scalpel blades.
- — Needle holder, foreps, scissors, clamps.
- — Special forceps for the removal of foreign bodies.
- — Sterile gloves.
- — Sterile covers as required.
- — Stethoscope.
- — Blood pressure cuff.
- — Auroscope and oththalmoscope
- — Tongue dipressors.
- — Rubber spatula for conversions.
- — Pocket torch.

Medications :

- — In addition to those quoted in above
- — Anti-inflammatory analgesics, for examples, neproxen, diclofenac, diflusinal.
- — Analgesics, for examples, morphine
- — Local anasthetics for injection, for example, lignocaine, bupivacaine, bupivacaine with adrenaline.
- — Local anaestheic eye drops.
- — Medications for haemorrhpodijal complaints.
- — Antibiotics.
- — Tranzuillizers and sedatives, for example, diazepam, nitrazepam.
- — Antimotion sickness drugs, tooth short-acting and long-acting.
- — Medications used against allergies and to reduce swelling in head injuries.
- — Anticonvulsants, for example, diazepam emulsion for dogeedbron.
- — Antidiarrhocal preparation for example, loperamide and fluid and salt replacements.
- — Medications for the treatment of gastritis.
- — Medication for used in acute constipation for example, enemas.
- — Eye ointment, for example, chloramphericol.

— Ear ointments, for example, hydro-cortisone with polymyxin B
— Diuretics for use in oedema, for example, bumetanicle.
— Medications used to treat cardiac arrhythmias (anti arrhythmics), for example, Lignocaine (Us : Lidocaine), adrenaline injection or inhalant.
— Medication for use in cardiac neurosis, for example, adrenergic beta-blockers.

CHAPTER 2
HEALTH & FITNESS

Q.1. What is Fitness ?

Ans. It is the state which characterises the degree to which a person is able to function efficiently. Fitness is an individual matter. It implies the ability of each person to live most effectively within his potentialities.

In other words, it may be said that 'the ability to carry out daily tasks with vigour and alertness, without undue fatigue, and with ampleenergy to enjoy leisure time pursuits and to meet unforeseen emergencies. It can be said that the physical fitness is the ability to last, to bear up and to persevere under difficult circumstances where an unfit person would given up. It is the opposite of being fatigued from ordinary efforts, to lacking the energy to enter bestfully into life's and to be exhausted from unexpected exercise demanding physical exertion.

Q.2. Name the components of Physiology of exercise & Physical Fitness.

Ans.
1. Metabolism-Production of energy for work.
2. The muscular system-performance of mechanical work.
3. Circulation and respiration-the oxygen transport system.
4. Nutrition, exercise, and control of body weight.
5. Chronic exercise training-physiological adjustments to regular exercise programmes.
6. Exercise training techniques-exercise programs designed to increase fitness levels.
7. Tests of fitness-evaluation of exercise training programmes.

Q.3. In the modern context what are the parameters of fitness ?

Ans. Thomas has identified the following parameters :
- — The ability to exert force-strength.
- — Along with optimum degree of joint mobility, the ability to react or move quickly-speed.

— To maintain function over time-stamina.
— To achieve sport objectives, the ability to select and execute by effective and efficient methods-skill.
— To have optimally motivated performance-spirit.
— According to him the Sports Medicine-The avoidance or minimising of injurious effects of competition and training stress.

Q.4. How can the sports stress be classified ?

Ans. It can be said as normal and abnormal streess.

The normal stress may be further subdivided into two i.e.

(a) Inherent in performance. Exacerbated by increased performance and catered for by increased fitness.

(b) Extrinsic to performance : Break down through lack of fitness and external unanticipated forces. To avoid abnormal stress is very difficult but general avoidance skill may be developed in training. It means development of awareness to danger, practice of avoidance manoeuvres and effective use of stress absorption techniques.

Q.5. How can be Fitness be explained ?

Ans. Fitness is the ability of an individual to live a happy and well balanced life. It involves not only physical but intellectual, emotional, social and spiritual aspects of an individual also. Interaction and interdependence of these phases of man's health or such that any deviation from normal in any aspect of these components of fitness will make an individual unable to meet the demands placed on him by his work or way of life.

Q.6. How can one assess his own fitness by asking certain simple question ?

Ans. A person who participates regularly in a well designed exercise programme should experience very few, if any, the following questions and should develop and maintain an optimum level of health, performance and appearance.

— Do you yawn regularly throughout the day ?
— Do you feel tired when you wake up in the morning?
— Do you Often not really want to get out of the bed ?
— Do you become fatigued from tasks requiring minimal energy, such as climbing a flight of stairs, walking

around a shopping complex ?

- Do you run out of energy by the middle of the day or early afternoon ?
- Do you experience a drowsy feeling during a long span of the day ?
- Do you fall asleep early in the evening while reading or watching television ?
- Do you experience difficulty in coping with daily pressures ?
- Do you experience nagging aches and pains ?
- Do you find it difficult to relax ?
- Do you have an irritable disposition towards others ?
- Are you vulnerable to variety of health problems, such as frequent cold and back pains ?
- Do you generally lack energy and vitality ?

Q.7. How will you explain the strength component ?

Ans. It is the ability of muscle or muscle group to exert force against a resistance. Strength is determined by measuring the maximal one time force that can be exerted. This is referred to as one repetition maximal.

Each person needs a certain level of strength. Without this, it would be impossible to carry out most of the simple tasks that are necessary each day. It is interesting to note that approximately 95% of average Indian college girls lack sufficient strength to do one regular pull-up.

Q.8. What do you understand by muscular endurance ?

Ans. It is the ability of a muscle or muscle group to apply force repeatedly for a period of time(isotonic) or to sustain a contraction for a period of time without movement (isometric). Here number of sittings may be counted for a given time.

Q.9. What is flexibility ?

Ans. The most important injury prevention tool is flexibility of the players. It is the capacity of a joint or joints to move through a full range of motion. The amount of movement possible is usually determined by the length of the muscles, ligaments, tendons and the structure of the joint Players must be able to bend, stretch, and twist and to possess a full range of movement if they are to function effeciently each day. It is interesting to note that people with poor flexibility tend to be accident-prone and to tire very quickly when performing simple task such as walking.

Q.10. How lack of flexibility harmful to body ?

Ans. Owing to exercise strain, most of the physical activities tend to shorten muscles and finally reduce the flexibility. Often this may result in muscle tear or strain and, as the body grows older, this becomes a more serious problem. It is, therefore important to include stretching, bending and twisting exercises to develop flexibility of an athlete.

Q.11. What are the components of Physical Fitness ?

Ans. It is understood that only those components related to the development of health and increase of functional capacity of the body will be classified as physical fitness components. There is now a general agreement that basically there are five physical fitness components.*

1. Cardiovascular endurance,
2. Strength,
3. Muscular endurance,
4. Flexibility, and
5. Body composition.

Some experts still consider the old time aspect of physical fitness such as-strength, power, flexibility, agility, endurance etc.

Q.12. What do you understand by Cardio-vascular endurance ?

Ans. It may be explained as the maximal amount of work an individual can perform continuously when the work involves large muscle groups. The 12 minute run test is a simple, practical test used to measure cardio-vascular endurance. When a person takes this test, the maximal amount of work he or she can perform is calculated by determining how far she or he can run in 12 minutes.

The capacity of heavy, prolonged physical work depends on the ability of the body to supply oxygen to the working muscles and on the ability of these muscles to use the oxygen. The more oxygen the body is able to take in and use, the more work the body should be capable of doing. The circulatory and respiratory systems must function efficiently if a high degree of cardio-vascular fitness is to be achieved. This, therefore, may be referred to as cardio-respiratory endurance.

Q.13. Give a brief idea of body composition.

Ans. The three basic structural components of the body are fat, muscle and bone. Determination of body composition shows what percentage of the total weight is fat and what percentage is muscle and bone (referred to as lean body mass).

In recent years, body composition has been included as one of the physical fitness components; people have come to realize that optimal functioning of the body depends on the percentage of fat as compared with lean body tissues.

Q.14. What is Cardio-vascular fitness ?

Ans. The ability of the organism to maintain the various internal equilibrium within the body as closely as possible to the resting stage during a submaximal task and to restore promptly after exercise, if any, equilibria which have been disturbed. It means a fit person will adopt more efficiently to the stress imposed by a specific game and will recover much faster after the game.

Q.15. What is the basic difference in fitness level of trained and untrained person ?

Ans. It can be explained in the following manner :

(a) The trained person has a slower heart rate in response to the same task. This indicates an increase in efficiency because less stress is placed on the heart.

(b) He also has faster recovery following the task, as the heart rate returns to its testing value much quickly.

(c) If this task is continued, the trained person would be able to perform more work before reaching exhaustion. Cardio-vascular fitness, as it is more commonly referred to, or physical work capacity, may be explained as the maximal amount of work an individual is capable of doing when the task is continuous and involves large muscle groups.

Q.16. What is Cardiac output ?

Ans. It is the amount of blood that the heart is able to circulate each minute. It depends on the stroke volume and the heart rate :

Cardiac output = Heart rate x stroke volume
= 72x70 = 5040 ml/minute
or 5.04 litres/min.

It means in resting condition approximately 5 litres of blood is circulated by the heart each minute. On an average an athlete will have about 5 litres of blood in his body.

Q.17. On how many factors does performance depend ?

Ans. Performance depends on the following six factors :

— The availability of sufficient oxygen in the inhaled air.
— The diffusion of the oxygen from the lungs into the blood.
— The chemical binding of oxygen with haemoglobin.
— A blood flow through the lungs geared to pick up and carry the amount of oxygen required by the body.
— The ability of the cells to pickup the oxygen from the capillaries in exchange for carbon dioxide and other waste products.
— The same complex mechanism just described is reversed for the elimination of carbon dioxide.

Q.18. What do you understand by aerobic and an aerobic work ?

Ans. (a) **Aerobic work :** A work in which the amount of oxygen taken in and used by the body is sufficient to provide the energy necessary for the performance of the task.

(b) **An aerobic Work :** A work in which the amount of oxygen that the body can supply is less than the amount necessary to perform the task An aerobic work can be performed only for a short period of time, since an oxygen debt is incurred, and there is build-up of lactic acid in the blood stream.

Q.19 Name the events of muscular contraction ?

Ans.
1. Rest
2. Excitation-coupling
3. Contraction
4. Recharging
5. Relaxation.

Q.20. What do you understand by maximal oxygen consumption ?

Ans. The ability of the total body to use oxygen for energy is called oxygen consumption. It is expressed as a volume of gas per unit of time and is abbreviated VO_2.

V = Volume (usually expressed in litres or milli-litres)

O_2 = Oxygen gas and per unit time is expressed in minutes.

An individual oxygen consumption may be divided by body weight (in kilograms) to standardize this value so that the comparisons may be made between individuals of different body weights. For example :

Subject's body weight	= 142 pouds = 65 kg
VO_2	= 3.21 litres/minute
	= 3200 ml/minute
VO_2	= 3200/65
	= 49.1ml/O_2/kg body weight/ minute is available.

Just as there is a maximal heart rate that can be attained during exercise, there is maximal amount of oxygen the body is able to use. This is referred to as the maximal oxygen intake, or aerobic capacity. This measurement is recognized by most authorities to be the best measurement of a person's cardio-vascular fitness.

Q.21. Mention the basic changes due to physical training?

Ans. Respiratory changes

Increased maximal minute ventilation.

Increased tidal volume.

Increased breathing frequency.

Increased ventilatory efficiency.

Increased static lung volumes.

Increased pulmonary diffusion capacity.

Other changes
Changes in body composition
Decreased total body fat
No change or slight increase in lean body weight
Decreased total body weight
Decreased blood cholesterol and triglyceride levels.
Decreased exercise and restoring blood pressures.
Increased heart acclimatization.

Q.22. On what factors does maximal oxygen consumption depend ?

Ans. It depends on the following physiological parameters :

(i) Ventilation : The volume of air that can be taken into the lungs per minute.

(ii) Pulmonary diffusion : The ability of O_2 and CO_2 to diffuse across the pulmonary membrane into and out of the blood.

(iii) Transportation of gases : The ability of blood to carry O_2 and CO_2 to and from the muscles.

(iv) Cardiac output : It is the amount of blood that can be circulated each minute.

(v) Distribution of Cardiac output : It is the ability of the body to circulate the blood to working areas.

(vi) Physiological state of muscles : It is the ability of the muscles to use the oxygen delivered to them.

Q.23. How can the maximal oxygen consumption increase?

Ans. With regular participation in a good aerobic exercise programme a person can increase maximal oxygen consumption by as much as 30% depending upon her or his initial level of fitness. The changes that take place in the body as mentioned below are possibly contributed by this phenomena :

(i) an increase in the amount of haemoglobin in the blood.

(ii) an increase in the maximal cardiac output as the heart becomes stronger and more efficient.

(iii) an increase in amount and/or size of capillaries allowing a more efficient exchange of gases, which enable the muscles to use more of the oxygen circulated.

Q.24. What are the major changes in ventilation during exercise ?

Ans. 1. A very rapid increase within only a few seconds after the start of exercise. This is probably related to nervous stimulation arising from the joint receptors resulting from the movement generated by the working muscles.

2. The rapid rise inventilation soon cease and is replaced by a slower rise, which is submaximal exercise tends to level off i.e., tends to reach a steady-state value. In maximal exercise this levelling off, or steady state, does not occur, rather, ventilation continues to increase until the exercise is terminated. These changes are thought to be caused by chemical stimuli, mainly from the carbon dioxide in the blood produced during exercise.

Q.25. What is fat-free weight (Lean body mass) ?

Ans. When the weight of body fat is subtracted from the total body weight the remaining weight is referred to as fat-free weight or lean body mass. The fat-free weight (FFW) reflects mainly the skeletal muscle mass, but it also includes the weight of other tissues and organs such as bone and skin. The muscle mass makes up about 40 to 50 percent of the fat-free weight. The average fat-free weight of college-age males is about 85 percent of their total body weight and that of college-age females, about 75 percent of their total body weight.

Q.26. What are the practical tests for measurement of cardio-vascular endurance without the use of costly equipments ?

Ans. The measurement of maximal oxygen consumption in a laboratory is not practical for large groups for want of time and equipment needed. For this reason several practical tests have been developed to estimate the measurements. The two most commonly used tests are the 12 minute run and the timed one and half mile run. Results from research clearly show close agreement between the objective criterion of maximal oxygen intake actually obtained and values obtained from results of field tests. In fact, the results from any running test between 10 to 20 minutes' period can be used to predict maximal oxygen intake reliably.

Q.27. What is 12 Minute Run Test ?

Ans. Run for 12 minutes as far as possible and try to maintain a steady pace until the last few minutes, when one should attempt to speed up slightly. The number of laps completed during this time is counted and recorded, and the actual distance covered is recorded.

Q.28. How can one find out his fitness category from the score ?

Ans. Fitness Category may be found out from following scores:

S. No.	Fitness Category	Men (Distance covered in miles)	Women (Distance covered in miles)
1.	Very poor	Less than 1.2	Less than 1.02
2.	Poor	1.20 to 1.23	1.02 to 1.19
3.	Average	1.24 to 1.53	1.20 to 1.27
4.	Good	1.54 to 1.84	1.28 to 1.42
5.	Excellent	More than 1.84	More than 1.42

Q.29. Can you explain, what is 1½ mile run test ?

Ans. Owing to administrative convenience one and half mile run test may be preferred to the 12 minute run rest. One should try to cover 1 1/2 miles in the shortest possible time. Elapsed time is recorded in minutes and seconds. From the following one can assess his fitness status.

S. No.	Fitness Category	Men (Time in min.)	Women (Time in Min.)
1.	Very poor	15 or more	17.3 or more
2.	Poor	14.30 to 14.59	15.15 to 17.29
3.	Average	11.45 to 14.29	14.15 to 15.14
4.	Good	9.45 to 11.44	12.45 to 14.14
5.	Excellent	9.44 or less	12.44 or less

Q.30. How can maximal oxygen consumption be estimated from running test ?

Ans. The results of the 12 minute run test or 1 1/2 mile run test can be used to accurately estimate maximal oxygen consumption. The average running speed can easily be determined.

Example : A person who runs 1.6 miles in 12 minutes has average velocity of 1.6 x 5 or 8 mph (multiply by 5 because 5 period of 12 minutes in 1 hour).

Example 2 : A person who completes the 1 1/2 mile run test in 10 minutes has an average speed of 1 1/2 x 6 or 9 mph. (Multiply by 6 because 6 periods of 10 minutes make up an hour).

Now the maximal oxygen consumption may be detected:

Speed	Predicated O_2 consumption (ml/kg body weight/minute)
5.0	30.5
5.5	32.9
6.0	35.3
6.5	37.8
7.0	42.6
8.0	44.9
8.5	47.2
9.0	49.7
9.5	51.9
10.0	54.5

Note : For speed between those designated, interpolation can be used to predict the maximal oxygen consumption value more precisely. For consumption value of approximately 41.1 ml/kg body weight/minute.

Q.31. Name a few other tests which can give adequate indication of cardio-vascular fitness ?

Ans. Following tests last for only a short period, there is evidence to suggest that they may give you an adequate indication of fitness :

(i) Step test,
(ii) 3-minute shuttle run,
(iii) 1-minute lateral jump test.

Q.32. How hard should one exercise to improve cardio-vascular fitness ?

Ans. It is an individual matter and depends upon the efficiency of heart and circulatory system. For instance, if two people of same sex and body weight run at the same speed, their heart rate responses may be quite different.

Q.33. What is the Target-Zone Heart Rate ?

Ans. For safe and effective work-out, the intensity of activity must be regulated so that the heart rate is elevated to a predetermined level. This level is referred to as the training heart rate, or, more commonly target zone heart rate. For detaining it first maximal heart rate is detected. This is not influenced by sex of individual or level of training; it is almost entirely dependent on age.

Example : Substract the age from 220. A 20 years old player's estimated maximal heart will be 200 beats/minute. The target zone heart rate ranges from 70 to 85% of individual's maximum heart rate. When heart rate is maintained in this range, then it can be considered that exercise is of sufficient intensity for development of cardio-vascular endurance.

Q.34. How do you count the pulse rate (heart rate) ?

Ans. Locate the pulse (commonly at wrist-radial artery) immediately after stopping exercise or at least within 5 seconds. Count the number of beats that occur in a 1st to 10th second, and simply multiply this value by six to convert it into beats per minute. Do not count for a longer period because heart rate begins to slow down as soon as exercise is stopped.

Q.35. How to calculate the Critical Heart Rate ?

Ans. This heart rate is located 60% of the way between resting and maximal heart rates and may be calculated as follows :

Critical heart rate = Resting heart rate + 0.60 (maximal heart rate-resting heart rate)

Example : If an individual has a resting heart rate of 60 beats per minute and a maximal heart rate of 200 beats/minute.

Critical heart rate = 60 + 0.60 (200-60)

= 60 + 0.60 (140)

= 60 + 84

= 144 beats/minute.

For such a person to improve his cardio-vascular fitness to must exercise above 144 beats/minute.

In practically every instance, the critical heart rate fall

somewhere near the lower end of the target zone heart rate.

Q.36. What do you understand by "Change in Exercise Heart Rate"

Ans. Exercise heart rate must be checked regularly because with regular participation, one will get a gradual reduction in the exercise heart rate. It is necessary to increase the intensity of task from time to time to maintain the heart rate at desired level. That is why there is a necessity for progression to be built in an exercise programme.

Q.37. What are the Doherty's general principles of basic fitness for a player ?

Ans. Basic sports training must be continuous in nature :

— This work should always be supplementary.

— The basic fitness work should always include the practices of skill of many sports, even though they seen unrelated to one's special month of 'active rest' from each year of training. Other sports are basic training in skill learning.

— The hard core of basic sports fitness develops gradually over a period of years.

— The hard core of basic sports fitness cannot be gained completely through the action of the event itself.

— The intensity of basic sports training must be varied (rising and rhythmic).

— Basic sports training must be individualized. It is said, "The amount of daily exercise at the highest attainable level; still determined mostly by observation or empirical methods. Experiments show that a daily amount of practice which is suitable for an individual is either too much or too little. It is also demonstrated that regardless of the physical capacity of a given subject, there is level of exercise which frequently repeated may lead to chronic fatigue."

Q.38. What are the characteristics of white muscle fibres ?

Ans. They are also known as fast twitch fibres which are rich in glycolytic enzymes. They contain comparatively fewer number of mitochondrias and work largely anaerobically.

Proportionally their cross sectional area is larger and also supplied by neurons of large size. They are responsible for work and high intensity type because they have fast contraction rate. Their concentration is more among weight lifters, throwers, sprinters etc.

Q.39. Mention the qualities of slow twitch fibres.

Ans. These are also known as red muscle fibres. Such fibres in a muscle have more mitochondrias and contain higher concentration of myoglobin and respiratory enzymes. Since they are capable of prolonged oxidative processes, that's why Vo_2 max is directly correlated with percentage of red fibres an athlete has. Cross sectional area of these fibres is smaller than that of to white ones. The neurons of these fibres are of smaller size along with low thresholds. Owing to these reasons they operate at low and moderate intensities with slower contraction rate. These facts justify the higher percentage of red fibres among distant runners.

Q.40. What do you understand by the term LSD ? Explain it.

Ans. It means 'long slow distance training' which is an activity of continuous low intensity for a longer duration of time. It may lead to muscle and joint discomfort. To avoid injury, the training sessions should be progressively lengthened as fitness develcps. Long work-outs should only be attempted when there is gradual built up without any soreness.

As a result of this there is no distressing effect on cardio-respiratory system. The better response may be seen in peripheral parts. The respiratory capacity of muscle fibres is related to their habitual contractile activity. The greater the number of contractions, the greater the improvement. Muscle mitochondria show increasing pattern and oxidation of fat and carbohydrate increases. The over-all training effect may be seen in the form of enhanced mechanical efficiency.

Q.41. Explain 'Fartlek type of exercise' ?

Ans. During normal routine when there is speed, play in the form of continuous fluctuating exercise of different intensity.

It is known as 'Fartlek'.
The exercise has spontaneous changeable work intensities from fast burst to jogging. Because there is freedom of time and distance, athletes enjoy it. Fartlek develops anaerobic as well as aerobic endurance. In this some advantage on speed aspect is also seen. Though mainly used for runners this type of training is also useful for cyclists, race waiking and cross country skiing.

Q.42. Is Pyramid training useful for swimmers ?

Ans. This training method was started by Russian distance runners. It is very useful for swimmers also. In this type of training work-outs of varying duration and intensities are practised along with recovery intervals. The speed and speed endurance are not neglected in the quest for greater endurance.

Q.43. Explain the 'Tempoluf' type of training.

Ans. It means high intensity efforts equalling or approaching competitive stress. The basic idea behind the training is to accustom the athlete to the tempo of competition. The player may take this training in the form of continuous of intermittent work as at time trials or brief repetitions of the competitive distance along with adequate intervening rest periods.
The demand of Tempolauf is harsh especially if frequently employed. Apart from its physiological effects it is likely to assist pace judgement and condition the athlete to the pain of competitions.

Q.44. Give the details about interval training ?

Ans. This type of training is used by most of the athletes namely rowers. cyclists, runners, swimmers etc. In this training method, short period of hard work with brief period of rest or diminished activity are practised. The duration of activity may vary from 0.5 minute to 5 minutes while recovery period is just kept as double that of the work-out.
The following variables are associated with training :
— number of repetitions;
— the duration of effort;
— work intensity;
— duration of recovery.

The number of repetitions can be systematically increased as conditioning develops, while the pace can then be accelerated. Lastly, the recovery periods can be shortened. If the period is inadequate for recovery, anaerobic endurance is also stressed. During recovery and intensive training among young athletes, the heart rate is allowed to fluctuate between 1200 to 180 beats per minute. These rates are considered fit to allow optimum stimulus for heart to expand and pronounced hypertrophy results.
The work speed may, however, be varied to put more or less emphasis on anaerobic endurance as peripheral, as well as central factors respond to interval type of training.

Q.45. Explain the continuous relay training technique.

Ans. It is also known as Parlauf training approach. This method is introduced periodically in the training schedule whenever club morale is to be stimulated. Generally two, three or four members, who are selected by the coach, take part. In the two per team format, rest periods do not allow complete recovery so that performance inevitably drops off. This type of training is particularly suitable for middle distance running and swimming but it can be incorporated into the fitness training of players of games.

Q.46. How you will summarise the various points for the development of muscle strength in an individual ?

Ans. It can be summarized into the following points :

1. Mere repetition of contractions which place little stress on the neuro-muscular system has little effect on the functional capacity of the muscles.
2. The amount of work done per unit time is the critical variable upon which extension of the limits of performance depends.
3. The speed with, which functional capacity increases, suggests that the central nervous system changes contribute an important component to training.
4. The ability to develop maximum tension appears to be dependent on the proprioceptive facilitation with which overloading is associated.

Note : In most athletic endeavours, the attainment of mere strength is not enough. The attainment of explosive power is often necessary.

Q.47. What do you understand by Co-ordination or Rhythm Training ?

Ans. This training is utilized to promote a more precise co-ordination of movement. The athlete learns a sense of pace and achieves confidence in his ability to continue work in spite of the pain and discomfort of his prolonged effort. Co-ordination training refers to the process of superimposing new movement patterns over habitual ones. Through improvement of form, extramovements are reduced, thus producing precise, direct, stronger, and more economical motor function.

Q.48. Explain the words 'Response training or Reaction training'.

Ans. This type of training is utilized to shorten the delay between a stimulus and response. This is done by exercises to eliminate cerebral decision,-making functions preceding the response. The objective in the process is to transfer the whole movement pattern from volitional to reflex control. Although some reflexes are developed prenatally, but most of them are learned. In order to improve the reaction time, the athlete must practice movements characteristics of the sport in which he or she plans to participate, and each of these movements must be performed as rapidly as possible.

Q.49. What do you understand by the word 'Heat training'?

Ans. Heat training is designed to induce favourable adaptation in temperature-regulating mechanisms. This improves resistance of endurance efforts to the high temperature and induces increased salt retention and sweating. The adapted individual perspires more, but the perspiration contains less salts. If the organism is unable to adjust rather rapidly to the increased heat produced by effort, then fatigue is rapidly to follow and performance is altered. Most of the Indians do not need extra salt as from the very beginning they get adapted due to climatic conditions prevailing in most of the parts of this country.

Q.50. What do you understand by 'Circuit Training'?

Ans. It is the scientific arrangement of known and proven exercises designed to elicit maximum overall training effectiveness. Total balanced development for all parts of the body is the objective of circuit training. This type of training is based on well-known physiological principles and aims at providing various activities and a continuous challenge. A circuit utilizing proper exercise equipment will improve muscular strength, endurance, cardio-vascular endurance and flexibility. It applies the principle of 'progressive overload', provides balanced development of the whole body, enables large number of the athletes to train at the same time, and all this is done according to his individual capacity. It allows each individual to acquire a maximum work-out in a short but adequate time. Circuit training inspires motivation through variety offered as well as by the application of new goals that become readily apparent almost daily.

Q.51. Describe in brief about 'Speed Training' ?

Ans. In this type of training, athlete performs the movements in a given exercise as rapidly as possible within a prescribed time. For each exercise a proposed range of 'sets' and a time interval are given. The time of exercising is gradually increased while the rest period is gradually diminished. As fitness improves, the number of sets of each exercise may be increased. Thus the effort-recovery cycle, referred to previously as interval training, is again utilized.

Q.52. What is Homeostasis ? Explain its relation to certain variables.

Ans. The human body cannot remain continuously active and it periodically requires rest, which amounts to a cessation of all voluntary activity. This enables the athlete to establish certain criteria of functioning for what is called resting state of the body. Players would naturally expect to find individual differences in these criteria, such as in the pulse rate, blood pressure, respiration etc. In fact, these values on the whole lie within rather a narrow range for those persons who are free from diseases i.e. for physically fit persons. It is also true because body maintains a system of automatic controls that tend to preserve these changes in spite of forces acting from outside and from within the body to change them. This principle is known as HOMEOSTASIS. This greater the stress laid on the body, the maore change will be there in the criteria that indicate the body's reaction to the stress, and the greater the effort must be for these criteria to be returned to their resting values.

Q.53. Can this principle be utilized for adaptation and physical fitness of an athlete ?

Ans. The repetition of stress increases the efficiency of the body in making and adapting the effort, and consequently also facilitates the recovery from it. The specific ability of adaptation with which one is concerned in the development of physical fitness helps the body in the following manner :

(i) to take more oxygen into the lungs;
(ii) to utilize it more efficiently;
(iii) to tolerate a greater than normal deficiency of oxygen during exercise;
(iv) to increase the force with which the heart pumps the blood into the circulation;
(v) to increase the size of the capillary bed in the lungs and the muscles;
(vi) to increase the size and strength of voluntary muscles.

Some adaptations of central nervous system is necessary for physical exercise. Extreme adaptation to permit highly skilled and co-ordinated motor performances is also possible, but it is not essential for physical fitness.

Q.54. Write four common methods which may be used to develop muscle strength in isotonic fashion ?

Ans. They can be listed in the following manner :

(i) Attempting to move a maximum weight at one time;
(ii) Making series of repitions against a resistance which is increased or decreased or decreased with each series;
(iii) Making two-third of a maximum number of repetitions against a fixed resistance.

Q.55. How can the word Balance be explained ?

Ans. Balance is regulated by impulses transmitted to the muscles from vestibular apparatus of ears and from the stretch reflexes. It is highly developed in the specific players (aerobat and juggler), but can be improved in any one by training. An athlete whose organs of balance are not functioning, can't maintain an erect posture even if all other systems are working normally. It is also dependent to some extent on visual input, but can be trained among handicapped (blind) by using other senses.

Q.56. What is 'Informal Training Programmes' ?

Ans. The general public, as a result of being stimulated by friends or teachers through the communication media, have embarked on their own personal training programmes. These may include a wide variety of activities or may concentrate on any one, such as walking, jogging, running, swimming, or cycling. Since these programmes are largely depend on self-motivation, they are more apt to be continued regularly over an extended programme and to be based on activities that is enjoyable in themselves to those who select them.

Q.57. Describe briefly the 'Kinesthetic Sense'?

Ans. This sense of the body comes from a system of receptors and effectors in the nerve supply of voluntary muscles which enables us to judge our position in space in relation to other objects, and to make comparisons of weights and pressures. This is highly susceptible to training. Where it is lacking, due to disease of the nervous system, the individual may be severely handicapped even if his other senses are in tact.

Q.58. Can physical fitness be attained by handicapped also?

Ans. Yes, even high level of physical fitness can be attained by persons with relatively severe handicaps. Athletes handicapped due to one or more limbs have been successful in amateur and even professional sports. Blind athletes have been excellent wrestlers.

Store Mandeville Games is an excellent example of it, where thousands of handicapped athletes from all over the world participated.

Q.59. Once the physical fitness developed, will it remain for ever ?

Ans. No, it cannot be maintained without a continuous effort. Any level of fitness can be maintained with less effort than is required to reach it. Regular vigorous activity, at least two three times a week, is necessary for the maintenance of fitness. Many persons find it more enjoyable to continue a daily programme of activity and can maintain their fitness with somewhat less intensity to work than those who exercise intermittently.

In the same way, various components of physical fitness deteriorate to a lesser or greater extent if exercise programme is not maintained.

Q.60. What do you understand by assessment of 'Running Endurance' by Balke's Method ?

Ans. Balke's 15 minute run is probably the simplest and reliable running test. The criterion of performance is the distance covered in 15 minutes. The individual makes his own pace. The raw score is compared to norms fixed for the age.

Q.61. What should be the optimum duration of exercise-session for an athlete ?

Ans. It may be divided into three sessions :

(a) 5 to 10 minutes warm up and stretching session so that the heart and circulatory system are not suddenly taxed.

(b) Sustained 20 to 30 minutes exercise-session in which the heart beat rate remains in the target zone.

(c) 5 to 10 minutes cool-down session in which the intensity of the task is lessened before exercise is completely stopped.

Q.62. What is the need of warm-up and cool-down ?

Ans. These phases are very important. A good warm-up gradually stretches the muscles and therefore reduces the chances of injury. In addition, it allows the heart to gradually adjust to the increase in work. It can significantly reduce the incidence of muscle soreness which often occurs as a result of a poorly planned exercise programme. In the same way, cool-down period is of equal importance. The blood on the contraction of the skeletal muscle, is returned to the heart from the lower extremities. If activity ceases abruptly and there is no contraction of these muscles, blood tends to pool in legs, and there may be left insufficient blood returning to the heart for circulation. Any type of body movement involving the legs will assist in the returning of the blood and will be beneficial.

Q.63. What physiological effects are there due to 'warm-up' ?

Ans. When muscles work for a few seconds, they need increased supply of oxygen and glycogen. The arterioles supplying the muscle dilate, the stroke volume and speed of the heart beats increases and the blood flow increases and respiration becomes deeper and faster. The cerebral blood flow remains constant, but to compensate the muscular vasodilation the splenchenic circulation diminishes, and process of digestion and absorption slows down. Glycogen, present in the liver cells, gets converted to glucose, and this is passed into the liver sinusoids, then to the general circulation. Vasodilation in the skin depends upon the excess of heat produced.

Q.64. Mention the sample programme for development of strength and muscular endurance ?

Ans. It can be planned in the following manner.

1. Basically all muscles may be divided in eight groups: chest, back, shoulders, extensors of the forearm (triceps), flexors of forearm (biceps) abdominal, quadriceps and hamistrings.
2. Exercises should be selected in such a way that desired muscle groups develop. Example : Bench press contributes to the development of the chest, the triceps and shoulders.
3. Now there is a need to determine the maximum lift which is possible or each exercise.
4. Start with the 70% of the maximum strength for each of these exercises. See whether one can perform 8 or 12 repetitions. If twelve then increase the weight, if less then eight times, then reduce the weight.
5. Start with the two sets of each per day. It may be done on alternate days also.

Always remember : Never overstrain yourself.

Q.65. What are the general guidelines for weight training programme ?

Ans. 1. Make sure that each training session is preceded by a 5 to 10 minute warm-up. It should include stretching exercise for each of the muscle groups involved in the programme.

2. While executing each exercise, it is important to breath normally.
3. The largest muscle groups should be exercised first. These are the ones that will require the greatest expenditure of energy.
4. Each exercise must be performed slowly, through the full range of motion, and with a steady, application force. This is important with the lowering phase (negative work) as well as the lifting phase (positive work). It is also recommended that the lowering phase should take approximately twice as long as (4 seconds) the lifting phase (2 seconds).
5. Progressive resistance must be placed against isolated movements at each joint. To develop maximal strength and endurance one must perform exercises for all movements of a particular joint.

Q.66. Does weight training reduce the flexibility ?

Ans. It is understood that weight training reduces the range of motion possible at various joints. This will not occur if exercises are performed correctly through the entire range of motion and if all major muscle groups are exercised. When a muscle is exercised through full range of motion, there should be an increases in flexibility rather than decrease. However, to ensure that adequate flexibility development has taken place it is important not to neglect any major muscle group and if it is so, due attention should be paid for stretching programme.

Q.67. What are the common weight training exercises for strength and muscular endurance ?

Ans. Following exercises are quite popular :

— Two Arm Curl
— Bench Press
— Lateral Machine pull down
— Upright rowing
— Quadriceps lift.
— Leg Curl
— Curl up

Q.68. What are the two common methods of developing flexibility ?

Ans. (A) Ballistic Stretching Technique : In this method there are bouncing and jerking movements, and the force of the movement stretches the muscle. Generally, it is not recommended, because of the amount tension it creates in the muscle and much more likely to develop muscle soreness or tendon damage. It repeated movements are to be used for the development of flexibility. It is important that they are performed slowly.

(B) Static Stretching Technique : Here the stretch position assumed slowly and gently and held for designated period. Care must be taken to move through the full range of motion until lightness is felt in the muscle or muscle group involved. However, this position is not forced to the extent that it causes pain. Flexibility exercises are designed to alleviate pain not to create it. This technique results in least amount of tension in the muscles.

Q.69. What common points should be kept in mind while performing flexibility exercises ?

Ans. Following nine points should be kept in mind while performing flexibility exercises :

1. Such exercises should be preceded by a mild warm-up designed to use the body temperature slightly. Activities that are continuous, rhythmic and involve large muscle groups are ideal for this purpose. Jogging in place, jumping across a line on the floor with both feet are examples of exercises that meet these criteria. Care must be taken to perform these exercises continuously but at a very slow pace. Warming-up first be allowed for a greater range of movement at the joint and will also reduce the likelihood of injury and soreness.
2. In static stretching technique, the movement takes place slowly through the full range of motion until tightness is felt. The position then should be held for a minimum of 10 seconds. Care should be taken not to force the joints beyond normal range of motion.

3. Exercises that are performed using only one side of the body must be repeated with the other side of the body also.
4. A minimum of five repetitions should be performed for each exercise.
5. Because flexibility is specific to various joints, exercise should be included for each movement at each joint for which flexibility is to be developed or maintained.
6. Exercises need to be alternated in the routine to stretch different muscle groups.
7. The correct execution of each exercise is most important. Unless movement occurs through the full range of motion, the exercise will be ineffective.
8. Relaxation must be a part of a good stretching programme. It must be emphasized that the more relaxed a muscle is, the less it is likely to be injured during the stretch.
9. In the beginning and at the end of each exercise session flexibility exercises should be included.

   REMEMBER : As progress occurs, and if time permits, it may be advantageous to increase the number of repetitons from 5 to 10 and to increase the amount of time that each contraction is held. There is evidence to suggest that maximal development will occur when each contraction is held for 30 seconds.

Q.70. Suggest some exercises for the development of flexibility ?

Ans. Following exercise may be used for development of flexibility :

— Straddle stretch — Groin stretch
— Achilles tendon and calf stretches
— Low Back Stretch — Lateral Leg Raises
— Sitting Hamstring Stretch
— Arm Circles — Hip Circles
— Quadriceps Stretch

Q.71. What do you understand by Cardiac Syncope ?

Ans. Let us understand what is cardiac syncope. The Cardiac syncope results in complete collapse, often with a short seizure and diaphoresis.

In this type of condition, the young athlete may complain

of 'passing out' or better described as sense of weakness and disorientation. The episodes often are repetitive and happen at the end of competitive event. The examination findings including echoecardiography, and exercise testing are normal. Careful questioning often reveals a potential psychological factor in these episodes. Treatment consists of full evaluation, attention to possible psychological factors, and reassurance.

Q.72. What are the common uses of exercise testing ?

Ans. Uses may be divided in three broad groups :

(A) Diagnostic or Prognostic :
- Evaluation of suspected heart disease.
- Evaluation of asymptomatic individuals with a risk of coronary heart disease.
- Post myocardial infection (pre-discharge)
- Dysrhythmia provocation
- Peripheral vascular disease.

(B) Functional Capacity :
- Exercise prescription for sedentary normal individuals.
- Post myocardial infraction.
- Post Coronary bypass after surgical repair of congenital or valvular abnormality.
- Chronic pulmonary disease.
- Chronic renal failure.

(C) Therapeutic efficiency :
- Anti anginal agents (nitrates, beta blockers etc.)
- Antidysrhythmic agents.
- Antihypertensive agents.
- Bronchodilators (exercise induced asthma)
- Vacillators (Congestive Heat Failure).

Q.73. What are the determinants of increased myocardial oxygen demand ?

Ans. A primary purpose of exercise testing is to evaluate myocardial function during condition of maximum performance. The major determinants of myocardial oxygen demand are given below :

(a) **Heart rate :** increased rate due to sympathetic stimulation and withdrawal of parsympathetic tone.

(b) **Afterload :** Increased impedance; systolic pressure; increased rate of arterial distension.

(c) **Pre-load :** Increased venous return, diastolic filling volume, and pressure.

(d) **Contractibility :** Increased contractile velocity and wall tension.

Q.74. Can E.C.G. help in screening cases ?

Ans. Exercise testing is an important clinical method for evaluation of cardio-pulmonary function. The diagnostic accuracy of exercise testing depends on the extent of disease process and sensitivity of monitoring methods. Electro-cardio-graphic recording provide a reasonable method of screening patients with probably ischemic heart disease. The addition of radio-nucleide perfusion or angiography to exercise testing greatly increases the sensitivity and specificity of exercise testing for coronary heart disease.

Functional exercise testing provides quantitative assessment of work capacity in patients and normal subjects. Periodic exercise testing is essential for accurate exercise prescription and training cardiac patients and others who require supervised exercise.

Q.75. What are the beneficial effects of training on human heart ?

Ans. There are some additional benefits of physical training. One is an increase in myocardial vascularization. This may be the result of an increase of collateral vessels in the coronary artery tree or an increase in capillary/myocardial fibre ratio from capillary proliferation. Another beneficial effect of exercise is on the other CHD risk factors. Exercise has a positive effect on lowering the blood lipids, particularly triglycerids, decreasing the percent of body fat due to obsity, lowering the resting blood pressure, and indirectly helping to abstain from cigarette smoking.

These combined metabolic and dynamic effects of training protect the heart against myocardiam even in the presence of some degree of coronary atherosclerosis. The greatest benefit of these protective mechanisms can be utilized for primary prevention. Owing to this reason, regular aerobic endurance exercise should start in childhood and continue throughout life.

Q.76. What do you understand by training senstivity zone ?

Ans. The "Training-sensitive Zone" Maximum heart beat rate for a specific activity can usually be determined immediately after 2 to 4 minutes of all-out exercise in that form of work. This level of exercise, however, requires considerable motivation and certainly is not advisable for adults without medical clearance or those predisposed to coronary heart disease consequently. People should consider themselves "average" and use the age-adjusted maximum heart rates presented in Figure 20-5. Although all people of a particular age do not possess the same maximum heart rate, the loss in accuracy due to individual variation (usual ±10 beats per minute at any age-predicted heart rate) is of small significance in establishing an effective training programme. As a convenient "rule of thumb", maximum heart rate is established as 220 minus the person's age. Figure 20-5 also shows the "Training-sensitive Zone" in relation to age. Conditioning of the aerobic system occurs as long as this exercise heart rate is maintained within this zone.

If a 40-year-old woman wishes to train at moderate intensity, yet still be at or above the threshold level, a training heart rate would be selected that is equal to 70% of the age-predicted maximum heart rate, i.e. a target exercise heart rate of 126 beats per minute (0.70 x 180). Then by trial and error (using progressive in cremates in lights to moderate exercise), The woman can arrive at a walking, jogging or cycling load that produces the desired target heart rate. If the woman wishes to increase her training intensity to 85% of maximum, her exercise heart rate would have to be increased to 153 beats per minute (0.85 x 180).

Q.77. What are the effects of exercise on cardiac function ?

Ans. These are given below in tabular form :

Decrease	Increase	Improves
Resting heart rate	Vegal tone	Oxygen transport system
Arterial Pressure	Peripheral shunt in of blood	Myocardial vascularization
Sympathetic tone	Lower function of the myocardium	Other risk factors.

Q.78. What criteria will you use for selection of candidates for exercise therapy ?

Ans. (A) Potential Candidates for Therapeutic Exercise : The healthy subjects who are coronary prone show the best response to a regular exercise programme. Alongwith physical activity, they should receive help in modifying their other risk factors. They should have a weight reduction programme with skinfold measurements to estimate percent of body fat. They should have diet counselling, especially if hyperlipidemia is present, and their blood lipid content should be periodically evaluated. An intensive anti-smoking programme should be started. Blood pressure records before and after exercise sessions should be kept in those who have hypertension. They should be encouraged to have regular medical followup examinations by their physicians. A change in risk taking behaviour patterns may change these persons from a high CHD risk status to lower one. The change is one of the primary objectives of a conditioning programme. Persons with clinically recognized ischemic heart disease and selected individuals with mild essential hypertension are also excellent candidates for exercise therapy.

(B) Contra Indication To Exercise Therapy : The contra indications to an exercise programme are listed in tabular form. Certain medical problems are absolute contra indications to physical conditioning while others are only relative.

A. Absolute Contra Indications to an Exercise Programme - No Exercise Programme Recommended
Recent myocardial infraction.
Changing patterns of angina pectoris.
Severe valvor heart disease.
Certain arhythemiss :-
Paroxysmal ventricular tachycardia.
Untreated aterial fibrillation.
Frequent ventricular premature beats with exercise, heart block, congestive heart failure.
Myocarditis or cardiomyopathy within a year.

B. Relative Contra Indications To an Exercise Programme - Exercise Under Medically Supervised

Rehabilitation Programme Only
Myocardial infraction after 3 to 6 months.
Angina Pectoris.
Moderate to severe hypertension (blood pressure greater than 160/100) massive obsessity.
These later cases, however, require careful medical supervision and frequent monitoring during and after the exercise session. There are a number of reported cases of cardio-vascular collapse. It is shown after the exercise session completed. A test-retest Protocol is necessary to follow the progress of these selected persons with relative contra-indications to exercise. If progress is not shown on regular testing, the exercise programme is discontinued and the medical problem revaluated. The improvement from physical recondition of these individuals is often rewarding.

Q.79. Give the brief comments on spasm hypothesis ?

Ans. The spasm hypothesis : Several experiment provide evidence to support the spasm hypothesis of muscle sorenees. In one study sorenees was produced in both arms by repeated wrist hyperextensions against a 4.3 kg. resistance. The muscles of the nondominant arm were streched by the static technique. This was beneficial because significantly greater levels of soreness occurred 24 & 48 hours after exercise in the dominant aims which was not stitched. In another study, the resting electrical activity of the anterior lower leg muscles was evaluated as a consequence of static streching procedures in subjects with shin splints, a musculoskeletal disorder involving severe pain in the anterior portion of the lower leg. Static stretching procedures brought about marked reduction in EMG activity. Symtplomatic relief with stetching was also occupants by a decrease in the amplitude of the EMG tracings.

Q.80. What are the problems of stress testing ?

Ans. They can be explained by mentioning;
Indications for termination of stress tests : Any test whether maximal or submaximal may need to be terminated. Conditions for terminations include hypertension, pallor, syncope, bradycardia, tachyarrhythmias, ventricular

premature beats and weakness. The incoordinaton ST segment depression in itself is not usually a reason for termination.

ST : T. changes on the Electrocardiogram :

The simplest method of observing myocardial is chemia is with the ECG during stress testing. A tracing with horizontal or down-sloping ST segment depression of one mm or more and of 0.8 to 0.12 seconds duration is considered significant. Persons showing such a phenomenon have positive electro-cardiographic evidence of myocardial ischemia.

Q.81. During exercise, what are the symptoms requiring medical review ?

Ans. The following signs and symptoms should be subject to medical review when they appear in any person on therapeutic exercise programme :

1. Any chest pain or pain referred to teeth, arm, jaw, ear or back.
2. Syncope, vertigo, light headedness.
3. Irregular pulse.
4. Persistent fatigue lasting more than one hour after exercise, Nausea and/or vomiting.

Q.76. What are the test for establishing intensity of rehabilitation programme during convalescence ?

Ans. After three or four weeks, if the evolution of disease seems favourable, the patient may undergo a more strenuous rehabilitation programme, either individually at home or collectively in a specialized centre : Most of the programmes involve rhythmic exercises (marching, cycling, etc.) of about 30 minutes duration. At Jaipur Medical College, it is being done by a physical educationist under the guidance and supervision of Dr. Sharma-Prof. and Head of Medicine Deptt.

Q.83. What is the prognostic value of exercise test ?

Ans. During the past 10 years, it is suggested that exercise E.C.G. obtained with gradually increasing load (bicycle or treadmill). In the interest of preventive medicine or life insurance or sports participation, one can detect the subjects in a population those who are likely, in the future, to show high moribidity and mortality from coronary disease.

The results seem to be conclusive, particularly in the middle-aged population and provided that the presence of a S.T. ischaemic response is taken as the only positive criterion. This seems to be only statistically valuable index. The frequency of S.T. depression shows the expected increase, proportional to age and to the intensity of effort; on the contrary, the frequency of T wave abnormalities do not change with age or intensity of effort.

Q.84. Give the importance and value of positive test ?

Ans. Subjects who show S.T. change ischaemic type during or after an exercise test seem to have higher probability of dying from coronary disease than the subjects who show no change. The magnitude of ischaemic S.T. depression during and after exercise is directly correlated with the severity of coronary disease.

Q.85. Explain, how exercise help in maintenance of myocardial oxygen supply ?

Ans. To increases the oxygen supply to the myocardium by the regression of delayed progression of coronary atherosclerosis among human beings, exercise also increases diameter of major coronary arteries and coronary collateral vascularization.

It is felt that exercise reduces ischaemia by redistributing myocardial regional blood flow, and thereby increases the volume of blood flowing to the ischaemic area.

Q.86. What are the common symptoms of Staleness ? How can athlete or coach identify the over-training syndrome ?

Ans. Staleness generally happens in endurance type of sports such as Marathon, cross country racing, swimming etc. 'Nonspecific' symptoms of staleness are fatigue, tiredness, sore throat etc. Most of the time, the physical findings of staleness are normal.

Laboratory studies may also be normal for athletes endurance activities.

In psychological area anxiety, depression and fatigue may develop.

Q.87. What happens if an athlete plays during febrile states ?

Ans. Episodic illness may occur in well-trained athletes in spite of apparent excellence in physical strength. However, symptoms of minor respiratory illness may be exacerbated as a result of perceived changes in airways function and work of breathing. Acute febrile illness may adversely affect cardiovascular and thermo-regulatory responses to exercise.

Training during illness is frequently understood as a fatigue producing illness. Psychological testing shows a characteristic pattern of altered mood state similar to 'burnout' in young professionals.

Q.88. What you understand by word 'Supplemental Oxygen'? Explain.

Ans. Supplemental oxygen is indicated by hypoxemia, either at rest or during exercise state. In healthy exercising individual, oxygen breathing gets little benefit. It has been demonstrated that breathing air enriched in oxygen during exercise improves performance. It also increases maximal oxygen uptake, and decreases minute ventilation at heavy work loads. However, the physical limitations imposed by the equipment necessary to supply the oxygen makes any form of supplementation impractical during exercise. Oxygen enriched air does not reduce recovery time from exertion because this phase is dependent upon the elimination of anaerobic metabolities. Therefore, any benefits that are derived from several breaths of pure oxygen after exercise are more psychological than physiological.

Q.89. What do you understand by the word 'Sports anaemia' among athletes ?

Ans. Haemoglobin or hematocrit levels in the trained athletes are slightly below normal. This condition is called sports anaemia. Certain researchers have found that a progressive decrease in haemoglobin concentration among runners participating in a 20 days, 312 mile road race was statistically significant. Couple of researchers, on the other hand, have quoted slightly or no decrease in haemoglobin percentage.

Q.90. What mechanism is involved in the development of Sports Anaemia ?

Ans. The differentiation of true anaemia (an absolute decrease in red cell mass) cannot be made from haemoglobin and haematocrit determinations alone, for this information on total red cell mass is required. Athletes have a more blood volume than the non-athleters. It is also observed that there was a 25 percent increase in total blood volume in male distance runners compared with a control group. However, there was a proportional increase in both red cell mass and plasma volume. In a similar way, when sedentary males were placed in a one month running programme, they developed 6 percent increase in total blood volume due to an increase in plasm volume without change in red cell volume. Therefore, decreased haemoglobin and haematocrit levels found in individuals participating in sports may be in some cases pre-present a pseudoanaemia because of expansion of plasma volume.

Q.91. What is the true anaemia of exercise ?

Ans. Anaemia may develop due to vigorous activity. The forces exerted on the red cells in the capillaries of the feet may rupture the cells after long brisk walk or running. Free haemoglobin s liberated into plasma. Heptoglobin is the principal plasma protein that binds the free haemoglobin during intravascular haemolysis. The heptoglobin-haemoglobin complex is rapidly cleared by the liver. When the haemoglobin binding capacity of the heptoglobin is exceeded, free haemoglobin may be found in the urine. Decreased heptoglobin levels have been noted in distance runners; this is consistent with the concept of running induced traumatic haemolysis.

Q.92. Mention the Pre-exercise response, also mention the activator for this type of response ?

Ans. Acceleration of heart rate; increased myocardial contractility, vasodilation in skeletal and heart muscle; vasoconstriction in other areas, especially skin, gut, spleen, liver and kidneys; increase in arterial blood pressure.

Activation of motor centex and higher areas of brain causes increase in sympathetic outflow and reciprocal inhibition of parasympathetic activity.

Q.93. What are the major causes of haematuria ?

Ans. Following causes may be listed for such condition :

(a) Kidney :	Ischemia Acute renal failure Increased vascular fragility Trauma Nephritis Stone
(b) Ureter :	Stone
(c) Bladder :	Contusion Stone Infection
(d) Urethra :	Contusion Stone Infection Trauma

Q.94. What are the common symptoms pointing to disease of Renal origin which should be investigated before permitting athletes to participate in games and sports ?

Ans. Some of the major symptoms which require further investigations are :

(i) Progressive symptoms-colicky or flank pain.

(ii) Persistence of Haematuria or proteinuria beyond 48 hours after exercise.

(iii) Urinary casts.

(iv) Positive urine culture for bacterial infection.

(v) Oliguria after prolonged, strenuous exercise.

Q.95. How emotional stress affect alimentary canal ?

Ans. Emotional Stress causes hyperfunction (spasm or hyperperistalsis), hypofunction (stasis, hypomotility) which impairs various smooth intestinal functions. About 60 to 70 percent gastro-intestinal complaints are found to arise from psychophysiological factors. There may be Gastritis and frequency of passing stools may increase.

Q.96. Explain the term - runner's trots ?

Ans. A number of G.I.T. symptoms may be there due to distance running. Commom signs and symptoms are : Periumblical abdominal cramping, bloating, and frequent watery stools, sometimes they may be complicated by malena (blood in stools).

These symptoms are most likely to occur after an episode of unusually sever exertion or during a period of rapidly increasing distance running. These symptoms usually disappear when malena is not present. Symptoms complex resembles lactase deficiency or an acute flare-up of irritable bowel syndrome.

Q.97. What do you understand by the word 'stitch inside' ?

Ans. Certain players complain about a sharp colicky pain in the left or right upper quadrant of abdomen during strenuous exercise. It may be due trapping of intestinal air 'Gas' in the hepatic or splenic flexure. Physical activity has been shown to increase propulsive movements in the human colon. These movements may cause intestinal air to move to the heptic or splenic flexure, where intraluminal pressure could cause symptoms. Another possible cause of this syndrome is intentinal ischemia brought on by a shift of blood from abdominal cavity to the large muscles during strenuous activity. When the pain persists, a rest period is usually sufficient to relieve the discomfort but continuous pain, even at rest needs medical examination.

Q.98. Mention the acclimitization responses due to heat and their effects ?

Ans.

Acclimatization Response	Effect
Improved cutaneous blood flow.	Transports metabolic heat from deep tissues to the body's shell
Effective distribution of cardiac output	Appropriate circulation to skin and muscles to meet depands of metabolism and thermoregulation. greater stability in blood pressure during exercise.
Lowered threshold for start of sweating	Evaporative cooling beings early in exercise.
More effective distribution of sweat over the skin surface	Optimum use of effective surface for eraporative cooling
Increased sweat output.	Maximize exaporatives cooling.

Q.99. Discuss the causes of Vertigo or Dizziness ?

Ans. If the player feels that room is spinning around him or he/she is spinning round the room, concomitant with nausea, vomiting, and possible sweating, these symptoms are most likely of true vertigo originating from disorders of the semicircular canals. However, disequilibrium is also called 'dizziness'. The athlete who is subjected to massive short duration fluid changes as a result of training may precipitate metabolic disturbances that potentially could cause disequilibrium.

If it is associated with concomitant loss of consciousness, than the cause is definitely with semicircular canals of vestibular apparatus.

In case of middle aged athlete atherosclerotic cardiovascular disease involving carotid arterial system must be considered especially when symptoms are exaggerated due to head, neck or trunk movements during exercise.

Q.100. Explain in brief the word "Thermo-regulation' ?

Ans. Normal comfortable body temperature may vary from 98°F in the skin; 98.6°F (37°C) in the mouth; 99.6°F (38°C) in the rectum: 100°F(38.5°C) deep in the liver. A diurenal variation generally causes a rise in temperature of 1°C from morning till evening.

Thermoregulation is maintained by a careful balance of heat production and heat loss. Sense of well being resists in losing at least 95 percent of all heat produced each day but not losing any more than that. Heat production and loss are regulated by a 'thermostat' in the hypothalamus, which is responsive both to slight changes in blood temperature and also to the impulses received from temperature sensitive nerves in the skin. The thermostat may be 'reset' by endogenous pyrogens, released by inflammation, resulting in fever. When the thermostat is stimulated by either cold or heat strees, it directs the body to alter both heat production and heat loss accordingly.

Q.101. Why hot and humid environment effects the body comparatively more ?

Ans. Exercise is hot, humid environments poses a challenge to temperature regulation because the large sweat loss high humidity contributes little evaporative cooling.

Q.102. In nut-shell, how do you explain the concept of Fitness ?

Ans. The degree of fitness required for sport must vary according to the desires of the participants.

It cannot be overstated that the physical stress of modern sports in considerable and that prolonged training is required to achieve the necessary standard for international competition. Nevertheless, it would be wrong to deprive those with medical histories of pulmonary or cardio-vascular disease of the joy and pleasure of games. For average man the game should be in the form of recreation and not with a view of ambitious performance. To an outstanding sportsman, fitness means : "Fitness is the ability of an individual to live a happy and well balanced life. It involves not only physical but intellectual, emotional, social and spiritual aspects of an individual. Interaction and interdependence of these phases of a man's health are such that any deviation from normal in any aspect of these components of fitness will make a man unable to meet the demands placed on him by his work or way of life."

Q.103. What precautions should be taken while doing exercise for cardio-vascular fitness ?

Ans.

1. Within a year of doing exercise. a complete medical check-up is a necessity.
2. Before starting exercise in full swing a gradual one to two minutes warm-up is a must.
3. Abrupt exercise is harmful. It should always begin slowly and later on increase the load and intensity.
4. Cooling down is equally important.

Q.104. What are the points to be kept in mind to avoid back problems and back-aches ?

Ans. Following points may be kept in mind:

— Never lift or carry heavy objects if they can be pushed or pulled efficiently.

— Get very close to the load before grasping or lifting it.

— When lifting, use the legs, not the back.

— While squatting or going down to sitting posture, the back should be kept straight and hips in tucked position.

— Exercises should be avoided which strain the back muscles.

Q.105. What type of muscles should be developed by exercises to prevent back problems ?

Ans. Strengthening or stretching exercises are suggested for the muscles. Couple of muscles need both stretching and strengthening exercises.

— Strengthening as well as stretching of low back muscles.

— Strengthening of gluteus muscles.

— Both strengthening and stretching of hamstring muscles.

— Stretching of ellipses muscles, and

— Strengthening of abdominal muscles.

Q.106. Write the common causes of blood in urine ?

Ans.

Kidney	Bladder
Ischemia	Contusion
Acute renal failure	Stone
Increased vascular fragility	Infection
Trauma	Urethra
Neproptosis	Contusion
Stone	Stone
Ureter	Infection
Stone	Trauma
	Cold.

CHAPTER THREE
SPORTS INJURIES

Q.1. How do sports Injuries occur ?

Ans. Following are the common causes for such type of injuries :

1. When rules and regulations of games are not followed.
2. Poor Knowledge-The ill-informed athlete does not know, that what he does is dangerous, e.g. unscientific weight training.
3. Faulty training techniques or equipments-Though the athlete is aware of the danger yet he must not know how to avoid it, e.g. defending punches in boxing.
4. Lacking in careful attitude-Though the athlete is aware of the danger and knows how to avoid it, yet since he is careless, so fails to take necessary action, e.g. close fielding in cricket, inadequate protective clothing etc.

Q.2. Give the step of ABC.

Ans. **i) A - AIRWAY**

— There must be a clear airway to allows oxygenated air to reach the lungs. You can gently tilt the head and lift the chin to pull the tongue clear of the airway. Take care if you suspect neck injuries.

ii) B - BREATHING

— The patient must be breathing so that the blood in the lungs can be replenished with oxygen. You should look, listen and feel for signs of breathing. If the casualty is not breathing, you should perform mouth to mouth ventilation after checking the carotid pulse (below).

iii) C - CIRCULATION

— The circulation of blood must be effective in order to distribute oxygen around the casualty's body. If you cannot detect breathing, you will need to locate the carotid pulse in the neck to check the circulation.

Q.3. How can you classify the sports injuries ?

Ans. Sports injuries may be divided into two groups :

1. Exogenous causes : Caused by edtenal agents like balls, sticks or by an action of the opponent.
2. Endogenous causes : Here example may be quoted as case of ruptured muscle fibres.

Injuries due to exogenous causes could be minimized by obeying the rules of the games. Endogenous causes are directly related to physical fitness of individual.

Q.4. What do you understand by protective clothing against heat and cold.

Ans. Out of necessity many contact sports require the participants protect themselves against on cold winter days it is important to keep warm. This does not mean wearing several layers of heavy clothing. Nowadays you can buy very light weight thermal tops and jackets that allow perspiration to escape. These are ideal to runners who train in all whether conditions. They keep then warm and allow their bodies to "breathe". On cold days, sweat cools quickly and you may soon get cold when you drop off the pace in running or slow down in a game of soccer, and cold muscles are more susceptible to injury and stiffness.

In summer you should opt for comfortable and practical clothing that will help take away sweat from your skin. The new coolmax material is particularly good at this and is preferable to nylon or cotton. As a general rule, make sure that no articles of clothing are too tight, that are not too prominent and thereby avoid chaffing of the skin.

Q.5. How to prevent the sport injuries ?

Ans. Prevention could be ensured through :

1. Fitness of the athlete.
2. Warm up exercises.
3. Cooling and warming.
4. Proper follow up of rules during games.
5. Killer instinct of optimum level.
6. Proper clothing and footwear for the specific game.
7. Protective clothing and equipment. Examples : Cricket : Legpads, thigh pads, abdominal guards, gloves, helmets.

Football : Gloves (for goal keeper), ankle strapping, shin guards, knee-guards.

Hockey : Shin guard, leg pads, abdominal guard, facial masks for goal keeper.

Boxing : Mouth guard, knuckle bandage, abdominal guard.

Cycling :

Car Racing : Halmet

Swimming : Goggles.

8 Proper equipment : Proper checking of the equipment is essential in contact games :

Boot	-	Football
Sticks	-	Hockey
Gloves	-	Boxing

9. Extremes of environmental conditions.
10. Fatigue,
11. Common sense.

Q.6. What do you understand by A.B.C. ?

Ans. A-Airway obstruction, B-Breathing (respiratory arrest) C-Circulatary or cardiac arrest.

Basic life support requries no instruments or supplies, and the correct application of the steps of CPR can maintain life until the patient recovers sufficiently to be trasported to a hospital or until advanced life support can be delivered.

Q.7. Explain with points 'jaw Thrust maneuver' ?

Ans. The methods described are effective for patients, if not, an additional forward movement of lower, jaw -jaw thrust- may be required. In this triple maneuver place the finger behind the angle of the patient's lower jaw and then :

1. Forcefully bring the jaw forward.
2. Tilt the head beckward.
3. Use the thumb to pull the patient's lower lip down, which allows breathing through the mouth as well as nose.

The jaw thrust is best performed with the trainer kneeling by the patient's head.

Q.8. What are the factors which affect conditioning of an athlete ?

Ans. They may be listed in the following groups :

1. Ability to play,
2. Mental attitude,
3. Determination,
4. Team work, and
5. Spirit of game.

Q.9. Name some basic events which develop selected aspects of physical fitness.

Ans. One should always keep in mind that :

— Short sprints develop speed.

— Distance running develop speed and endurance.

— Running in circles and figures of eights develops strength of ankle, knee, hip etc.

Q.10. What are the points to be kept in mind for prevention of injuries among players ?

Ans. Following points may be listed as important for prevention of injuries :

1. Medical check-up and medical history should be taken at the beginning of each session before allowing a young man to participate in vigorous activity.
2. All personnel concerned with training the youth, should emphasize physical conditioning. It should always be gradual and complete.
3. A sports physician or well trained coach having good knowledge in prevention of sports injuries should be present during all active sessions.
4. Health Education regarding the problems and safety measures related to physical activity is a must.
5. There should be strict enforcement of games rules and administrative regulations in order to protect the athlete from injuies.
6. There should be continued emphasis on employment of well-trained athletic personnel, and provision of excellent facilities and the safest possible equipments.
7. Last but not the least is that there should be continued research especially on preventive aspects of sports medicine.

Q.11. Explain the importance mid sole and heal counter in a sports shoe.

Ans. Mid sole : If the sport involves a heavy landing then plenty of pedding is required. Most shoes now use artificial materials which regain their shape after compression. A football player landing on soft turf requires less mid sole padding as opposed the road runner or hard court tennis player.

Heel counter : This is the curved heel of the shoe which supports the human anatomy. It should grip firmly, but not tightly to prevent calcanlal bursae and bruised heel fat pads.

Q.12. What is the rule of Thumb for initial treatment of injuries ?

Ans. It can be explained in the form of following points :

(i) Elevation : It may help because elevation of injured part above the level of heart, uses the force of gravity to drain excess of fluid.

(ii) Compression : Following trauma, blood and fluid from the surrounding tissues leak into the damaged area and distend the tissue Swelling is sometimes useful since it brings antibodies to kill germs, but if the skin is not broken, antibodies are unnecessary and swelling will only prolong healing.

(iii) Ice : The most important, Preferably it should not be applied directly, but crushed kept in a towel, cotton or bandage and than applied for atleast 15 to 30 minutes over the part. Frequent ice application according to severity of injury for first 48 hours helps to a great extent. It decreases the bleeding from injured vessels because it causes them to contract. If ice or cold water is not applied at an early stage, more blood collects - more swelling - delayed recovery.

(iv) Rest : It is necessary because if exercise or game is continued, it will extend the injury. Stop using the injured part, the moment it is hurt. But in certain cases after ice application passive stitching is beneficial.

Q.13. What are the factors responsible for recovery from an injury?

Ans. Factors responsible for recovery are :

(i) Adequately and timely ICE is received.

(ii) Level of training, better conditioned athlete will have better healing.

(iii) More extensive injury, longer duration of recovery.

(iv) Proper and timely diagnosis of the athletic injury.

Q.14. What do you understand by word 'Muscle Soreness ?

Ans. A runner when doing painful work may develop muscle soreness of arm. At one time or another, everyone experiences muscle soreness, which usually sets in 8 to 24 hours - after any exercise or work. If the discomfort is localized, the muscle may be injured to some degree. However, all muscle soreness is not due to injury. If diffuse, it is probably the result of swelling of the muscle fibres, which are stretched with each muscle contraction Such soreness is very common. Rest for a day reduces it. The treatment consists of application of ice and aspirin preparations relieves pain but does not hasten healing.

Q.15. Will you mention something about 'pulled muscles' ?

Ans. It is an acute tear of skeletal muscle fibres and is characterized by sudden, localized and persistent pain in a muscle. For example, swimmers get it in the shoulder and horse riders on inner thigh. There are hundreds of muscles in the body but only less than five percent are commonly injured. There are the muscles which are used or involved to the maximum during game situations.

Q.16. Why does muscle pull occur ? What are common factors responsible for it ?

Ans. Muscles pull result when more tension is applied to a muscle than the tolerable limits of that muscle. As a general rule, the more severe the pain, the more severe the injury (extension injuries.)

There are certain common factors responsible for it :

* Insufficient warm-up before game or exercise.
* Poor flexibility,
* Over Training,

* Muscle imbalance,
* Mineral deficiency,
* Structural abnormality,
* Poor training methods,
* Trauma, and
* Lack of an adequate endurance programme.

Q.17. How to treat such conditions ?

Ans. (i) There is no medication that will make the muscle heal faster. So, first go for ICE.

(ii) Discontinue the ice and compression within twenty four hours. As long as swelling is there, elevation may be continued.

(iii) Heat applications of any kind are suggested only after Ice application, and it brings more amounts of nutrients to the injured area. Nutrients are the muscles building bricks and also provide energy for healing. Heat may also increase the rate of healing process itself.

(iv) Strengthening exercises : It may be continued as a long term treatment which will help the muscle to stand better to stress. But they may not be useful at early stage.

(v) Stretching exercises : It is now well known that pulled muscle will aways feel tight when it is healing because healing process causes it to shorten but these exercises are more helpful after ice application.

Q.18. What do you understand by word tennis-elbow ?

Ans. The condition of elbow is common among tennis or badminton players. It is usually caused by excessive strain on the muscle of the forearm which is attached at the elbow. These muscles produce forward and backward movements at the wrist. The pain usually is at the medial or/and lateral condyle of humerus bone. It may be of two types :-

(a) Forehand tennis elbow,

(b) Backhand tennis elbow.

Beside the players this condition can be developed even in a mechanic or housewife i.e. whenever there is too much use of these group of muscles i.e. mechanic using screw drive.

Q.19. What are the common causes ?

Ans. (i) Using too heavy a racket. The heavier the racket, the more stress on the arm.

(ii) Playing on grass. The ball bounces off on such surfaces with a greater velocity, hitting the racket with a dreater force, which is transmitted to the elbow.

(iii) Using heavy balls : The heavier the ball, the greater the force against the racket.

(iv) Having too much tension on the strings. If the strings are too tight they transmit greater force to elbow.

(v) Using oversize grip : If the racket is held insecurely, the ball will be hit with a wobby stroke and the elbow absorbs the shock.

Certain sports medicine experts are of the opinion that an aluminium racket is superior to a wooden one because it bends more when the ball hits. Wooden rackets are stiffer. But on the contrary certain experts suggest the use of wooden rackets of good quality. Stress to elbow may be due to any condition, i.e. housewife may get it from opening jars.

Q.20. How to prevent the development of Tennis Elbow ?

Ans. Prevention : For the first time when tennis elbow develops, stop playing game After waiting for two to seven days for pain to disappear, start the following exercises. Perform each exercise twice a day :

(i) Forehand tennis elbow : Lay the arm flat on the table, keeping hand extended over the edge, palm should face upward; With 3 to 5 pound weight flex the wrist ten times. Repeat till hand gets tired. Increases or decrease the weight according to the need of optimum requirements.

(ii) Back hand tennis elbow : Keep the hand in the position desirable above except that hand should face downward. Dorsiflex the wrist ten times. Repeat it upto just tiredness.

Q.21. What are muscle cramps ? Mention their common causes.

Ans. Muscle Cramps : They are painful, sustained contractions of all the fibers in a muscle. They can last for just a few seconds or continue for several hours.

Following five common causes are listed here :

(i) Salt deficiency, especially when athletes are suddenly exposed to hot environment.

(ii) Low levels of other minerals such as potassium or magnesium.

(iii) An injury or strain on the muscle.

(iv) An obstruction of the muscles blood supply by sustained muscular contractions.

(v) Hyper-ventilating - breathing too fast when it is not necessary, which prevents the body from using calcium.

Q.22. How to treat such patients ?

Ans. Try to avoid the cause, stretch and squeeze the muscle. If it is the calf, squeeze the muscle with one hand and stretch it by pushing the front part of the foot up with the help of hand or other foot.

If it is the biceps, squeeze the muscle with one hand and have a helper straighten the elbow.

Q.23. Will you explain the word 'Stitches.' ?

Ans. The sudden, sharp pains that athletes sometimes experience in the upper part of abdomen are a form of muscle cramp. Medical experts are of the opinion that mostly stitch is due to a cramp of the diaphragm - the large flat muscle that controls breathing.

(i) It is caused by the blood supply to the diaphragm being shut-off due to pressure from lungs above and abdominal contents below.

(ii) Another cause of stitch, particularly in novice athletes, is gas distending the colon. As a result of the degradation of food, gas is formed throughout the entire intestinal tract. Exercise speeds up intestinal contractions and pushes gas towards the rectum, but if due to hard stools gas moves, upper side may press the diaphragm.

(iii) Eating just before games or exercise programme just after meals.

(iv) An intolerance to milk or wheat protein.

The prevention is possible by trying to avoid the mentioned causes.

Q.24. What to do when one gets the stitch ?

Ans. Slow down and push fingers up into the site of pain, usually just below the last rib on the right upper part of belly. Bend forward and exhale pursing the lips. The pain will disappear soon and it will be possible to continue playing or running.

Q.25. What do you understand by the word tendinitis ?

Ans. It is an inflammation of the tendon which causes the tendon fibres to swell, and is caused due to tight or shortened muscles - the pulling at the tendon even when it is not being used. Generally pain is more severe when one gets up in the morning. Because the pain decreases with exercise, the player won't stop the game. This causes further harm to the tendon.

Each sport has its most common site for tendonitis. In running sports - basket ball, football and track events - Achilles - tendonitis; in swimming - shoulder tendonits.

Q.26. What should be the line of treatment of tendinitis ?

Ans. For all such conditions, it is the same line of treatment as mentioned earlier (Ice). Stop that game. After few days when pain is not there, stretching is suggested. Always remember that the cause of damage to the tendon fibre is muscle tightness caused by hard exercise or vigorous games. Stretching should be done slowly and gently and position may be kept for thirty seconds or longer. Quick, jerky stretches may cause further damage.

Never have steroid injections to relieve pain or for the purpose of recovery. These drugs prove to be more harmful when activity is continued along with the medication.

Q.27. How can you prevent the knee injuries in contact sports ?

Ans. Following points may be kept in mind to avoid the injuries :

(i) Run with short, choppy steps : The less time foot is on the ground, the less likelihood of knee injury. If there is likelihood to get hit from somebody, shorten the stride.

(ii) Protect the knee from a hit towards back or sides. At these places knee is most susceptible to injury.

(iii) Exercise the muscles around knee. Research has proved that exercise may also thicken ligaments and make them more resistant to injury.

Q.28. What are the important tips for treatment of injuries ?

Ans. Remember the following points :

(i) Muscles are treated with strengthening exercises.

(ii) Tendons are treated with stretching exercises.

(iii) Bones put usually heal themselves after a surgeon has aligned them so that they will be put together properly.

(iv) Joint therapy is complex and should be treated by sports.

(v) Ligament injuries can be severe and should be treated by sport medicine expert.

(vi) Facial injuries of the feet are treated with mechanical support or tapping to relieve the pressure. Surgery may be required for some cases of facial injury.

Q.29. What are the factors which should be kept in mind for the prevention of injuries ?

Ans. 'Cure is the whisper of past but to prevent is the divine voice of today.'

Once the damage occurs, it takes lot of time to recover and complete cure normally may not be possible. In any training or game programme it is advisable that one should take care of oneself so injury is avoided. Following are the common factors which may lead to the injuries in games and sports :

(a) Overtraining,

(b) Poor training methods,

(c) Lack of flexibility, and

(d) Muscle imbalance.

Q.30. What do you mean by overtraining ?

Ans. Overworked is most common cause of sports injuries. The important warming signals are persistent pain in muscles, bones or joints.

Beginners are more likely to get injury than known players;

conditioning counts a lot; too much motivation leads to the habit of ignoring pains.

Rest : Time or rest is the best healer. When stress is applied to an injured tendon, muscle or ligament, further injury usually results. This is something known as over-training syndrome which can be explained in the following points :

(i) In the beginning, during a hard work-out dull pain is felt at muscles, joints or ligaments. Here treatment is to reduce the intensity of work.

(ii) If pain continues during and after a work-out also and if it does not improve in a week, see for structural abnormality, muscle imbalance etc.

(iii) Pain : When one is at rest it suggests the need of change in biomechanics of activity or consultation of a sports medicine expert.

Q.31. Explain the meaning of' change in bio-mechanics of activity?

Ans. Rapid increase in work load, speed, and resistance, or adding new training methods on same muscles often puts more strain on the athletes, than their bodies can endure and they injure their concerned muscles.

Example : Football player complaining about shin splints gives history that a week before, he has added running up the stadium steps regularly as extra training after playing routine football. Here the player should do other type of exercises which gives rest to the concerned muscles. If at all, activity is to be done it should be done in the form of pool running.

Q.32. How structural abnormality causes injuries ?

Ans. It puts extra strain/stress on muscles, fasciae, bones, joints, tendons and ligaments and results in injury to these structures.

(i) 'Flat feet' can cause injury to the arch, ankle, hip and lower back.

(ii) Too high an arch can cause stress fractures of the foot and may also lead to pain on lateral part of knee joint.

(iii) injuries.

(iv) Bow legs can cause low backache.

(v) Knock knees can cause pain in the ankle, knee and hip.
(vi) Exaggerated curve in back may also cause low back pain.
(vii) Lack of flexibility.

Q.33. Why are the stretching exercises considered as important injury preventive measure ?

Ans. During games when athletes exercise vigorously, their muscles are injured slightly. With healing, the affected muscle becomes stronger, shorter and tighter. A tight muscle is more susceptible to injury. This is the reason why athletes who do not stretch regularly before games (lack flexibility) are injured more frequently.

The sports where running is the main component, the two muscles are most commonly victimized by pulls and strains. They are the hamistrings, in the back of thing, and the calf muscles.

Research work has proved that stretching if done regularly and properly, will reduce these injuries by 80 per cent.

Q.34. What do you understand by word 'Muscle Imbalance'?

Ans. When a muscle moves in one direction, another muscle relaxes in the opposite direction (Antagonist). The ratio of strength between opposing muscles is delicately balanced. If one of the muscles is much stronger than the other, the imbalance exists. The stronger muscle can overpower the weaker one, causing damage to its fibres and tendons. The treatment of such a condition is to strengthen the weaker muscle and to stretch the stronger one.

The most common victim of muscle imbalance is Hamistring group of muscles.

Q.35. What is Tibialis Anterior Syndrome ?

Ans. Generalized pain in front of the lower leg is particularly common among runners. It is due to injured muscles, and should be differentiated from a crack in the bone. (Doctor should always be consulted.) Later on this pain may become very severe type after activity.

Q.36. Will you give another example of muscle imbalance in leg ? Write its treatment also.

Ans. The calf muscle which pulls the forefoot down, overpowers the shin muscles which pulls the forefoot up. As the athlete continues training, the calf muscle becomes proportionally much stronger than the shin muscles.

In this situation treatment is to strengthen the weaker muscles (shin) and stretch the stronger muscles (calves).

(i) To strengthen the shins, run upstairs, to stretch the calves, either use the inclined plane or wall push-ups.

(ii) Always remember that warming up before any game is a must and also the best prevention against injuries.

(iii) Sometimes there are vague impressions the athletes explain. They describe pain over the front and sides of the leg, especially lower inner side. It may be just nagging type and associated with running. It is often difficult to remember how the pain started - unaccustomed walking long distances; triggered by an accident; may be a kick or direct blow to the leg. Remember rest, ice, compression and elevation may be applicable here also. Use them according to the condition, need and time.

There may be a need to stretch the affected muscle also. Kneel down with top of foot flat on the floor, gently sit back on heel, a pulling sensation will be felt - count for 10 seconds.

(iv) If the anterior tibial muscle strain may come as a pain in central ridge of the shinbone, the periosteum may be damaged. The bony ridge will feel sore to touch and the problem will take longer time to clear up.

Q.37. In the same contest, will you explain the word 'Stress fracture' also ?

Ans. Stress fracture generally develops in the upper central part, due to excessive pull on bone by anterior tibial muscles. Here the muscle pain is a secondary reaction. The stress fracture gives rise to protective spasm to the muscles. Here sports medicine expert is to be consulted. Point tenderness is an important feature for diagnosis :- Fork Test with clear sciagram may be indicated to support the diagnosis.

Q.38. What is Anterior Compartment Syndrome ? Mention its management also.

Ans. Pain usually starts gradually, but may come quickly also. It is due to over expansion of anterior tibial muscles and their containing sheath (sheath is being comparatively inelastic). The muscles may tend to swell due to injury or simple overuse. Each time muscles overswell and exert pressure on sheath (pain when starts during exercising). This may lead to reduction in blood supply.

Treatment : ICE as mentioned for previous conditions also. Try to identify the cause - change in activity or repition. If faulty mechanics are contributing, correct it. Strengthen the feet muscles (arch of foot), here exercise is to press toes down into the floor. Rarely posteriorly tibial muscle strain may be there and it can be treated more or less on already mentioned principles.

Q.39. Will you mention in brief about ankle-sprain ?

Ans. The unstable weight bearing joint is most likely to suffer and needs immediate attention also. Slightest strain on ankle may be very painful (mostly if it is on lateral side). Mostly the damage is more severe in the form of bore fracture, ligament rupture but it may not look that alarming in the first instance. Owing to this reason such conditions should always be ruled out before diagnosing a simple sprain.

— The wet cold towel method will be the most suitable; wrap the cold towel around the joint.

— Foot should be kept up. Patient should not be allowed to sit or stand. Use a pillow. This will help the swelling from gathering and increasing around the ankle.

— Bandage from toes below toward upper side may be applied as a support. Crape bandage is the best. If needed, etestoplast bandage may be used.

— Look for the colour of the nails - watch tight bandage but it should not stop the circulation.

— After a couple of days try to move if pain is not there. Avoid circular movements.

— To keep fit, do other types of exercises as for example cycling where only heel may be used.

Q.40. How to strengthen the ankle joint ?

Ans. By doing movements like alphabets i.e. A to Z such type of movements of ankle joints will strengthen all sides of joints.

Q.41. How does the injury to abdominal muscles occur ?

Ans. These muscles may be injured suddenly or gradually. A direct blow to stomach while the muscles are contracting, or over contraction of the muscles, may cause a sudden tear. This kind of accident may happen in sports like boxing, football where a missed kick may damage the muscles.

More gradual strain can happen if excessive movements or overuse is there (fatigue and insufficiency).

Rarely it may be due to repeated twisting movements, say during long sessions of discuss throwing or tennis serving (strained oblique muscle of abdomen).

Q.42. What are the common signs and symptoms ?

Ans. Gradual or sometimes sudden pain may be present on front side of abdomen. It may be noticed as discomfort only. Initial symptoms of pain may be there. This pain may be felt during games or even during coughing and sneezing. Local tenderness may also be noticed. Pain is directly related to the damages to the muscle fibres and its extensiveness. The initial severe pain of a sudden injury should subside within a few days, if there are no complications, but as the muscles tighten up to protect themselves from further harm, pain of stabbing type may also be there.

Q.43. What is to be done in such type of injuries ?

Ans. During a sudden injury, rest should be given to the trunk by bending forward. Signs of bruising and swelling need doctor's attention (blood collection due to ruptured blood vessels). If rest is given in the form of 'three quarters prone position' is the best.

(i) Minor strains may be helped with ice compression,

(ii) When pain subsides, passive stretching should start.

Dhanurasan for 10 seconds every time (5 times a day)

After regaining flexibility of abdominal muscles, strengthening exercises are useful. Always remember that pain should not be there while doing stretching or strengthening exercises.

After this stage, the concerned sport may be started. Practise the appropriate trunk movements, as shadow practice in the first instance, and then have a practice session regularly.

Q.44. How can you classify the injuries ?

Ans. Most of the athletic injuries can be classified into two broad groups: Intrinsic and extrinsic. Intrinsic injuries are derived from the athlete's own actions and most of the time due to faulty techniques while extrinsic injuries are due to causes outside the athlete's own immediate control. Common injuries for convenience may be divided into three broad groups :

(a) Soft tissue injuries - muscle, tendons etc.
(b) Bone injuries - fractures.
(c) Joint injuries - dislocations.

Q.45. How will you manage the sprain, strain and tendon injuries?

Ans. 1. First aid,
2. Immediate management
3. Later management.

1. Most common symptoms are pain, swelling tenderness at the sit of injury, so place the injured area in a comfortable position. Give cold compression for 20 to 30 minutes. It is a must. Do not give massage or formentation for 48 hours because this procedure aggravates the bleeding and also increases the damaged tissue.
2. Immediate Management :

(a) Effective control of bleeding in the area of injury by ice packs and pressure bandages is of great help.
(b) Relieving pain : Cold compression also reduces pain sensation. Elevation of part and rest are important. Local painkillers as ethyl chloride spray which may be useful in case of severe sprains. But ice remains the corner stone of treatment.
(c) Minimising the reaction of injury, mainly the inflammatory swelling:- Cold compression causes vasoconstriction of capillary bed, reducing the inflammatory exudation. Rest and elevation of part

helps in reduction of blood flow to the injured area.

(d) Care of the associated damage, if any, to other structure : Nerve, artery, organ etc. Proper assessment is always done to find out the damage to associated area.

3. Later Management : Here comes the repair and restoration of the injured part to normal function. It can be planned on the following principles.

(a) Promoting the drainage of the products of inflammation:

Application of heat, using a wide spectrum of thermo-therapeutic measures, hot baths or hot packs, paraffin bath, infrared rays therapy, short wave diathermy and electro-therapy of other types are useful. Similarly different types of massages to the part are specifically beneficial. Specific manipulations would help in the drain age of the selected pockets of exudates in the injured area. Manipulations should only be practised in consultation with the medical doctor.

(b) Preservation of strength in the non-injured segments and promotion of strength in the injured area :- Early exercises are prescribed to maintain the muscular fitness of non-involved segments.

(c) Early joint mobilization and progressive improvement of range of movement is also necessary. This is only done when the required strength and the muscular balance is re-established.

(d) Protective padding, support and use of the specific safety aids are of great help.

Q.46. How will you manage a bone injury ?

Ans. Following points may be kept in mind while handling the bone injuries :

(i) The mobility of damaged fragments of bone should be prevented by cautious splinting of the bones. As long as bones of the extremities participate in two joints usually, the principle of splinting should be to include both the joints of function. For example, for Radius - the splint should include the elbow, and for the wrist joint, the splint should extend from the middle of the upper arm to the level of the knuckles of the hand.

(ii) Support of splinted segments is done with proper slings and bandages. This helps to keep the fragments immobilised during transportation to the hospital, as well as to counter considerably the action of gravity.
(iii) Careful transportation is planned in a position of comfort.
(iv) Handling which would either aggravate the damage already caused, or involve the other structures in the vicinity, making a simple type of fracture to a complicated fracture, should be avoided.

Q.47. What points are kept in mind during Immobilisation?

Ans. During the period of immobilisation, the following procedures are adopted:
(i) Prevention of wasting in the muscles included in the immobilisation.
(ii) Prevention of functional limitations of the joints due to stiffening and consequent adhesions.
(iii) Prevention of decalcification of bone tissue in normal sites due to inactivity.
(iv) Prevention of vasomotor alterations.

Q.48. What are the immediate symptoms of 'dislocation' ?

Ans. Following are the immediate symptoms of dislocation:
(a) Intense pain amounting to agonizing pain.
(b) Joint is fixed in a particular position, according to the type of dislocation, and the bony part getting out of the anatomical position.
(c) Deformity of the limb or segment due to the protrusion of the bony part out of alignment.
(d) The function is totally lost.
(e) Swelling of the joint, due to traumatic effusion into the joint.

Q.49. What are the 'Delayed symptoms of Dislocations' ?

Ans. The delayed symptoms of dislocation may develop like this:
(i) Pain may be actually aggravated by any attempt to move any of the bony structures.
(ii) Swelling is pronounced and is due to the periathritis as a result of the injury to the particular soft tissue

structure. The effusion into the joint is also increased, the effusion is the inflammatory exudation, a reaction to the trauma by the lining of synovial membrane. Threre may be damage to the other structures also :

(a) there may be parses or paralysis of muscle or muscles due to nerve compression.

(b) Vasomotor effects may be in the form of ischaemia-deprivation of blood supply, resulting in tingling and numbness and other sensory alterations, or congestion-stagnation of venous blood due to the injury to the veins, and the resultant inefficient and inadequate drainage.

Q.50. What First Aid can be provided to such type of cases?

Ans. The patient is kept in a comfortable position, as he wishes to assume and all movements are restricted in the neighbourhood of the joint, to prevent the complications. Protective strapping is provided and the part is supported by the use of slings and bandages. Ice-packs or cold compression could help to relieve pain, or to minimise bleeding or to reduce inflammatory swelling.

Q.51. Will you mention the basic principles of immediate management of dislocated joints ?

Ans. (i) For clinical evaluation sciogram should be taken.

(ii) Reduction (Closed Method) :- The dislodged bony participant of the joint is allowed to retrace the actual pathway of its exit out of the joint capsule, by special skilled manipulatory manoeuveres. Anaesthesia may be used, if necessary. This procedure is done usually in operation theatre.

In case, the closed reduction fails or is not possible or in case of repeated and troublesome recurrence of the dislocation, open methods or reduction and surgical correction of the defect are attempted. This aspect of injury is generally handled by the orthopaedic surgeons.

(iii) Absolute rest to the affected joint by immobilisation with strapping or plaster cast, for specified period of time is to be given. This all is done according to the type of joint, the nature of injury and the involvement of other structures in the vicinity.

Q.52. Can physiotherapy be of any help in such type of cases ?

Ans. Yes, During the phase of immobilisation, many physiotherapeutic measures judiciously incorporated in the management would help to a great extent in maintaining the joint supple; this happens by lessening the secretions and reducing the chances of adhesions. It also helps in preventing the setting-up of the tissue atrophy of the muscles as the muscles are included in the immobilisation schedule.

Q.53. What are the common physiotherapeutic measures helpful ?

Ans. Physical methods, specifically, thermo-therapy using radiant-heat-shortwave diathermy-would help in the healing process as well as in facilitating the absorption of the exudates of inflammation. Certain types of massage also assure adequate drainage of the area by promoting function of the lymphatics and the venous channels.

Q.54. Will you also mention the exercise pattern for such conditions ?

Ans. The isometric series of exercises for the muscles included in the immobilisation regimen, would maintain the muscle tone, and help in the maintenance of muscular strength to a certain extent.

(a) The non-involved joints and other segments of the body should be kept active to enable them to maintain fitness. At the same time, exercising the contra-lateral segments would result in the cross-education effect and help in promoting muscle tone.

(b) Once the joint is ready for re-education and resumption of the routine range of movements, the muscular strength should be built up in all the groups to re-establish the muscular balance. The specific movements which would cause the recurrence of the injury should be carefully attempted at this stage. All other movements are practised actively.

(c) Once the routine joint movements are perfected with the re-establishment of muscular balance, the special sports skills helping the convalescing joint alone, or in combination with the other joints, are tried. The harmonious and sequential co-ordinated joint movements are practised under guidance and supervision.

All through the entire period of re-education, reconditioning and resumption to routine range, psychological guidance should be provided motivation, encouragement and building confidence will be of great help.

CHAPTER FOUR
SELECTED SPORTS INJURIES

Q.1. What do you understand by forehand tennis elbow ?

Ans. This condition may be more common in professional players because they stem from the wrist snap in booming service. Serving in this way may strain the muscles that bend the wrist. These muscles are attached on the inner side of the elbow and consequently the pain occurs at this side (flexor group of muscles).

Q.2. What is cerebral contusion (Cerebral Contusion) ?

Ans. Cerebral confusion is a bruising of the brain. When a small area of the brain is involved, a contusion is difficult to distinguish from a concussion and no permanent effects occur. In more severe contusions, cerebral edema, with brain swelling results in increased intracranial pressure. If a generalized contusion with bruising of the brain stem occurs, decerebrate regidity follows and the patient may die or have permanent deficit after a long illness. The usual treatment is medical and is aimed at reducing increased intracranial pressure with good oxygenation, dexametha sone and mannitol.

Q.3. Write the 5 age of concept of treatment.

Ans.
(1) Accept athletics
(2) Avoid expediency
(3) Adopt the best method
(4) Act promptly
(5) Achieve perfection

Q4. Discuss with details the concussion ?

Ans. Concussion is a syndrome in which there is an immediate impairment of neural function following a blow to the head. The deficit is usually noticeable in the degree of consciousness but may also involve memory, visual disturbances or equilibrium problems. In third degree concussion patient is unconscious for more than five minutes with moderate retrograde amnesia. No treatment is required because there is no permanent deficit, although a decision does have to be made concerning a participant's ability to return to play. Multiple concussive episodes may result in permanent sequelae, and individuals reflecting this pattern need to be evaluated by a neurological surgeon to determine whether they should continue in athletics.

Q.5. Explain the 'Backhand tennis elbow' ?

Ans. It is generally developed in novice or weakend players, it comes from hitting backhand strokes incorrectly. A backhand stroke stresses the muscles that straighten the wrist. These muscles are attached on the outer side of the elbow (extensor group of muscles).

Q.6. What is the basic reason for development of this condition ?

Ans. Besides many other factors which are already discussed, it develops in the people who try to hit the ball with a wrist movement rather than using their entire upper arm. Such type of beginners are generally more susceptible to the complain of tennis elbow. A wrist wing puts tremendous stress on the muscles of the forearm. If the player has stronger forearm muscles, the more protected he is from these conditions.

Q.7. Will you mention the additional factors which are responsible for aggravating the condition ?

Ans. Other factors which may predispose this condition are once again mentioned here :

(a) Heavier the racket, the more stress is on the arm.

(b) Playing on cement. The ball bounces off these surfaces with a greater velocity and thus hitting the racket with a greater force, which is ultimately transmitted to the elbow.

(c) Heavy balls : The heavier the ball, the greater the force is felt against the racket.

(d) Too tight strings : If the strings are too tight, naturally when the ball hits with a greater force and ultimately it is transmitted to the elbow

(e) Over-size grip : If the racket is held loosely, the ball will hit with a wobbly stroke and the elbow absorbs the shock directly.

(f) There is controversy regarding aluminium racket. It

is considered superior to a wooden one because it bends more when the ball hits if wooden rackets are considered as stiffer.

Q.8. How is tennis elbow to be treated ?

Ans. In a few cases friction massage may help. As a rule stretching exercises after Ice application gives the best results. It is worth mentioning that in a case of severe pain and tenderness over the epicondyle of humerus, suggested treatment is to inject locally 4 ml of 1 per cent Xylocaine along with one ml. of a steroid combined in the syringe. After injection activity is to be totally stopped otherwise there is risk of damage to the patient. Ice should be used on thefirst day followed by formentation and whirlpool therapy. In exceptional cases surgery may be indicated.

Note: Remember hydrocortisone therapy should be used with caution and as far as possible should be avoided and if it cannot be avoided then no exercise of the part is to be done.

Q.9. Will you suggest strengthening exercises for prevention tennis elbow ?

Ans. Once again it is being explained.

(a) Forehand tennis elbow : Lay the arm flat on the table, letting hand to extend over the edge, patient's palm facing up with a five pound weight (adjust it according to developed elbow muscles) weight, flex the wrist ten times and repeat it until you feel tired (Wwight may) be adjusted according to the type of individual and number of repetitions).

(b) Backhand tennis elbow : Lay the arm flat on a table, letting the hand extend over theedge of table, palm facing down with a five pound weight, flex your wrist ten times. Repeat until tiredness is felt. Remember never over-strain the muscles.

Q.10. Explain injury to rotator cuff in brief ?

Ans. The rotator cuff, a group of small muscles and tendons which are attached to the upper arm bone and hold it in the shoulder socket. The tendons may be torn or over reptured by sudden forceful injuries, whereas repetitive movements in throwing and racket sport, swimming and weight-lifting can all cause swelling and inflammation.

Q.11. What do you understand by bicipital tendinitis

Ans. Where the long head of biceps passes through a groove in the humerus (upper arm bone) inflammation can occure which is painful and can prevent throwing or which causes pain when putting the arm into the sleeve of a coat. Testing for this injury can be performed by opposing elbow bending which will cause pain. If physiotherapy and anti-inflammatories fail to settle the condition a cortisone injection may be successful. But rest to the arm is a nacessity.

Q.7. Can you calssify the lower leg pain, popularly known as 'shin splint' in Runners ?

Ans. Following classification is self explanatory :

(A) Posteromedical pain is the commonest one. Here pain and tenderness is seen on posteromedial aspect of tibia.
   - (i) Tibial stress reaction if not treated and exercise continued may develop into stress fracture for tibia. It develops in same mechanism as march fracture develops among soldiers due to continuous stress.
   - (ii) Inflammation, tendinitis, muscle and periosteal irritation of the ppsterior tibial area are the common structures when involved causes shin splint.

(B) Tibial pain directly on bone (This condition may be diagnosed by tuning fork test).
   - (i) Tibial stress reaction may develop into fracture if not treated with proper rest and change in biomechanics and lower limb movements.
   - (ii) Pes anserive tendinitis or bursitis or in players where both conditions are present.

(C) Pain and tenderness within the anterior tibial compartment.
   - (i) Here muscle strain, tenderness, inflammation and tendinitis may be there.
   - (ii) Anterior compartment compression syndrome.

(D) Pain in the lateral compartment of leg.

(i) Again muscle strain, inflammation and tendinitis of concerned muscles.

(ii) Lateral compartment compression syndrome.

(E) Pain and tenderness directly of Fibula.

(i) Fibular stress reaction or stress fracture of lower end of fibula.

(ii) Pain at or around the head of fibula which may be due to biceps tendinitis.

(F) Pain on posterior aspect of lower leg : Here you will find the same common conditions such as

(i) Tendinitis, inflammation, strain of adjacent structure.

(ii) Superficial or deep posterior compartment compression syndrome.

(iii) Thrombophlebitis is a rare condition.

(G) Miscellaneous conditions which may rarely cause pain in lower limb.

(i) Fascial Hernia.

(ii) Vericose veins.

(iii) Pain referred from lower back.

(iv) Interosseous membrane calcification.

(v) Popiteal artery entrapment syndrome.

'The mentioned conditions are more of the theoretical importance.

Q.13. How to differentiate between tibial stress fracture and soft tissues inflammation of the earea ?

Ans. (A) Soft tissue inflammation of adjacent structures will produce the following signs and symptoms :

(i) Tenderness mainly over the soft tissue area.

(ii) Tuning fork test-negative.

(iii) Percussion of tibia may not increase the intensity of pain.

(iv) Swelling is usually present over the soft tissue area.

(v) If stress put on involved muscles may cause further increase in pain.

(B) Tibial strees fracture :

(i) Tenderness may be at the area devoid of muscles, i.e. lower third of tibial or on tibial shaft.

(ii) Tuning fork test may be positive.

(iii) Percussion on tibia increases the intensity of pain.

(iv) Swelling may be present over the bone.
(v) Stressing the muscle may not increase the pain.

Q.14. Should player with an osteochondritis of the lunate be permitted to participate in sports ?

Ans. No. Especially during early stages, "Klenbock's Disease" which is a late involvement of lunate, may well result in compression fracture of this bone. In this condition, there is definite involvement of the lunate with bony changes, the bone going through various stages of atrophy followed by sclerosis and later calcification.

How to prevent this condition ? It may be prevented by adequate protection in the from of reinforce wrist and forearm splint.

Q.15. How does the Sprain Fracture occure ? Write its management.

Ans. Avulsion of the ligament from the bone results in a sprain fracture Such fractures require a longer period of time for union in comparison to simple sprain, when painful non-union develops between the flake of bone and the parent bone. In such cases, it is necessary to remove the fragment by operation and suture the tendon to its original bed.

Q.16. Where there is Avulsion of the Styloid, can you help the athlete ?

Ans. In such cases, the styloid process of the ulna may be pulled off. Healing occurs with fibrous union without instability. If the area is painful on movements, the styloid should be removed and the ligament may be sutured to the lower end of ulna bone.

Q.17. How to manage if Aulsion of the Radial Styloid is there ?

Ans. Since in such cases fracture involves the articular surface of the radio-carpal joint, so the fragment must be perfectly reduced and then firmly held until union is secured. If the fragments involve two-fifth of the articular surface, it should be totally replaced.

The main problem is recognition of the nature of the injury. It will be futile to try to replace the fragments and maintain fixation by any bizarre position of the wrist. Internal fixation is an absolute necessity.

Q.18. How will you treat a case of bite to 'knucle' during games ?

Ans. The following points should be kept in mind while treating a case :

(a) Infection of human bite is most difficult to treat. There may remain defect in capsule. The irregularity of metacarpophalangeal joint is also there.

(b) Treatment is to retract the would edges carefully; to ravage the wound thoroughly and to clip away any obviously necrotic tissue but be careful about sacrificing tissue.

(c) Tendon should be examined carefully by flexing the tinger. If needed, the wound may be enlarged to permit careful suture of the tendon. When the skin is ready to be closed, the contused, devitalized edge may be trimmed away very sparingly. It is important to keep well demarcated skin edges. The wound may be closed without drainage but must be watched very carefully for any swelling or infection. Prophylactic broad spectrum antibiotic is always helpful.

Q.19. What do you understand by the world 'Felon' ?

Ans. It is an abscess located within the fat pad of the finger tip. Here the pus creates pressure in the closed septal spaces, which exist primarily to provide a cushioning effect from the fat on the palmar side of the finger. When these spaces become infected, abscess pressure builds up, as it is not easily decompressed by expansion of the skin. The abscess continues to invade tissue adjacent to it, gradually enlarging until the whole finger tip may become involved. If not treated timely osteomyelitis of the distal phalanx may develop.

Q.20. How will you treat this condition ?

Ans. Incision and drainage is the only answer. Incision should be given along either the medial or lateral border of the phalanx. Fish mouth type incision is not necessary. All involved compartments should be decompressed. The wound should be closed when inflammatory reaction has subsided.

Q.21. What do you understand by 'Boutonniere Deformity'?

Ans. In this type of deformity there is avulsion of the central slip of the extensor mechanism at the proximal interphalangeal joint.

(a) Inability to actively extend the proximal interphalangeal joint is not the sign of correct diagnosis.

(b) The injury is seen after a flexion contracture of the joint takes place.

(c) X-ray may be of great help in diagnosing the condition at an early stage.

How to help the patient ? A demanic splint will be of great help. The simple splint can also be used to prevent deformity while healing takes place in the incompletely avulsed tendon for which surgical repair is not elected. An untreated boutonniere deformity will require reconstructive surgery.

Q.22. What do you know about Arterial Injuries of Hand ?

Ans. These are rare conditions. When there is direct trauma to the palm of the hand, an occasional case of thrombosis of the palmer arterial arch and its tributaries occurs. It is most prevalent in aged athletes. It may also be found in younger age groups. It is generally due to the direct trauma on the ulnar border of the hand.

Q.23. How will you diagnose this condition ?

Ans. There may be point tenderness and swelling over the hand, most commonly on the ulnar border of the hand. The fingers may be cool and pale in comparision to the other hand. These symptoms are more evident during winter season. On examination, tenderness, swelling and evidence of decreased circulation may be present. Allen's test should be performed in cases where thrombosis of the palmar arterial arch is suspected. Such test should be performed by obliterating both the radial and ulnar arteries at the wrist by pressure from doctor's finger. Patient now opens and closes his hand repeatedly until blenching occurs. At this stage pressure from ulnar side is released. If ulnar artery is an almost immediate erythema develops throughout the palm and finger.

Q.24. How does the fracture of scaphoid bone occur ? Please write its management also.

Ans. A fall on outstretched or dorsiflexed hand may cause fracture of scaphoid bone. There will be pain in the anatomical snuffbox and a weak grip will be present. The line of treatment for such a condition is immobilization for 2-3 weeks even if X-ray does not clearly show the fracture.

Q.25. If sciagram shows clear fracture of Scaphoid bone then what will be the line of treatment ?

Ans. In such cases, wrist is immobilized for 12 weeks. The persistent tenderness usually indicates non-union and onset of avascular changes in the proximal part of the bone. If fractured ends do not unite, a bone graft can be carried out by an orthopaedic surgeon.

Q.26. What do you understand by Bennett's Fracture ? How will you treat this condition ?

Ans. It is Intra-articular fracture dislocation which often requires internal fixation. In this condition, a small screw is used into the medial fragment across the fracture line. However, the small size of the fragment and obliquity of the articular surface of the trapezium often require the fracture to be reduced by pulling on the thumb, adducting and extending. Now it is transfixed by crossed kirschner wires, which can pass into either the adjacent second metacarpel or the carpel bones. These wires are removed after 3 weeks. Plaster may also be applied for 4 to 6 weeks. Sports can begin after 6-8 weeks but in boxing and similar sports, a 3-6 months lay off may be needed.

Q.27. Explain the Strain and its management giving the examples of deltoid muscles ?

Ans. Since the deltoid muscle attachment encompasses the entire outer clavical and the acromion, strain may be a problem. However, contusion of the deltoid is much more common than strain. The deltoid has a broad attachment without any particularly well localized areas of stress. If muscle tendon injury occurs, it is usually in the muscle belly. The most common site of this in the whole deltoid mechanism is at the attachment of the deltoid muscle to the shaft of the humours.

Treatment should be that of muscle strain elsewhere i.e., rest, application of heat, protection and gradual resumption of active motion, with no passive stretching. Complete rupture of a segment of the deltoid is unusual in the athlete.

Occasionally the deltoid of the throwing arm may be subject to chronic strain and may require treatment. This is much more common around the glenoid humeral joint, in the biceps, in the rotator cuff or in the attachment of the triceps to the glenoid.

Q.28. What mechanism causes 'rotators cuff' injuries ?

Ans. The following mechanism may cause injuries :

(a) During the event of throwing the whirling, head of the humerus is applied to the anterior capsule, with subsequent labrum losening and finally subluxation and rupture of the capsule occurs.

(b) Rotators cuff injury occurs when a direct fall on shoulder may tear the capsule as well as cause a fracture of the humeral tuberosity. This displaced fragment can disort the normal overhanging arch leading to subacromial bursitis and interfering with shoulder mobility.

(c) Lastly, a vertical thrust through an extended limb can be transmitted to the capsular structures. Normally, the arm is held in abduction and flexion during a fall and the forces are transmitted through the bony structure. When arm is kept by the side of soft tissue it suffers most; such an accident occurs when in skiing or skiers tend to hold the poles close to the body.

(d) A cuff injury may accompany a shoulder dislocation also.

Q.29. Explain in brief frozen shoulder ?

Ans. This describes the condition where the shoulder is frozen after some form of over use. Initially, it is most comfortable to rest the shoulder, but a loading dose of anti-inflammatory drugs, ice and mobilization under the guidance of a physiotherapist should limit the time to recover. In many cases this may take a long time in spite of all the therapies that medicines has to offer.

Q.30. What is painful arc ?

Ans. When the arm is elevated, the inflammed supraspinatus tendon is pinched between the humerus and the over hanging acromion process thereby causing pain. This over use injury affects players in contact sports, throwers, racket players and weight-lighters.

Q.31. How to manage such conditions ?

Ans. The repair of rotator cuff by using either axillary approach or anterior, superior approach is the answer. The first one is comparatively bloodless and avoids damage to tendons and muscles. However, access may be limited and the anteriosuperior incision is to be preferred in the presence of bulky muscles. The coracoacromial ligment can be divided to allow full inspection and mobilization of rotator cuff. All adhesions are divided and the torn surfaces trimmed; the edges are sutured. If the tubersity of humerus has been avulsed, the small piece of bone is removed and the cuff is laid over the defect so that it lies flush with the bone and does not impinge on the arch during an overhead swing.

Q.32. What do you understand by 'Bateman operation'?

Ans. It is the repair of anterior capsule and muscle subscapularis using facial strips darned across the defect; they are anchored in the scapula just anterior to the labrum and into the humerus just lateral to the insertion of the subscapularis. An abduction splint is worn for 3 weeks but gentle abduction exercise begins after 7 days with lowering of the splint.

Q.33. In throwing events how does the fracture of Olecranon process occur ?

Ans. When there is a sudden jerky forceful throw the triceps it may tear a small flake of bone from the tip of the olecranon. Example : Javelin or other strenuous throwing events. This injury settles in a broad arm sling for 2-3 weeks. Tension band wiring has added advantage in early immobilization. If the condition is bilateral and if there is forward slip of the upper vertebral body, the defect may c heal by fibrous tissue.

Q.34. What is Spondylolisthesis ?

Ans. Usually it is a slip of 4th lumber on 5th lumber or 5th lumber on 1st sacral vertebera. Symptoms are aggravated by exercise and pain radiates to the buttocks and legs. A disc tension may also occur but it is very rare.

Q.35. How will you diagnose this condition ?

Ans. Following points may help in the diagnosis of Spondylolisthesis :

(a) Paraspinal muscle spasm and tight hamistrings with a marked dimpling of the skin over the slipped spinous process. This feature may help in diagnosing the condition.

(b) X-ray may show the upper border of involved vertebra as too low (on level of transverse process).

(c) A gap in pars-inter articularis or an elongated lamina.

Q.36. What can be the line of treatment ?

Ans. Following approaches may be made to help the patient :

(a) Direct surgical repair provided there is little vertebral slipping. The fibrous tissue is exercised exposing the defect and after this with the help of a screw cancellous bone chips added. Both sides are treated. The player stays in bed for a few days and begins light training after 4 weeks, may start the games after 3 months.

(b) Inter transverse grafting of the slipped vertebra to the one which is situated below.

(c) The bony defect may be grafted with cancellous bone. Owing to operations (b) & (c), player has to lie prone in bed for 4-6 weeks and later he or she can get up remain in plaster jacket for another 4-8 weeks. At this stage a lumbosacral support will be of great help. Sports can start after 6-12 months. Training should be gradual at initial stages and weight training is to be avoided.

Q.37. What are the stable fractures of Spine ?

Ans. Such type of fractures involve the spinous processes, transverse processes and laminae; they also include compression fractures of the vertebral body. Treatment may be taken at an out patient basis using analgesics, lumbar supports or plaster jackets or a collar but during the acute phase, a few days of bed rest may be required. But rest is rarely needed for more than 1-2 weeks. Sports can begin with light mobilization exercises at 3-4 weeks and full activity may be joined after 2 weeks. Some discomfort may persist for several weeks; it also gradually subsides.

Q.38. Will you describe the unstable fractures of spine also ?

Ans. Such fractures may be common between C5 to C7 and T12 L2. The reason seems to be the maximum mobility. In all unstable fractures, there is soft tissue disruption of the posterior spinal ligaments, sometimes there may be separation through a disc. This soft-tissue injury is a key factor in the treatment of unstable fractures.

Q.39. What do you understand by term 'Spondylolysis' ?

Ans. This condition is found commonly in lumber vertebra where a break in the continuity of the parts interarticularis of the neural arch. It is probably a stress fracture which develops in athletes. It is common among defenders who head the ball frequently. Such problems may also develop among fast bowlers, weight lifters, javelin and hammer throwers. Though asymptomatic, it usually produces lumbar pain referred to the buttocks and legs. Players may also complain of lower abdominal discomfort especially in the region of rectus abdominis insertion.

Q.40. What do you understand by slipped disc. ?

Ans. Sudden backache is as likely to be due to aligament tear or muscle spasm as to a slipped disc in which the inner gelatinous core of the flattened disc between vertebral bones slips out to cause pressure on a nerve root emerging from the spinal canal. Sudden backache should be assumed to be from this cause until proved otherwise. The game must be stopped and the sufferer made to lie down in a comfortable position.

Q.41. How should this condition be treated ?

Ans. Rest is quite important, pain relieving drugs and plaster of lumbar support are effective. Rest may be provided by avoiding game for 2-3 months.

Q.42. There is a common word 'sciatica'. Explain it in your own word ?

Ans. This is the pain which rediates down the leg mainly as a result of a slipped disc and the psoas position may be found to be most comfortable. Back injuries need assessment to find a cause, though fifty percent of back pains will get better within a week in spite of medical help with bedrest and anti-flammatory durgs. Recurrent or continuing pains need full assessment, including X-rays and scans if appropriate, and a planned mobilization with a physiotherapist. Those that fail resolve may need traction, manipulation or even surgery.

Q.43. What may be the common signs and symptoms of trauma to abdomen ?

Ans. In all such cases, localized pain, abdominal rigidity and vomiting are present. Pain may be referred to the shoulders as abdominal contents or blood irritates the diaphragm. Blood may also appear in the urine or in stool. Kidney injuries of mild type may be treated conservatively and a precautionary intra venous palaeography is suggested.

Q.44. What is about the Heamatoma and Sprains of Abdominal wall ?

Ans. These injuries are of minor importance and may heal with rest of 1-2 weeks. Sprains of the pelvic insertion of rectus abdominis may require local infiltration with hydrocortisone and ligocain if they become chronically painful. Here vigorous activity is to be avoided otherwise otherwise athlete may damage his rectus abdominis muscle.

Q.45. Will you mention about abdominal hernias ?

Ans. Events like weight lifting, weight training, wrestling etc. may be considered as common sports for hernia development in unconditioned players. As a known procedure, surgical repair is the answer. After 6-12 weeks gradually sports may be started.

Q.46. What are the avulsion fractures ?

Ans. Violent muscles which cause avulsion fractures are the sartorius, rectus femoris and the hamstrings.

Q.47. How will you treat them ?

Ans. Rest to injured muscles in a relaxed position of comfort is a necessity. The normal activities are resumed after 4 weeks or so depending on local discomfort.

Q.48. What is subcutaneous Emphysema ?

Ans. When the air escapes from a damaged lung or air passage and finds its way into the chest wall, mediastinum and subcutaneous tissues by way of a tear in the parietal pleura. It is occasionally associated with the open chest wound; and when there is a rapid accumulation, a torn bronchus should be suspected. This condition should be immediately controlled otherwise there may be risk to the life of patient.

Q.49. What should be the treatment for such type of condition ?

Ans. For such type of condition, no specific treatment is required but attention should be directed to treat the underlying cause. If there is an open sucking wound of chest wall, it should be immediately closed with a clean handkerchief or vaseline pad.

Q.50. What are the possible cardiac injuries in sports ?

Ans. The great vessels and heart may get injury as result of trauma to the chest while contusion to the pericardium can result and there may be E.C.G. changes in heart. There may be ST segment depression and T wave inversion. Arrhythmias are not uncommon but usually transient. Treatment is by complete bed rest for several days and sports is not recommended upto 3 months. A further E.C.G. may be required before activity is resumed.

Q.51. What can happen when there is a direct 'Blow to the Abdomen' ?

Ans. There are rare chances to injure the contents of abdomen because of protection by the strong abdominal muscles and the mobility of many of the viscera. Relatively fixed organs are the most frequently damaged.

Sometimes liver injury may follow a blow to right lower ribs, when there is direct blow to left lower ribs, the spleen may be damaged. The common organs which may be damaged are kidney, testis, urethera and intestines.

Q.52. How will you diagnose 'Osteitis Pubis' ?

Ans. Ostetis Pubis may be diagnosed from the following :

(i) Discomfort in groin which will gradually increase especially during and after exercise by sprinting, jumping etc.

(ii) In the next stage, the pain extends over the whole of the pubic area, perinium and down the inner aspect of the thigh (along the distribution of the obturator nerve).

(iii) Tenderness is found over the sumphysis, the whole of the pubic bone.

(a) on compression of pelvis; during full flexion of the either leg;

(b) on passive adduction at the hip;

(c) on resisted contraction of the adductor muscles of the thingh.

(iv) X-RAY shows fraying of the corners of the symphysis. Osteoporosis and moth eaten erosions may also be seen.

Q.53. How will you treat this condition ?

Ans. (a) Activity is to be stopped for 4-8 weeks. In the initial month the suggested treatment is anti-inflammatory drugs with short wave diathermy. After reclassification, gentle mobilization and at a later stage running may be permitted. Full sport is allowed after three months.

(b) Very rarely surgery is needed for bone block grafts.

(c) Refractory cases may take 9-12 months to become symptoms free although most of the players return to game in six months.

As far as possible, natural healing process should be allowed to work and local injection, ultra-sounds should be avoided as they may hinder the healing process.

Q.54. What are the rider's and hamstring origin strain ?

Ans. It may occur in two ways :

(a) The adductor origin strains (rider's strains) are found in cyclists, horsemen, runners, footballers and fast bowlers. Pain and stiffness are felt in the groin and there is local tenderness and pain while adduction action is performed.

(b) Hemistring origin strains are common among sprinters and footballers. The sudden severe pain in the buttock may predispose to sciatica. Tenderness may be found at the insertion of the muscle. Treatment is by heat, and gentle stretching. If pain is too much, it may be done under local anaesthesia. This type of stretching under anaesthesia is rarely needed.

Q.55. What will be the treatment for rider's strain ?

Ans. Here the treatment is by manipulation under general anaesthesia. Massage or local steroids are also suggested. When calcification in the adductor longus tendon is seen (horse riders) they need local excision. Heat and analgesics are also helpful during an acutely painful episodes. Remember, in breast stroke swimming, with its usual leg action chronic adductor tendinitis may be produced.

Q.56. What is to be done when there is a fracture of Sacrum Bone ?

Ans. Generally the displacement is not there and pain relieving drugs will help. However, sitting may require a rubber cushion for several weeks. Chronic pain after this type of fracture is treated by local anaesthetic injections; persistent coccygeal tenderness may warrant excision of the coccyx.

Q.57. What do you understand by condition 'Osteitis Pubis' ?

Ans. Osbtetis Pubis is a self limiting condition of sportsmen, often in their thirties, and common in professional footballers, but may be found in runners and long distance walkers.

Q.58. Explain in brief the condition 'Spina Bifida Occulta'.

Ans. In this condition there is failure of fusion of the arch of one or more of the vertebrae posteriorly. This common finding has no significance. The player should not be unnecessarily alarmed or be told that spinabifida is a dangerous condition. Exceptionally, a wide open spinabifida involving several vertebrae may be of importance to require the additional support. A well placed sacral pad may provide some protection. If at all needed, the player who has wide open spina bifida may avoid vigorous activities.

Q.59. Describe the 'Pellegrine - Stieda. Disease'.

Ans. This disease develops due to formation of a plaque of calcium on adductor group. Along the medial femoral condyle in the vicinity of the adductor tubercle, there is separation from the tibia by a band of radiolucency. In a few cases a reaction to sprain occurs, in which there has been a forcible detachment of the medial collateral ligament at its attachment to the femoral condyle while in certain players there is evidence of partial avulsion of the adductor longus tendon. The symptoms are those of the knee with the tenderness on the condyle in the one case and of adductor strain in the other. The presence of the mass is not necessarily of any consequence, the significant factor being the degree of pain. Frequently the area remains painful even after the injury has healed.

Q.60. What is the management of this condition ?

Ans. As per decision of the surgeon, if needed, the removal of the plaque is necessary. It is done if the surgeon is too eager and removes the mass before it is entirely mature, it will form again. If it is necessary to remove it, great care should be taken that there is no interference with the attachment of the ligament to the femur. In majority of cases, removal of the plaque will not be necessary because the condition may mature and become quite insert with the passage of time. The anterior edge of the shoulder pad usually extends to about this level and edge of the pad itself may well contribute to the damage rather than protection to the area. The haemorrhage that occurs generally is not extensive and, indeed, is not enough to be palpable as haematoma.

Treatment : Treatment at an early stage is by adequate protection with a simple fibreboard pad. This pad prevents recurrence of injury. Suitable injunction in the area and timely cold and hot applications may give prompt relief.

Q.61. What are the other conditions which should be ruled out, before diagnosing a tennis elbow ?

Ans. Following important conditions of related structures should be kept in mind :

(a) true epicondylitis of the extensor supinator aponeurotic attachment to the lateral epicondyle;
(b) radial ulnar sinovitis;
(c) strain in the aponeurosis itself, often it develops directly over the radial head;
(d) radial humeral bursitis and a rare condition ulnar neuritis.

Q.62. Explain in brief the 'Kienbock's Disease'.

Ans. It is a late involvement of the lunate bone, may well be the result of compression fracture of this bone. This condition is called osteitis, osteochondritis or malacia of the lunate. It is most common in the adolescent. There is a definite involvement of the lunate along with bony changes, this bone goes through various stage (atrophy followed by sclerosis and layer decalcification, often with fragmentation resulting in marked change in shape of the bone). This deformity may be prevented by early recognition and protection. Now the question arises whether an athlete should be allowed to participate in sports. Certainly, he should not participate during early stage. Without protection of reinforced wrist or a forearm splint athlete should not play. Generally the period of resolution of this bone may be a couple of years. If other carpel bones are also involved same treatment should be given to these carpel bones.

Q.63. What are the basic principles of fast running ?

Ans. The following points should always be kept in mind while running.

(a) Relax. The body must be supple to attain best performance.
(b) Run on the balls of the feet.
(c) Point the toes straight ahead. Athlete loses at least half an inch on each step if toes are not kept straight ahead (Remember P.T. Usha missed her bronze medal by. 001 seconds. So every inch is important for an athlete.)

(d) Always try to run in a straight line. It is the shortest distance between two points.
(e) Develop proper stride. The average stride should be of the light of the athlete's body in any case, muscle shortening should not be developed).
(f) Remember : never overstride, it is worst than an understride as it may reduce the speed.
(g) Running angle is also important; body leaning, head up; ankles, hips shoulders and head in a straight line. Do not bend too far backward with proper running angle. Proper stride should be maintained.

Opposite arm and leg should move in an order. Arm should be relaxed, not allowed to go out of the centre of body. A relax piston like movement should be there for both arms. (It is especially needed for middle distances and long distance running.)

Q.64. What are the basic things for approaching an athlete for treatment ?

Ans. Remember 5 A's. viz.

— Accept athletics.
— Avoid expedience.
— Adopt the best method.
— Act promptly.
— Achieve perfection.

Q.65. For treating a haematoma, what point should be kept in mind ?

Ans. Diagnosis should be prompt because delay will cause more collection of blood. Aspirate if necessary.

— The volume of contained blood should be reduced by aspiration, hyaluronidase, pressure, first ICE, then heat, and later on closely controlled activity.
— Resorption should be encouraged by exposing the haematoma to a larger surface area of circulation and by maintaining the general circulation.

Note : Excessive haematoma formation enhances chances of ossification or calcification which may be prevented by using needed procedure timely. It is always done according to size and site of the haematoma.

Q.56. What do you understand by the term 'Tenosynovitis'?

Ans. It may be defined as inflammation of the synovium surrounding a tendon. Such type of inflammation is usually due to strain from unaccustomed overuse but also may be due to a direct blow. It is very rare when infection may be the underlying cause. Normally the vascular synovium reacts with increased blood supply over secretion of synovial fluid and increase in fibrin content, causing 'sticky' adhesions between the tendon and its surroundings.

Q.67. What are its common signs and symptoms ?

Ans. Signs and symptoms depend on the tendon involved pain on movement or even during rest; crepitation is frequently present. As the tendon with movements slides up and down, it adheres to the sinovium, causing so called 'snowball crepitation', later on due to adhesion formation gliding movements stops.

Q.68. What is the possible treatment of this condition ?

Ans. These conditions are treated by rest, heat and local injection Specific treatments are given according to site of involvement.

Q.69. What do you know about the 'Blocker's Exostosis' ?

Ans. This condition may be defined as :

"It is a contusion of the middlethird of the arm in the vicinity of, and actually just over, the attachment of deltoid muscle on the lateral aspect of the humerus." Here the bone approximates the skin quite closely, particularly in sulcus it is between the anterior distal portion of the deltoid and the biceps. This coincides with the area most frequently struck by the blocker as the throws his arm up to check the impetus of the charging, opposing player. A direct blow by the hard head-gear or repeated light blows in this areas will result in contusion of the tendon of the deltoid and of the periosteum of the humerus where the deltoid inserts.

Q.70. Can you describe the word 'stitch' in relation to athletic activities ?

Ans. Though this condition is not directly related to injury or muscle strain yet it is quite common among sportsmen.

The pain is felt on one side of abdomen during excessive training or exercise. It subsides when exercise is stopped. Mostly it is present on right side of abdomen, but it may also be on left side or all over abdomen. There may be many factors responsible for it :

(a) Spasm of diaphragm wall.

(d) Ligaments linking the diaphragm to digestive system get tense due to exercise and put vibrating stress through abdomen. Example : running in basket ball etc. (Player bends and runs, so more intra abdominal pressure.)

(c) Gas in large bowel or liver congestion.

Until or unless it is quite severe, on should not worry about it. Stretching helps the, athlete. Though this condition is partially explained in previous questions yet the above mentioned aspect is important and should be clearly understood.

Q.71. How to identify 'acute abdomin ?

Ans.
1. No evident abdominal injury.
2. Abdominal pain, local or diffuse.
3. Abdominal tenderness, local or diffuse.
4. A quiet patient who does not want to move because it hurts.
5. A patient who is breathing rapidly and not deeply because a deep breath hurts.
6. Rapid pulse.
7. Low blood pressure.
8. A tense, often distended abdomen.
9. Referred pain.
10. Fever.

Q.72. After the examination, how acute abdomen can be suspected ?

Ans.
1. Determine whether patient is restless or quiet, whether motion cause pain, or whether any characteristics position, distention or abnormality is present.
2. Feel the abdomen gently to see whether it is tense or soft.
3. Determine whether the patient can relax the abdominal wall on command.
4. Determine whether the abdomen is tender when touched.

Q.73. What do you understand by 'Back problem' ?

Ans. Besides games and sports, a variety of medical conditions may hurt the back by affecting the spinal joints. Apart from joint problems in the spine, problems of the various internal organs in the abdomen may give rise to low back pain. In most of the athletes, it is observed that it is due to inflammation of connective tissue of muscles, fascia, ligaments, nerve sheaths, tendons and periosteum. Regarding etiology, there is no proof that it is due to infection the intestine or in other sites such as the teeth, tonsils, sinuses or gall bladder. Exciting causes are strain, cold and damp climate.

Q.74. What is the basic pathology behind common type of Low Back-ache ?

Ans. Small nodules are formed in some cases in the muscles, lipomatous masses between the superficial and deep fascia which are vascular and become oedematous. They constitute trigger points for referred sciatic pain, and in this condition inflammatory changes occur in the connective tissues also.

Q.75. What are the common clinical findings in such cases ?

Ans. The clinical findings may be divided in three broad groups :

(a) The patient is usually an adult. There may be history of cold exposure, or of muscular strain. The lumbar muscles are commonly affected. The attack comes usually after making a violent movement with the leg, or spine, or arms.

(b) In sub-acute case, there is less severe pain, felt in the back, which is intensified on stooping, lifting, sneezing and coughing On deep palpitation nodules which are very tender, may be felt.

(c) Sometimes the inflammatory process may extend to involve the sheath of the sciatic and other nerves. Generally the patient recovers from an acute attack in 3 to 4 weeks, but he is liable to get recurrences of the problem.

Q.76. What are the causes for back problems ?

Ans. Detailed lists of the common causes for back problems are :

(A) — Urogenital problems,
— Gynaecological problems,
— Digestive problems,
— Muscle strains,
— Chronic strains,
— Ligament strains,
— Sprung back,
— Prolapse intervertebral disc,
— Sacro-iliac sprain.

(B) The Skeleton may cause back ache due to the following conditions :
— Fracture and Dislocation,
— Spondylosis,
— Spondylolisthesis,
— Congenital abnormalities (Spina-bifida)

(C) Disease of the Spine :
— Tuberculosis,
— Ankylosing Spondylitis,
— Vertebral Epiphysis,
— Osteoarthritis.

Q.77. Mention in brief the anatomical structural support to back.

Ans. It may be divided into the following groups :

(A) Anatomical consideration : Lumbar vertebrae with cartilaginos cushions (discs) between them, and the fused bones, of the sacrum and coccyx that forms the back of the pelvis. There are also ligaments, thick dense strains of connective tissue that attach one bone to another. Following ligaments have some elasticity and thus provide the back with mobility.

Ligaments of Lumbar Region :
— Inter-spinous,
— Inter-transverse,
— Ligamentum flavum,
— Anterior and posterior longitudinal ligaments,
— Annulus fibrosus.

(B) Muscles : There are four groups of muscles essential for support of the back and play major role in back pain. We may think of the low back as a pole held erect by four guy-wire muscle groups :

Muscle groups :

(a) Anterior guy wires - rectus abdominis, internal and external oblique, transverse abdominis,

(b) Posterior guy wires - all muscles of back, tendons and ligaments,

(c) Side muscles or two lateral guy wires - guadratus lumborum, psoas major.

(C) Besides this hips and other muscles have very significant effect on the back. They may be divided into four groups viz.

— Flexors (lifts hip up)

— Adductor (turns hip out),

— Adductors (turns hip in),

— Extensors (lifts hip back) - most massive and important support for back.

Q.78. Can you explain about low back pain among athletes ?

Ans. Most of the athletic injuries to the low back involve contusion, a bruise from direct blow; strain, pulling with stretching and tearing of the muscles or their tendons; or strain, tearing of aligament. In general strain is more painful especially when the back is forced in opposite direction. This produces a strain produced pain when the effected muscle is contracted. Because of the intricate relationship of the muscles, tendons, and ligaments of the back, most of the injuries involve two or all the three entities together. Trying to separate them is of academic value only.

The cause of most back sprains and strains in the athletes and non-athletes are generally due to weak muscles. It is especially true with the abdominal muscles and hip flexors. One aspect is of importance, i.e. tension or lack of flexibility especially in the hamstring-hip extensor muscles. But how could national level and even world class athletes have weak muscles ?

Answer is during intensive training for specific requirements of their sports, they neglect anatomic areas (the back-abdomen-hip). It is the wrong notion that these structures do not require development for specific game and here lies the main fault.

Q.79. Will you explain it with few examples or game situations ?

Ans. Here are a couple of examples to make it more clear :

(1) Weight lifting accounts for proportionately more injuries than any other sport, though exact figures cannot be quoted in view of the frequent adaptation of weight training by participants in other sports.

(2) Field events in athletics-the hammer, Javelin and putting the shot, high jumping and long jumping are particularly proved to cause muscle strains.

(3) Gymnasts repeatedly dismount with a hyper-extended low back as their feet hit the mat. Something happens when diver hits the water in extension with foot entry dives.

(4) Lack of training may be additional factor in strain of muscle, while the degenerative changes of middle age are more likely to predispose to ligament tears.

Q.80. So, what preventive steps should be taken ?

Ans. To prevent an injury is more beneficial than to cure it. Some of the rules which apply particularly to the back are enumerated below :

(1) Elimination of the basically unfit, i.e. Scheuermann's disease.

(2) Gradual training to attain the necessary fitness.

(3) Correct technique in training and performance.

(4) Applying the techniques of training to everyday life. Correct posture at work and adequate support during sleep are equally essential. The ligaments of the lumber spine may be subjected to constant irritation from a habitually flexed position at work, or due to sleeping on a soft bed at night.

(5) Recognition of the early signs of degenerative changes in the tissues and adjustment of the athlete's demands on his own body accordingly.

Q.81. What is the line of treatment of low back pain ?

Ans. The successful treatment of low back pain in athletes involves a three-step programme. First is relief of pain and spasm; Second of an appropriate exercise programme that includes both stretching and strengthening exercises; Third, an educational programme that takes into consideration one's training program and is tailored to preventive future injuries.

(a) Relief of pain and spasm : Ice, analgesics, muscle relaxants, anti-inflammatory agents and rest are used in acute stage.

(b) Heat, muscle stimulation and/or ultrasound, physical therapy, and the same pharmacologic agents are used 12 or more hours after injury. Ultrasound and gentle muscle stimulation seem more helpful to dissipate muscle spasm, point tenderness, and general soreness. This is probably due to enhanced muscle circulation and exchange at the cellular level of prescribed pharmacological agents. It also nelps in elimination of toxic cellular products.

(c) Actually, while modes of pain relief exist, no one treatment has been clearly demonstrated to accelerate actual tissue healing.

Q.82. Mention the management if backache is due to prolapsed inter Vertenral disk ?

Ans. The treatment of prolapsed intervertebral disc should be conservative at the initial stage with complete bed rest advisable for a severed ligament sprain. Early operation shouid only be recommended when extensive neurological signs are present. Very marked paralysis or sensory loss may never recover fully if the nerve roots are not decompressed within a matter of two or three days. Besides already mentioned points for backache traction proves to be of great value.

Q.83. What is the role of manipulation in backache ?

Ans. Manipulative treatment is controversial in the problems of lumbar spine. The success rate in relieving symptoms is 85 per cent. In chronic muscle injury or ligament sprain resulting from old injuries may have more success but it is very much less in acute sprains.

Q.84. Will you mention about operative proccedures for back problems ?

Ans. It may be described in the following groups :

(A) Exploration of the spine is occasionally indicated in dislocations in the presence of a progressive paraplegia, or a partial paraplegia when it is felt that additional recovery may follow decompression of the spinal cord. After exploration, the opportunity will usually be taken to fuse the affected area.

(B) Prolapsed intervertebral discs may require operation when there are gross neurological changes. It may also be advisable in relapsing case or following failure to an adequate course of conservative treatment.

(C) The removal of a disc through an inter-laminar approach (Posterior rhachotomy) is quite feasible. It is of importance particularly in the young adult, and does not interfere in any way with the stability of the lumbar spine. It is, therefore, a relatively minor procedure and there is no contra-indication afterwards to an active athletic life.

(D) Spinal fusion for instability is mostly required at the lumbosacral joint. An athlete subjected to spinal fusion should be warned against taking part in further violent exercise or competitive sport. Not only does he run the risk of fracturing or stressing the graft, but the remaining joints of the lumbar spine are subjected to extra strain and will wear out all the more rapidly.

Q.85. What type of instructions should be given to the athlete ?

Ans. The detailed education may be given in the following ways :

Health Education Programme : The final link in the low back pain elimination triangle involves educating the athlete how to avoid back problems, both in training and in daily life. Good posture is achieved by rotating the top of the pelvis backward, which, which flattens the curve in the low back. Common every day tips to avoid the occurrence of low back pain include the following :

(a) Standing and Walking : Stand with low back erect and as flat as possible. By squeezing buttocks and sucking in and tensing abdomen, the lower back is straightened. Walk, stand and sit as tall as possible.

— Bend knee when leaning, as whenever a wash basin is used. Avoid leaning whenever possible.

— Avoid high heeled shoes. They shorten the Achilles tendons and increase lordosis.

— Avoid standing for long periods of time, but if it is necessary, alternate leaning on the left foot and right foot, and if possible use the bent knee position as on a stool. This flattens the lower back.

— When standing, do not lean back and support the body with the hands. Keen in fron of body and lean forward slightly.

— When turning to walk from a standing position, move feet first and then body.

— Open doors wide enough to walk through comfortably.

— Carefully judge the height of curbs before steeping up or down.

(b) Sitting : Sit so that lower back is flat or slightly rounded outward, never with a forward curve.

— Sit so that knees are higher than hips; this may require a small footstool for a short person sitting in a high chair.

— Hard seat backs that begin contact with back 4 to 6 inches above the seat and provide a flat support through the entire lumbar areas are preferable.

— Do not sit in a soft, or overstuffed chair or sofa.

— Do not sit with legs out straight on a footstool.

— Never sit in the same position for prolonged periods, get up and move around.

(c) Bedrest : Sleep or rest only on a flat firm mattress. If one is not available, place bedboard of no less than three-quarter inch plywood under the mattress. A board of less thickness will sag, preventing proper spine alignment.

— When sleeping, the preferred position is lying on the side, both arms in front, and knees slightly drawn up toward chin.

— Do not sleep on stomach.

— When lying on back, place a pillow under knees, as raising the legs flattens the lumbar curve.

— When lying in bed, do not extend arms above head, relax them at sides.

— If the doctor prescribes absolute bedrest, stay in bed. Raising the body or twisting and turning can strain the back.

— Sleep alone or in an oversized bed.

— When getting out of bed, turn over on side, draw up

knees, then swing legs over the side of the bed.

(d) Lifting : When lifting, let the legs do the work, using the large muscles of the thighs instead of the small muscles of the back.

— Do not twist the body, face the object.
— Never lift with legs straight.
— Do not lift heavy objects with jerks.
— Do not lift from a bending forward position.
— Do not reach over furniture to open and close windows.
— Tuck in the buttocks and pull in the abdomen when lifting.
— Only lift holding the object close to body.
— Lift a heavy load no higher than the waist, and a light load no higher than the shoulders, as greater height increases lumbar lordosis.
— To turn while lifting pivot feet turning the whole body at one time.

Q.86. Give few tips on running ?

Ans. 1. Short sprints develops speed.
2. Distance running develops endurance.
3. Running in circles and figure 8's streng thens ankles, knees, hips and back.

Q.87. What is the role of warming up and warming down in back-ache prevention ?

Ans. In training, to minimize back injuries, the athlete should always warm up slowly up slowly and cool down after the main work-out. Both the warm-up and cooling-down periods should include backstretching exercises. Calisthenics that involve hyper-extension of the back such as back bends, straight leg sit-ups, or straight leg raises should be avoided when possible.

By faithfully carrying out a daily programme of back exercise, the athlete can pursue a variety of potentially hazardous sports with minimal risk of back injury.

Q.88. Name a few sports and games where chances of getting backache are less.

Ans. The sports less likely to result in back injuries include basket ball, golf, soft ball, water skiing, rowing, cross-

country skiing, badminton, and archery.
Sports least likely to result in back injury include bicycling, hiking, swimming, fishing, sailing.

Q.89. Please enumerate certain important positions of selected games which may lead to backache.

Ans. The athlete can best prevent back injuries by daily execution of appropriate back and abdominal muscle stretching and strengthening exercises. For any sports, the athlete should always warm up slowly and include back stretching exercises. In specific sports, the most hazardous manoeuvers, those carried out with the low back in extension can be modified. The serve and the overhead are the two tennis strokes most strenuous to the back. By tossing the serve slightly forward, legs back extension is required and, thus, less back strain. For those who play a serve and volley game, it will also aid in gaining forward momentum toward the net. When hitting the overhead, up to the ball hitting it slightly in front of the body. When trying for a low ball, whether tennis, handball, volleyball and softball, whenever possible bend the knees rather than the back. Most gymnastic sports, including diving, stress good posture. The athlete at all times should sit and stand as tall as possible. The runner, equestrian, diver and gymnast alike should keep their low backs flat by tensing their buttocks and abdominal muscles whenever possible.

Q.90. Wow can exercise therapy help the low back problems ?

Ans. Medications, Electro-therapy, massage, hot and cold applications do not strengthen weakened muscles or ligaments. Once the heating process has occurred, it is essential to embark on an exercise programme in a progressive manner to rebuild the back and abdominal muscles.

Q.91. What peculiarities Lumbar vertebrae has in relation to their anatomical structures ?

Ans. The human spine is a phenomenal structure that can withstand the force of thousand pound pressed by a weightlifter, yet is flexible enough to nearly bend itself.

In the Laboratory, the lumbar disc in the young adults will tolerate force about 500 kg. prior to injury to the vertebral plate. The lumbar disc behaves similar to a universal joint and allows for a great deal of flexibility because of the plastic qualities and high liquid contents of the disc. It functions according to the principles of hydrodynamic. The disc flexibility allows Lumbar Motion in all axial planes. The fluid properties of the muscles distribute the forces applied to the disc uniformly on the end plate of the vertebral bodies. However, if the torsion is too severe then the distribution of forces become unequal and disc herniation or vertebral body fracture will occur.

In the Lumbar Area, the facets are located more posteriorly than in the remaining spine. Therefore, the excess of rotation is posterior to the disc and excessive rotation exerts a shearing stress (small forces acting on the surface of the structure on a plain parallel to the applied load) on the disc. The disc fails mainly in torsion (rotatory forces in opposite direction-a frequent stress in athlete.) The Lumbosacral Junction is the area of motion in the Lumbar Spine. Pain frequently has it origin from this level.

Q.92. How is the flexibility of this spine maintained ?

Ans. The stability and flexibility of the Lumbar Spine depends upon intrinsic structures. The disc and ligaments are the initial support while the extrinsic influencing structures are the thoraces and abdominal cavities with their associated muscles. The thoracic and abdominal cavities as act as cylinders composed of air liquid with rigid muscular walls to diminish the stress on the spine during strenuous activity.

In the Lumbar area, the disc in between, push the vertebrae apart while the supporting ligaments pull the bodies together, thus creating a strong but flexible bond. The erector spinal muscles are the major muscles of the lumbar spine. They are the primary muscles injured in lumbar muscular strain. The abdominal and the iliopsoas muscles also play a significant role in low back problems. The abdominal muscles are responsible for positioning the lumbar spine of the athlete in a position of flexion to diminish the forces of shearing, bending and torsion, frequently encountered in sports activities. These muscles function to position the spine for maximal power and efficiency.

The iliopsoas muscles is a strong hip flexor due to the upright position of the human, this muscle is in constant contraction and pulls the lumbar spine into lordosis. The cause of most of the lower back pain/sprain and strain is due to lumbar lordosis and weakness of the abdominal muscle Back and abdominal strength diminish stress and fatigue on the spine.

Q.93. What is the need and importance of strengthening exercises?

Ans. Strengthening exercises have an important role to play. Do these exercises comfortably, never push body forcefully :

(a) Back extension exercise : All these exercises are carried out lying on stomach, Except where otherwise stated, do three sets of ten, for each exercise.

(i) With your hands resting at your sides, lift your head and shoulders backwards, just a little, hold for a count of three, then gently lower.

(ii) With your hands clasped behind your back, elbow straight; lift your head and shoulder backwards just a little, hold for a count of three, then slowly lower.

(iii) Lie over the end of your bed, so that your trunk bends forward (fix your feet if necessary). With your hands by your side, lift your head and shoulders backwards until you are arching back slightly, hold for three, then slowly lower down again.

(iv) With your arms stretched out straight forward, above your head, lift your arms, shoulders, head, together with both legs, just a little way backwards, so that your whole trunk arches slightly. Hold to three, then slowly lower.

(v) With your hands behind your head, finger touching or interlocked, elbows bent, lift your elbow, head and shoulders, together with your one leg, then lower and lift again, this time raising your another leg backwards a little way. Repeat in quick succession.

(b) Abdominal Exercises : All these exercises are carried out lying on back. Except where otherwise stated, of three sets of ten for each exercise.

(i) Lying flat, with your hands resting on your things, lift your head and shoulders forward a little way, sliding your hands down your thongs towards your knees. Do not sit right up, but just enough to see your feet. Hold to three, then gently lower back.

(ii) Lying on your back with your knees bent, feet flat on the floor, with your hands clasped behind your head, elbows bent, lift your head and shoulders then slowly lower back.

At the same position, now lift your head and shoulders to touch your left elbow to your right knee, then lower back, and lift forward again to touch your right elbow to your left knee.

(iii) Lying flat, with your hands, behind your head, lift both legs back, bending your knees and bring your head and shoulders forward to touch your elbow to your knees. After this slowly lower back.

Q.94. Will you further explain the mobility exercises ?

Ans. These exercises are done kneeling on hands and knees.

(i) Keeping your arms and legs still, arch your back to hump it upwards, while you bend your head downwards.

The curve your back to hollow it out, while you raise your head up. Repeat the sequence in quick succession ten times.

(ii) Bend your one knee forward as you bend your head down, so that you touch your forehead with your knee, then stretch your leg straight out behind you, as you raise your head so that your back arches slightly. Repeat in quick succession three times on each leg in turn, up to ten sets on each leg.

(b) Lying on your back : These exercises are done with your knees bent and your feet resting on the floor. Flatten your back, then keeping your feet and shoulders still, push your set up, then lower it, quickly ten times.

Q.95. How are the stretching exercises performed ?

Ans. These exercises can be done in the following manner :

(1) Lying on your stomach with your arms bent close to your sides so that your hands rest just under your

shoulders, push your arms straight to arch your back, lifting up your head so that your whole spine curves back. Hold for a count of ten, then gently relax.

(2) Lying on your stomach, holding your ankles in your hands, stretch your shoulders and ankle upwards and backwards to arch your back.

(3) Lying your back on a cushioned but firm surface, rest your weight on your shoulders, Gently take your legs over your head, keeping your knees bent at first, and gradually straightening your knees as you become more flexible with practice. (Do not do this exercise if it hurts your neck, or if you have blood pressure problems.)

Q.96. What is the importance of these exercises ?

Ans. The athlete can best prevent back injuries by daily execution of appropriate back and abdominal muscle strengthening, and stretching exercises. Poor posture or lumbar lordosis should be prevented by keeping the low back flat by tensing the buttocks and abdominal muscles. There is no substitution for the faithful daily back exercise programme. The ultimate responsibility for eliminating the risk of back injury, therefore, lies with the athlete.

Q.97. What do you understand by word locking of knees ?

Ans. Although a torn certilage may cause locking of knees. They also became solidly locked if a piece of loose bone or cartilage prevents normal flexion or extension of the knees. Osteochondritis dissecans is a condition which can particularly affect young footballers where trauma causes fragments to break off from the articular surface of the bones to float about within the joint causing pain and disability. The diagnosis can be confirmed by X-ray. It is some times possible to surgically reattach the loose body, but as osterarthrits is more prevalent in sports person who have suffered from steochondritis dissecans they are advised to reduce their sporting activity.

Q.98. How does better muscular development around knee joint reduce incidence of injury ?

Ans. It can be explained in the following three groups :

(a) The muscles constituting the thigh and surrounding

the knee joint are of extreme importance in preserving the stability of a basically unstable knee joint. It has been shown that athletes who conditioned all the muscles around the knee have a far less incidence of injury than those who do not.

(b) The quadriceps are the prime knee extensor but also control flexion by antagonizing gravity and the hamstring muscle. It also enhances the patellar stability. Contraction of the quadricep muscles has been shown to reduce strain the medial collateral ligament, regardless of the degree of knee flexion.

(c) The hamstrings are situated on the posterior aspect of the thigh and are nearly as important as the quadriceps in preserving the stability of the knee.

Q.99. What are the major functions of the Hamstring muscles ?

Ans. The major functions of Hamstring muscles are :

(1) To flex the extended knee.

(2) To control the extension of the knee by acting as a break to the quadriceps. If the quadriceps are too powerful relative to the hamstrings a strained hamstring can result.

(3) To extend the hip.

At the clinical level, one observes a relatively high incidence of hamstrings strains at junction of the long and short heads, a fact explained by many Orthopaedic surgeons and bio-mechanical experts that the cause is due to two separate innervations.

Q.100. What is Hoffar's syndrome ?

Ans. Many sports-men, particularly runners, are concerned by pain and swelling which can occur below each side of the kneecap. This is fat rather than fluid and occurs following overuse. It is one of the causes of anterior knee pain and is normally 'settled using Rice, anti-inflammatries, physiotherapy and occasionally a cortisone injection. The player should reduce his training to the amount that was comfortable before the condition occurred.

Q.101. What is Charley House ?

Ans. It is nothing but the contusion to the quadriceps. It can be one of the most disabling injury to an athlete. This is generally caused by a severe blow to the front of the thigh causing bleeding and variable amount of muscle is crushed. This injury is also known as Charley House. Swelling and tightness of the thigh musculature are observed soon afterwards together with loss of knee flexion.

Q.102. Explain in brief ITFB syndrome ?

Ans. As well as the muscles which stabilise the knee there is a sheet of rough muscular running minning down the outside of the leg known as the ilio-tibial band. This normally rides without friction over the outer side of the lower end of the femur, but if sportsman are at all bow-legged this band may rub against the bony prominence causing a clicking discomfort when the knee is slightly bent though it does not occur when the knee is fully straightened. It may be possible to correct the gait with shoe build-ups to prevent the exaggerated bowleggedness, but some sports-men require steroid injections between bone and ilio-tibial tract if ice and phystotherapy fail to settle the condition.

Q.103. How to manage such an injury ?

Ans. Following procedure is to be adopted for management of Charley House :

(a) Application of cold and a wet elastic wrap to the thigh at the level of the contusion. The ice should be kept on the spot for a longer time.

(b) Mild Quadriceps Stretch : The athlete should lie prone, keeping the knee flexed. This can be achieved if an elastic bandage is tied around the ankle and the knee is flexed until minimum discomfort is felt. The athlete holds the elastic bandage over the shoulder to maintain the desired amount of knee flexion. Force should not be applied in flexing the knee. This procedure helps to maintain the flexibility of the knee and the quadriceps. If the leg is kept straight, marked stiffness will occur.

(c) Analgesics are of use but may decéive the athlete regarding recovery. Ice should applied for 20 minutes. The knee should be kept in flexion. If there appears to be pain and inflammation then the same procedure should follow for at least 12 to 24 hours.

(d) Icing should be continued with the knee flex for 30 to 60 minutes at a time once or twice a day.

(e) Quadriceps drill should be started provided no pain is caused.

(f) Isometric exercises should start. The contraction should be held for at least 5 to 8 seconds and such exercises should be done 10 times in each hour. When full contraction of quadriceps is achieved, straight leg raising can be started.

A period of 4 to 8 weeks is necessary before the athlete can start using rehabilitated leg.

Q.104. What is Myositis ossificans ? Explain it in relation to knee joint.

Ans. A severe injury may cause mysositis ossificans (Calcification within the muscles at the site of the injury). This is a serious type of injury and massage should not be applied on the site. Mysositis ossificans can permanently limit the amount of knee flexion and also produce a hard, painful limp especially commonly in the thigh injuries. If this occurs the athlete should not participate in an activity and an X-ray should be taken. This generally involves surgical treatment.

Q.105. What is the common cause of strain of the quadriceps ?

Ans. The Quadriceps strain can occur due the tight musculature. This may be precipitated if there is imbalance between the quadriceps and the hamstrings or between the quadriceps strength of two legs. In most of the cases, there is a pain in the entire length of rectus femoris. The knee flexion is usually limited.

Q.106. How will you manage this condition ?

Ans. Ice therapy and compressed bandage. The doctor may prescribe anti-inflammatory medicine or any other type of pain reliever. If crutches are used by the player, the response is found to be better.

Once the bleeding has totally stopped, cryotherapy should be applied along with gentle controlled stretching exercises.

However, such exercises should not cause any pain. As healing continues and strenght returns a full quadriceps rehabilitation programme may be started.

Q.107. Write the cause of Hamstring strain.

Ans. Hamstring strain is common among sprinters, hurdlers and jumpers. There is usually generalised pain and localized tenderness. Passive straight leg movement is limited and there is inability to fully contract the hamstrings against resistance.

Q.108. Write the common points of its management.

Ans. Again Ice and compression are of paramount importance. Gentle retching of the hamstrings during cryotheraphy will prevent decrease of exibility. If the athlete cannot walk, crutches may be advised.

After a few days of cryotherapy, isometric contraction of the hamstrings should be started. Ultrasound, gentle frictional massage and control hamstring stretching should be continued. Once sufficient strength and flexibility have been achieved, jogging may be started by athlete. Backward running is considered as a very good exercise. After this stage, straight running should be gradually increased.

Q.109. What do you understand by the word groin stretch explain.

Ans. Assume a stance with feet planted about double shoulder width and feet pointing forward and flat on the floor (keep them this way throughout the exercise). Now lower your body to out side so that your fingertips support your balance by being placed on either side of your supporting leg. The opposite leg will experience a stretch from the inside of the knee clear into the groin area. Release and stretch the other leg.

Q.110. Describe in brief anatomical and bio-mechanical structure of knee joint.

Ans. The knee joint bears the full body weight. It is also subjected to tremendous bending and torsional forces via the body's longest body leavers. It also represents the athletes most massive, yet most vulnerable joint.

Functionally it may be considered to be comprised of three joints-the medial and lateral tibiofemoral and the patellofemoral joints.

The Knee is capable of motion in two planes, namely the transverse axis which governs flexion and extension and the long axis controlling rotation. The poor degree of interlocking of the articular surfaces which favours mobility renders this joint liable to various kinds of sprains.

Ligament function is most important in stabilising the knee, but joint topography, the menisci and muscle function are all contributing factors.

Q.111. Write in brief Knee Ligament Injuries.

Ans. It can be divided in two broad groups :

1. Medial Ligament Injuries : Such an injury is caused by a valgus force. If the valgus force is applied to the knee while the foot is fixed, an injury of the medial ligament can occur. The injury to the medial collateral ligament is more common than the lateral ligament. At times, in severe sprain there is an injury of the medial menisus.
2. Lateral Ligament Injuries : The lateral ligament is injured less than the medial ligament as it is not so vulnerable to injury. Usually the lateral capsular ligament and the fibular collateral ligament are the first structure to be injured. If the injury is more severe, the biceps tendon and the iliotibial band may be injured.

Q.112. Will you mention, how anterior cruciate ligament injuries occur ?

Ans. Let us discuss it in relation to right leg. The anteriorcruciate ligament is normally injured when the right tibia is internally rotated. The food is fixed, the femur and body rotate exernally as the athlete cuts to the right side. This can also be caused through hyper extension. It can also be injured when a force which drives the tibia in an anterior direction when the knee is flexed at 90° angle.

Q.113. Explain in the same manner about posterior Cruciate ligament.

Ans. This can be injured when a forceful landing on the tibial tubercle may drive the tibia backward on the femur, rupturing the posterior cruciate ligament. It can also occur in severe hyper-extension injury.

Q.114. Explain how injuries to medial and lateral ligament occur. Also write the management of injuries.

Ans. These injuries are generally divided into three degrees :

(a) First degree sprain : In this injury, the integrity of the ligament is undisturbed and there is almost normal tensile strength. The athlete usually complains some pain on twisting the leg. There is usually no swelling.

Treatment : Ice therapy followed by Isometric quadriceps and hamstrings contraction. Exercise on a stationary bicycle is considered to the an excellent exercise. Stretching exercises may also be undertaken.

(b) Second degree sprain : There is some tear of the medial or lateral ligaments and some decrease in tensile strength. The athlete might be able to play for some time but afterwards complain of stiffness and pain. There may be slight swelling and localized pain.

Treatment : The treatment is same as first degree sprain. It does not require surgical treatment but is treated by immobilization in most instances. After immobilization right type of rehabilitation should be given.

(c) Third degree sprain : In a third degree sprain, there is complete disruption of the ligament. In such a case, the treatment is surgical within the first three or five days. Rehabilitation should begin soon after operation.

Anterior and Posterior Cruciate Ligament Injuries : The treatment of anterior cruciate ligament is controversial. There are many surgical procedures and it is only the orthopaedic surgeon who can decide the best method. The posterior cruciate ligament tears are usually repaired through surgical means.

Q.115. Give steps for rehabilitation (Exercise therapy) for knee injuries.

Ans. Rehabilitation of knee injuries may be explained in the following steps :

1. Quadriceps sets (hold contraction-5 to 10 seconds) 20 times every hour. This exercise should be avoided for 6 to 12 weeks in case of anterior cruciate injury. Always remember that contraction of quadriceps puts an extra stress on the anterior cruciated ligament.
2. Hamstring set.
3. Combined quadriceps and Hamistring Exercises.
4. Straight Leg Raise : Raise the leg 60 0 , hold for three seconds and slow lowering. Repeat 30 to 50 times twice or thrice a day. Concentrate on vastus medialis contractions.
5. Straight Leg Abduction and Adduction against resistance, and knee rotation in flexion are advised at this stage.
6. Stretching of the Achilles Tendon. Elastic tubing exercises for inversion, eversion, dorsiflexion and planter flexion of the ankle.
7. Hip flexion with knee bent against resistance. This will improve knee flexion.
8. Isotonic hamstring exercises.
9. Running in water, provided the facilities exist.
10. High speed cycling on Ergometer for 20 minutes.
11. Rope jumping : It is the most convenient exercise, can be performed anywhere.
12. Half squat jumping. Side to side running and jumping, for three minutes.
13. Figure of eight running should be started in slow wide circles Gradually increase the speed.
14. Backward running, specially useful for hamstring injuries.
15. Running with sudden turn, also found to be useful at this stage. Knee strength test should be done by the sports.
16. When the athlete has achieved sufficient strength of the knee, he should be prepared for the specific activity.

Remember that

When the knee is free from pain and sufficiently strong, increase the speed and endurance part in exercises.

Q.116. What is 'jumper's knee' ?

Ans. This is a tendinitis of Patella and Quadriceps. This condition is peculiar to jumping and landing activities such as Backetball, High Jump, Long Jump and Triple Jump.

The cause is Microtrauma due to repeated jumping and also due to heavy squats with weights. There is pain in the localised area. There is a feeling as knee has given way. Wasting of quadriceps may be there.

Q.117. What should be the line of treatment in such a case ?

Ans. Sciagram should be taken and Cryotherapy should start at the earliest. The activity should be modified. Any aggravating exercise and heavy squat is to be avoided. The massage may be indicated after activity. Ice massage and moist heat should be applied before activity. Quadriceps exercises should be undertaken. As a support, the doctor may prescribe anti-inflammatory medicine. Ultra sound can be given with 10% cortisone. Lastly, in case the athlete does not improve, surgical treatment may be necessary. It should only be decided by a senior orthopaedic surgeon. Movements should be restricted if cortisone is used with ultra sound therapy.

Q.118. Expiain the word 'footballers ankle'.

Ans. Multiple trauma and kicking impacts at the front of the ankle may cause repeated strain and inflammation. As a result little bony osteophytes may develop within the ankle joint and limit its range of movement with increased pain. The footballer will need to cease play and possible subject himself to surgery to prevent chronic pain from a young age. Common injuries to the back of the heel have been dealt within the achilles tendon section, but the rim and underneath of the heel, as well as the bony and muscular structures of the foot, are particularly prone to sporting injury.

Q.119. Classify the various types of Sprain.

Ans. Sprains can be classified into the following manner :

1. Inversion sprain : Over 80% of all ankle injuries are inversion sprain. They occur due to the anatomical construction of the two malleoli. Owing to sudden twisting of the ankle inwardly while running inversion

sprain may develop. Generally Tibiofibular ligament and the interosseous membrane are injured. In some cases there may be a fracture of the fibula.

2. Eversion Sprain : It is not as common as inversion sprain. The foot is everted abnormally and may injure the deltoid ligament.
3. Dorsiflexion sprain : The Achilles tendon may be injured and the sudden force may cause fracture of the talus (which is very rare).
4. Planterflexion : Such sprains are extremely rare.

Q.120. What is the common line of treatment for sprained ankle ?

Ans.

1. RICE for at least 20 minutes every hour. It may continue for 12 to 24 hours. It should be combined with compression and elevation. Sciagram should be taken.
2. First or second degree sprains treated with compressed bandage or tape. Elevation is important.
3. Start stretching and eversion exercises. These movements should be very gentle. Slightest paint warrants stopping of movements.
4. Active dorsi and planter flexion without pain may be done.
5. Stretching may be done in the cold whirl-pool.
6. Always remember that contrast bath should start with ice and also finish it with ice cold water.
7. Isometric peroneal exercises. Sitting heel fixed on the ground, evert the feet against resistance. Maintain contraction for 5 seconds.
8. Eversion exercise should also be performed like this.
9. Balancing on one leg - maintain for two minutes.
10. Toe curling using a towel end.
11. Picking up marbles may be interesting among children. These two methods will also control the tendency of foot drop.
12. Bycle Erogometer exercise while tapping the ankle and heel may be used for padding.
13. Running in swimming-pool is best, provided facilities exist.
14. Icing the ankle and elevation for 20 to 30 minutes at the end of the exercises helps in draining the oedema.

15. Heel raise and tendo-achilles stretch should be performed.
16. It has been observed that at times gluteus muscle become weak after ankle sprain. Straight leg abduction exercises will strengthen the muscle.
17. Once the ankle joint has achieved sufficient strenght, after this more stress should be paid on isotonic exercises for this joint.
18. Now at this stage, balancing on the Tilt board may be practised.
19. The final functional exercises should consist of jogging, backward running, sideward jumping, figure of eight running etc. The trainer or the coach may prescribe more and more of sports specific pattern exercises according to the need of the player.

Q.121. What do you understand by heel angle pain ?

Ans. Sporting youngesters may suffer form an osteochondritis (like osgood schlatter's disease) of the heel, known as sever's disease. The pulling tendon is usually too painful to permit running or jumping though with RICE and heel padding some activity may be possible. This area may also be affected in the older runner due to some traction by the achilles insertion, but this can also be confused with bruising of the heel caused by frequent impact. The bruising may be helped by fitting a heel cup, which condenses the fat pad under the heel, the increased thickness making it more able to absorb trauma. Performance of gentle achilles tendon stretches regularly will also help to prevent and eliminate the problem.

Q.122. What is the functional approach of Rehabilitation of sports injuries.

Ans. The functional approach is nothing but the modern approach to rehabilitation of sports injuries. In functional approach, the muscles and the ligaments are sufficiently strengthened. The function of the movement should be regained and more specific type of exercises should be done in relation to particular sports. This is the only way to achieve specific type of movements involved in a particular sport.

Q.123. Why is prevention of injuries more important ?

Ans. The prevention of injuries should be the major goal of any one responsible for the physical and mental conditioning of players.

O'Donogue has pointed out that "We should spend much time devising ways and means to relieve the effects of injury. If we spend even a small percentage of this time in striving to prevent the injury from securing, a major portion of problem is solved."

Q.124. What are the common methods of prevention ?

Ans.
1. Responsibility of coach, sport-physician, Sports Physiotherapist, the Athlete, and the Administrator should be specified.
2. Attitude towards taking steps for prevention of injuries to be developed.
3. Physical conditioning with special reference to preventive conditioning exercises gets due importance.
4. Stretching exercises : It should be a slow and gentle stretch which can be used during warm-ups, this is particularly necessary for those who have tight muscles and those engaged in sporting activities. The tight muscles tend to produce muscle imbalance such as in long distance runners (tight hamstrings) and sprinters (tight quadriceps) are mainly injured. Stretching of these muscles should be a regular feature.

   During stretching programme, stretching, bouncing or rapid movements should be discouraged. In the beginning, the athlete should gently stretch in a comfortable position for about 10 to 15 seconds and later on it can be continued upto 1 minute. There should be no straining and breath-holding, and it should have no feeling of pain or discomfort. The athlete should concentrate on muscles - contraction and relaxation.

Q.125. What are the common stretching exercises ?

Ans. The following stretching exercises are quite commonly used:-

1. Hamstring stretch.
2. Quadriceps stretch.

3. Groin stretch.
4. Achilles and calf muscle stretch.

Q.126. Suggest basic principle of planing.

Ans. 1. Relax. The body must be supple to attain best performance.
2. Run on the balls of the feet.
3. Point the toes straight ahead. You lose at least one-half inch on each step if toes are not straight ahead.
4. Run in a straight line. It is the shortest distance between two points.
5. Develop your proper stride. The average stride is in relation to the height of your body. Lengthen your stride as much as possible but do not overstride. It is worse than an understride.
6. Running angle is important; body leaning, head up, ankles hips, shoulders, and head in a straight line. Do not bend too for backward. You should be in the proper running angle and with the proper stride 12 to 15 yards from the starting point.
7. Arm action is very important; opposite arm and leg move in union. Keep arm relaxed and shoot uppercuts to height of shoulder and not beyond centre of body. Bring arm back so hand does not go beyond crest of hip, a relaxed position like movement.

Q.127. Justify the statement 'Proper shoe prevent injuries.'

Ans. Most of the knee injuries occur when the foot is planted and fixed. This position will injure knee ligaments. If an athlete is wearing a shoe with a low co-efficient of friction, there is definite chance that the foot will move with the blow and eliminate the force.

Studies have shown that the soccer style shoe with a relatively large number of cleats (i.e.14) that are low (e.g.1/8" high and 1/2" in diameter) is probably the safest. This type will reduce the incidence of injuries. The type of shoe sole in contact with the playing surface is particularly important. For artificial turf the soccer style shoe with low wede cleats and a poly urethrae sole is recommended in comparison to the rubber sole shoe. It is further recommended that the same soccer style shoe, i.e. used for artificial surface be used for grass.

There are certain features to be noted when examining a running shoe. The heal counter should support the heel and Achilles tendon adequately. The sole at the heel should be built up about 3/4" (1.8 cms). The material used for heel should not be soft so that, it is easily compressed, but it should not be rock-hard also. There should be adequate cushioning for the ball of the foot, because much force is directed through that area. There should be some flexibility of the front sole - otherwise the foot and the lower leg are strained during the push-off phase of gait-but it should not be so flexible that the shoe can easily be bent into a U shape.

An athlete should not run in shoes immediately after purchasing them, but should walk in them for a day or two, to allow them to adopt the feet. After a few days of walking around, he or she can go on a short run of about 30% of normal distance, gradually increasing the length of time.

A very thin layer is all that is usually required. If the outside of the sole is built up too high, the foot tends to tilt inward, resulting in increased promotion, which could easily lead to new injuries, Before the shoes wear down completely, it is prudent for the athlete to obtain a new pair, so they can be slowly broken in before the old ones are discarded.

Q.128. What is terosynovitis ?

Ans. Terosynovitis may be defined as inflammation of the sinovialm surrounding a tendon. This inflammation is usually due to strain from unaccustomed overuse but may be due to a direct blow or infection. The result is that the normally a vascular synovium reacts with increased blood supply, invasion by inflammatory cell, oversecretion of synovial fluid and increase in fibrin content, causing "Streky" adhesions between the tendon and its surroundings.

Q.129. What is chondromalacia Patellae ?

Ans. This condition is seen commonly among adolescent girls. It may be found in cyclists and occasionally in sports such as hockey when blow to the knee has been an aggravating factor. The articular cartilage loses its normal smooth glistening appearance; in one or more areas it becomes oedematous, dull and soft. Fine irregular fissures or a small erupting area (like a blister) are found at surgery, and not uncommonly a 'kissing' lesion is found on the femoral condyle.

Q.130. How can you diagnose this condition ?

Ans. Pain in knee while sitting or climbing and the knee may give way. Grating and tenderness are found when the patella is pressed against the femoral condyles. There may be other associated conditions like : valgus knee, external tibial torsion and 'squinting' patellae.

Q.131. So, how to treat such condition ?

Ans. Quadriceps exercises are performed and sport is stopped for 2-3 months. If pain is too much, analgesics may be given. Surgery may be done in the form of lateral setinacular and if needed arthrotomy may be carried out. Very severe cases need patellectomy. After retinacular release sports can begin at 8-12 weeks.

Q.132. What is 'Jumper's knee' ?

Ans. There is a pain over the infrapatellar or suprapatellar regions. It is gradual in onset and disappears with rest. The description which athlete gives, is a sensation of weakness, giving way and fullness of knee. In games where repetitive activities are involved, and when it is continued then an acute episode (giving way) is experienced. The games in which jumper knee is common are basketball, volleyball, football, tennis and long distance running. Though effusion is rare but there is sometimes a snapping sensation of the patella on full knee flexion. The athlete usually tall and having other disorders, too i.e. chondromalacia patellae, patella alta, osgood Schlatter's disease, genu valgum external tibial torsion.

Q.133. What can be the line of treatment of this condition ?

Ans. Rest is most important. It should be associated with elastic support to knee and anti-inflammatory drugs.
Following surgical procedures are generally practised :
— drilling of involved poles;
— excision of any degenerated tendon;

— reattachment of patellar tendon;
— retanacular reinforcement.

Q.134. How will you diagnose and treat the condition of 'Osteochondritis Dissecans' ?

Ans. Athlete, generally between the age of 15 to 20 years, complains of vague knee pain. There may be swelling and a tender medial condyl, knee may get looked. Sciagram shows ovoid segment on the medial condyl close to the anterior tibial spine, while somethimes loose bodies may be seen.

Initially, treatment is conservative, later on surgery is performed. The fragments where-ever they are (talus, femoral head, capitellum or metatarsal head) fixed with small pins or excised.

Q.135 Explain in details the meaning and role of team physician ?

Ans. Team physician directly supervises the athatic trainesand advises on the overall conditioning program. He is responsible for performing or collecting and reviewing the pre participation physical evaluation and making the final determination of fitness participation.

The team provides medical coverage for competitive events especially contact sports, supplying emergency wvaluation, treatment and triage of atheletic injuries and illnesses. He also will provide primary care of athelcticinjuries or arrange referrals to the family physician or qpesialist consultants as indicated additionaly,he oversees or eastablishes the guidlinesand procedures for trainer personnel to respond to emergencise and can suggest emergency equipment needed.

Following injury or illness the team physician is responsible for insuring that rehabilitation has been adequate. He should assess the athelete for readiness to returns to activity.

Finally the team physicain should educate coaches, trainers, administrators, athletes and parents regarding the medical aspects of sports.

Q.136. What are the suggested exercises for 'Chondromalacia Palettae'?

Ans. If the condition is mild and there is no similar involvement of the underlying femur, then a continuation of straight leg raising exercise beyond the usual period of time is usually all that is necessary for rehabilitation.

However, in more severe cases or in those complicated by femoral involvement, the following exercises should be performed :

(a) Straight leg raising,

(b) Isokinetic exercise using a 'self adjusting resistance' so that undue pressure will not be placed on the patella during maximum patellofemoral contact.

(c) Isometric exercises performed at varying degree of knee extension against a fixed object or the uninvolved limb.

(d) Negative resistance exercise performed by lifting the weight with the uninvolved extremity.

(e) Modified 'Bench technique' is suggested so that starting position of the exercise permits only 10 to 15 degrees of knee flexion. As the legs are straightened, the major action of patella is upward in line with the quadriceps mechanism, and little pressure is placed on the patella against the femur in the terminal phase.

Q.137. What is bursitis ?

Ans. Bursitis is an inflammatory reaction within a bursa. It may vary in degree from very mild irritative synovitis with discomfort to supporative bursitis with actual abscess formation. A bursa is specifically designed to facilitate motion between contiguous layers of the body, and the athlete with his violence of motion is particularly prone to bursal involvement resulting from repetitive local trauma due to tissue friction or from direct blows.

Q.138. Will you also write about the 'Home Knee Exercises' ?

Ans. Following are the home knee exercises:

(a) Lie on back. Keep the knee absolutely straight and lift it to 45 degree. Lower it slowly. Do not relax the leg, but repeat 45 times. As one gets stronger, add weights by means of putting weight as sand bags etc.

(b) Standing front leg raise is done exactly as the

preceding exercise, but one should stand to do the lift. Perform 15 repetitions. Add weight when athlete is in a position to do more.

Standing side raise is done exactly as the preceding exercise, only the weight is lifted to the side.

(c) Be seated on the floor. Place couple of rolled towels under the knee. While pushing the back of the knee down into the towel as hard as possibie, attempt is made to keep the entire surface of the leg incontact with the floor Hold 5 seconds, repeat 10 times.

(d) Sit on a high table, with the back of the knee just at the edge of the table. Towels may be used to pad the back of knee. From the fully bent position straighten the knee as much as possible and hold for 3 seconds. Repeat 15 times, as one gets stronger, add weight by means of a weight bag. Continue using this exercise only as there is no increased pain or swelling as a result of exercise.

(e) Stand erect and balance by holding on to a stable piece of furniture bend the exercising knee backwards. Use the weight bag or sand bag as mentioned earlier. Do 15 repetitions.

Q.139. What is Isometric Ankle 'Wrestling' ?

Ans. In this type of exercise, sit and place one ankle over the other (half way through switch ankles). Exert an outward force with both ankles so that the feet are firmly pressing against each other. Hold for 10 seconds, release, and repeat 10 times.

An ankle becomes stronger and less painful or stiff, allow it to move in and out against each other as one exerts the outward force. Make each full movement last 10 full seconds. Repeat 10 times.

Q.140. What are the common running induced injuries to knee ?

Ans. There can be the following common conditions :-

(a) Medial Patellar Pain,
(b) Pes Anserine Bursitis,
(c) Patellar Tendinitis,
(d) Retropatellar Pain,
(e) Lateral Patellar Pain,
(f) Lateral Knee Pain,

Q.141. What do you understand by medial patellar pain ?

Ans. Medial patellar pain is the pain related to medial aspect of patella. In it, the medial joint line or the medial tibial plateau is usually associated with excessive promotion during the mild-support and take-off phases. One theory about the occurrence of this pain relates to the excessive internal rotation of the tibia which accompanies a prolonged pronatory phase. When the knee starts to extend after reaching its maximal point of flexion, the tibia and femur start rotating externally. As a result of excessively prolonged pronation, the tibia stays in internal, rotation. Owing to all the mentioned movements stress is thus placed on the medial patellar structures because patella tends to follow the external rotational movement of the femur.

Q.142. So, how can this condition be treated ?

Ans. As a routine Ice and aspirin forms the initial phase of the treatment. It is to be done at least 4 times a day. Next step is to improve musculature particular of vastus medialis, the posterior tibial, and flexor hallucis longus muscles. Orthotic devices are often used and they show improvement in fairy high percentage of cases, while the athlete is revcovering, it may be necessary to decrease the mileage and perhaps change the running shoe and/ or the surface.

Q.143. Illustrate the common causes of overuse injuries of lower limb in runners ?

Ans. Following are the common causes of overuse injuries among the lower limb of runners :

(a) Lack of flexibility-especially of achilles tendon and that of the hamstring muscles.

(b) Muscle weakness of intrinsic muscles of the foot, the anterior and posterior tibial muscles, and the quadriceps muscles.

(c) Impact force : While running, impact force is three to five times in comparison to walking, it may lead to 'stress fracture' or 'stress reaction' of bone. The symptoms of stress fracture may develop gradually in a couple of weeks.

(d) Hard surface - Again it increases the impact force.

(e) Change of surface-Particularly from soft to hard, but it can be due to reverse order also.
(f) Down hill running-This may also especially be associated with illotibial tract irritation, popliteus tendinitis and patellar tendinitis because it puts direct load on concerned area.
(g) Overstriding-Results in hamstring pulls and knee pain.
(h) Poor Posture-Especially leaning too far forward and hyperlordosis of the lumbar spine.
(i) Overdistance - There is relatively high incidence of injuries in runners running over forty miles a week. Heavy schedule of training does not allow adaptation to develop.
(j) Anatomical Factors-Malalignment of the lower extremity or foot.
(k) Shoes-Should prove control and shock absorbency. Most of Indian athletes cannot afford standard quality shoes.
(l) Side of the road-Running on the same side of a sloped road for a long time can produce knee pain.

AND MOST IMPORTANT IS TOO MUCH, TOO SOON.

Q.144. How to relieve the athlete from retropatellar pain ?

Ans. The most important aspect of the management is vastus medialis and quadriceps exercise. The shoe orthotic device will further help it. Gentle quadriceps stretching should be performed as long as this is not painful. High doses of aspirin along with vitamin C may be helpful. Ice gives symptomatic relief from discomfort. Along with this heavy running schedule or hill running is to be avoided till retropatellar irritation subsides. For cardiovascular fitness pool running is advised. Rarely surgical intervention may be needed.

Q.145. What do you understand by lateral patellar pain ?

Ans. Either it may be related to feet or due to an alignment defect involving the patella. There may be a muscle imbalance of the vastus, the vastus lateralis being more powerful or tighter than the medialis. Athlete may complain of pain and tenderness on the anterolateral aspect of patella. The lateral patellar structure may be tight, allowing little medial movement of the patella when pressure is applied to the lateral facet.

Q.146. How to give relief to the patient in case of lateral patellar pain ?

Ans. Here basices are again ice and aspirin. In such cases quadriceps exercises are to be carefully controlled, emphasizing the vastus medialis. It is important to attend to gentle stretch of the quadriceps over a period of time. Orthotic and cortisone may be helpful but should be sued with care.

Surgery performed rarely by lateral retinacular release.

Q.147. Why does the runner's get lateral knee pain ?

Ans. The common cause may be due to soft tissue problem, which is due to tendinitis or friction of Iliotibial tract as it runs over the lateral femoral condyle. Occasionally the popliteal tendon or the lateral ligament become inflamed. Irritation of these tissues appear to be related to increased mileage beyond normal and poor shock absorbency either through the shoes or through the body alignment, and it, therefore, shows up quite frequently in runners with rigid feet.

Q.148. How to diagnose this condition ?

Ans. In this condition pain occurs during running and may be localized to the lateral epicondyle or run diffusely along the iliotibial tract. It may not be there when patient runs uphill but pain develops while downhill running. At the origin of the popliteal tendon (Gerdy's tubercle) at epicondyle patient has pain. Inflammation and credpitus may be there alongwith iliotibial tract.

Q.149. Will you mention the line of treatment for lateral knee pain ?

Ans. For management of lateral knee pain, the following points are mentioned here :

(i) Patient should be asked to run on soft surfaces with shoes having good shock absorbency.

(ii) Ice aspirin, anti-inflammatory alongwith use of orthotics are of great help.

(iii) Stretching of iliotibial tract is a necessity.

(iv) Strengthening exercises may have added advantage.

(v) Surgery and corticosteroids may be of use only when they are of utmost importance.

Q.140. Please explain the condition 'Pes Anserine Bursitis'.

Ans. Whether running is the only cause of this condition is uncertain. Possibly, it is related to an attempt by the pes to compensate for excessive tibia-varum at heel strike. Frequently, a week vastus medialis muscle is found in association with this condition.

In this condition there is pain and swelling of the pes anserine bursa, which lies in close promimity to the insertion of the pes anserine tendon. This condition needs to be differentiated from a stress fracture of the upper tibia, whichcan be present with the same findings.

Q.151. What is the line of treatment for this condition ?

Ans. First ice and anti-inflammatory drugs are used along with exercise to improve vastus medialis muscle and pes anserine muscle groups. Orthotic devices are often useful. On occasion, a local injection of cortioosteroids may help.

Q.152. What are the common signs and symptoms of Patellar Tendinitis in a runner ?

Ans. Pain and tenderness are localized at the interior angle of patella at the origin of patellar tendon, and sometimes further down the tendon. An excessive Q angle may also be found.

Q.153. How should this condition be managed ?

Ans. Initially start with ice and tablet of aspirin. Also use orthotic device. Neoprene with a patellar support can be used on those with an excessive Q angle. The quadriceps muscles should be strengthened. Anti-inflammatory drugs will be of great help.

Q.154. How you will diagnose retropatellar pain ?

Ans. Pain occurs behind the patella when the athlete runs. It may also occur when he or she walks up and down stairs, cycle (after cycling), or sits for some time with the knee bent at 90°. Frequently there is an extensor mechanism malignment related to the hips, tibia, feet.

Q.155. How will you diagnose and treat the condition of Biceps tendinitis ?

Ans. As just proximal to the insertion of biceps tendon in fibula there is pain and tenderness which may be associated with swelling. Ice, anti-inflammatory and reduced intensity of activity will cure this condition.

Q.156. Please, also explain Acute Sinovitis of Ankle.

Ans. It may follow an injury or an infection, or a metabolic disturbance such as gout, the ankle is painful, swollen, and hot and has all the appearance of an acute inflammatory reaction. Aspiration is not the answer but this condition may be treated on the following lines :

(a) Systematic treatment of underlying condition-antibiotics for infection, general condition should be corrected.

(b) Local treatment is rest, elevation, support and local heat. Although it is difficult to aspirate the fluid, but ankle may be injected in local anasthetic. An the acute symptoms subside, it is important to protect the ankle against stress and strain until healing is complete. Always keep in mind that sinovitis has great tendency to recur.

Q.157. Describe in brief the exostosis of Tibia.

Ans. They are managed as exostosis anywhere in the body except that a much smaller exostosis will be symptomatic in a subcutaneous bone than in one surrounded completely by mussel. If the condition is symptomatic and cannot be handled by a simple protective pad, surgical excision is the answer.

While a player is running, one of the tendons of pes may snap over the exostosis and in fact may catch over it and simulate rocking or catching knee.

Careful attention to the location of the tenderness and to the absence of knee symptoms will prevent an embarrassing error in diagnosis. Last resort is the surgery.

Q.158. What do you understand by the word 'Heel Walking' ?

Ans. Athlete walks, keeping the toes as far off the ground as possible Short 'choppy' steps are taken, shoes are used with good solid heels; one should always walk on firm surfaces. After covering a distance of 100 feet, progress to carry weighted objects or one may walk on inclined surfaces or hilly area.

Q.159. Will you describe the chronic Sunovitis of Ankle ?

Ans. The sinovitis be identified by pain, swelling and disability and it is secondary to a primary condition which may not reveal any particular etiology, but treatment of this condition must be local. Rest is again important. Stirrup splint should be used if swelling is marked. When swelling subsides, a walking boot cast may be substituted. It will take several weeks of adequate protection followed by a period of strapping in order to permit the condition to heal and athlete endeavour to resume. Until or unless underlying cause in near joints is treated, this type of sinovitis is likely to occur.

Q.160. Give brief account of halluxrigidus.

Ans. Pain at the junction between the first metatarsal and the big toe may well be due to immobility as the result of premature arthritis. Any attempt on examination to stretch the toe through its full range induces sharp pains. It may be associated with plantar fascitis. Initially the condition can be relieved with the use of anti-inflammatory drugs and self help physiotherapy to enlarge the range of improvement. Padding in the shoe or a softer landing surface may help, but altering the fulcrum by means of a metatarsal bar behind the heads of the bones may again relieve the condition provided the sports man's shoe is not too overcrowded. Resistant cases may eventually require surgery, though the loss of leverage may severely handicap the competitive player.

Q.161. What exercise programme will you suggest for an athlete suffering from Chondromalacia Patella ?

Ans.
(1) Straight leg raising.
(2) Isokinetic exercise using a 'self adjusting resistance' so that undue pressure is not placed on the patella during maximum patella femoral contact.
(3) Isometric exercises performed at varying degree of knee extension against a fixed object or the uninvolved limb.

(4) Negative resistance exercises are performed by lifting the weight with the uninvolved extremity and lowering the weight with the involved extremity.

(5) 'Bench technique' modified so that the starting position of the exercise permits only 10 to 15 degrees of knee flexion. As the legs are straightened, the major action of patella is upward in line with the quadriceps mechanism, and little pressure is placed on the patella against the femur in this terminal phase.

Q.162. Will you explain in brief the 'Home Knee Exercises' ?

Ans. (a) Lie on the back. Keep the knee absolutely straight as one lift it to 45 degrees. Lower it slowly. Do not relax the leg, but repeat 15 times. As one gets stronger, add weights by means of putting weights in a bag and wrapping them over the ankles.

(b) Standing front leg raise is done exactly as the preceeding exercise. Only athlete stands to do the lift. 15 repetitions are performed. Weight is added when one is able to do with previous weights comfortably for more than three days.

(c) Standing side raise is done exactly as the previous exercise, here the weight is lifted to the sides. Same as previous exercise. 15 repetitions are made.

(d) Place a couple of rolled towels under the knee. While pushing the back of the knee down into the towel as hard as possible, attempt is made to keep the entire surface of the leg in contact with the floor. At this stage, one should hold the leg for 5 seconds. Repeat this exercise 10 times.

(e) One should sit on a high table, with the back of the knee just at the edge of the table. From the fully bent position, straighten the knee as much as possible. One should remain in this stage for 3 seconds. This exercise is repeated 15 times. Gradually weight may be added.

(f) Stand erect and balance by holding on to a stable piece of furniture. Bend the exercising knee backwards. Use the weighted bag, as in preceeding exercises. Do 15 repetitions.

Q.163. Will you mention the rehabilitation of a case of Myositis ossificans ?

Ans. Following points are kept in mind during the rehabilitation of such cases :

(a) The inflammatory stage should be protected from further injury. Immobilization is usually helpful, and limitation of motion at adjacent joints is usually beneficial. No active exercise should be given to the involved area at this stage. ICE application is the best.

(b) For Proliferative stage quadriceps setting exercises for the thing are suggested. If arm is involved, hand grip or upper extremity setting exercises are helpful. When pain and soreness subsides active range of motion exercises are suggested. Forcible motion should never be increases.

(c) In repair stage, It is usually possible to begin light resistive exercises through the available range of motion. Joint motion should be monitored daily. If pain or reduction movement is there, the exercise should be stopped. Always remember that exercises should be pain free. Pain in involved muscle indicates overload.

Q.164. How you will stretch the quardriceps muscle in sitting as well as standing position ?

Ans. (I) Sitting Quadriceps stretch :

Kneel with one knee on the ground and the other bent in front of you with your foot flat on the ground. Raise the foot behind you as far as it will go and clasp it in both hands. Hold the stretch for a few seconds, then lower your foot, and repeat to the other side.

Kneel with your toes pointing backwards away from the body behind you. Slowly lean back with your hands placed on yours feet and lifting the pelvis up and out. Repeat 5 times.

(II) Standing Quadriceps Stretch

Stand up holding on to a bar or chair back feet shoulder width apart. Raise your right knee and grasp your right ankle in your right hand take your leg back until the heel is close to your bottom. Hold for a count of 10 and repeat with the other leg. Be sure to keep the knees together when you take your leg back.

Q.165. What do you understand by the word 'Neuromuscular Re-education ?

Ans. It primarily involves development of a proprioceptive awareness. Normal function in most cases will return more quickly. The athlete is allowed to continue with activities that permit near normal function but such activities should not interfere with the normal healing process.

Q.166. What points are to be kept in mind while rehabilitating a case of 'Rotator Cuff Injuries' ?

Ans. Following points should be kept in mind during rehabilitation of such cases :

(a) Early Rehabilitation :-

— Gripping exercises;

— Pendulum exercises;

— Bench press supports;

— Hanging from chin bar position.

(b) Intermediate Rehabilitation :-

— Light Dumbbell circles;

— Bench presses;

— Upright Rowing

(c) Advanced Rehabilitation :-

— Alternate dumbbell presses; or presses behind the neck;

— Dumbbell bench press; incline presses; parallel bar dips;

— Bent arm pullovers;

— High pulls with a snatch grip, or repetition 'cleans';

— Straight arm pull-overs across the width of a bench, using a progressively wider grip, the weight is kept at a permanently tight setting;

— In the last stage, a cable is held in the back of the shoulders, with the palm facing forward at shoulder height;

— The cable is worked forward and backward, stretching pectoral girdle and rib cage.

Q.167. What is SAID principle in reconditioning for vigorous sports activity following an injury ?

Ans. The letters SAID stands for : Specific Adaptation to Imposed Demands. This means that the training programme must attempt to adapt the individual to the demands that may be made upon him during athletic performance. Adaptation is specific and refers to the alternation of the structure or functions of an organ or part as a result of an altered environment. Function increases with use, and that which we do not use, we lose. The intensity, duration and frequency of activity are all related to the functional capacity that is developed.'

Rehabilitation of the athlete deals primarily with the restoration of muscle function, i.e. the missing quality of muscle function must be identified and restored (muscle, strenght, endurance and flexibility). Strength is general, but the application of strength is selective. The proper use of strength in any activity comes only from the practice of the particular activity.

In formulating the exercise prescription, exercise should be applied selectively, depending upon the sport in which an athlete is involved.

Q.168. In the sequence of exercises what basic principle should be kept in mind ?

Ans. The largest muscle group is worked first, proceeding down to the smallest group. Working largest muscle group first causes the growth stimulus. Also, it is sometimes impossible to reach the required condition of momentary muscular exhaustion while working a large muscle group if the system has been previously exhausted by exercises for other smaller muscles.

Q.169. Give brief description of sky stretch and groin stretch and also explain the adductors strecth.

Ans. (I) Ski Stretch:- Stand with one foot forwards and one foot behind you in a lunge position. Slowly lower your body, bending the front leg until your weight is resting on your hands. Keep the back leg straight with the heel off the floor. Hold for account of 10 and then change legs.

(II) Groin Stretch:- Stand up straight and place one leg about one stride in front of the other with your hands resting lightly on your hips, bend the front leg, transferring your weight on to it, keep your back leg straight and hold for a count of 5, Repeat 5 times with each leg.

(III) Adductors stretch :

— Sit on the ground with the soles of your feet pressed together and clasp your feet in your hands. Gently try to lower your knees towards the floor, leaning forwards from the hips. You will feel the stretch in your adductors.

— Stand with your legs as far apart as possible. Grab your right thigh with both hands and gently and slowly slide your hands down your right leg as far as they will go and feel comfortable. Hold the stretch for a count of 5 and then return to the original starting position. Repeat 5 times, and then change legs. Note that this stretch is for the more advanced sports person who has a supple body. Do not attempt it unless you are fit.

Q.170. What is 'tennis leg' ?

Ans. Popularly known as 'tennis leg' is rupture of plantar is muscle. Usually the medial head of gastrochemius when dorsiflexed foot gets extension of knee joint. This may also occur when in extended knee position foot is suddenly dorsiflexed. This condition is more common in middle aged player and those who have some degeneration of muscle or musculotendinous junction.

Because this condition usually developed among tennis players named 'tennis leg'.

Q.171. How to diagnose the tennis leg ?

Ans. The shooting pain in leg or sudden sharp pain in calf region is the symptom which suggests to look for the condition 'tennis leg'. Ecchymosis alongwith swelling in leg may be seen alongwith localized tenderness. Warning predisposing symptom of this condition is aching or dull pain at musculotendinous function of gastrocnemius after activity or tennis game.

Q.172. What is the first line of treatment for this condition ?

Ans. Ice with crepe bandage and the leg should be elevated in planter flexed position. Use of crutches, anti-inflammatory drugs and analgesics are always helpful.

Q.173. Will you also mention the definitive treatment of this condition ?

Ans. For severe cases, surgery is the answer but mild cases may be treated by raised heel and limited weight bearing, ultrasound, muscle stimulation, Achilles stretching and gastrocnemius strengthening exercises are beneficial to the patient. For sports activities a heel lift of half an inch is of great help.

Generally the prognosis of this condition is better provided if the athlete takes advised rest (if needed even plaster cast) and attends activities after complete rehabilitation. Unnecessarily one should not try to get back to the game within a short period.

Q.175. Explain with details the procedure of various types of hamstring stretch.

Ans. (I) Raised hamstring stretch- Above. Stand with your foot on a raised surface at hip level. Lean forwards and try to put your head on your knees. If you are not really fit, do the alternative exercise (left) instead: left; stand with your foot on a raised surface at knee height. Place both hands on your raised thigh and slide them gently down your leg as far as feels comfortable. Repeat with the other leg.

(II) Hamstring stretch-Again, you should only do this if you are very fit. Sit down with legs outstretched and close together. Slowly bend forwards from the hips and clasp your feet in your hands.

(II) Hurdler's hamstring stretch- Sit down with one leg stretched out in front and the other leg bent at the knee at 90 degrees to the body. Lean slowly forwards from the hips, sliding your hands down of your outstretched leg as far as feels comfortable. Repeat on the other side.

Q.176. Give the method of cuff stretch with bend knees & straight knee.

Ans. (I) Stand about 2 feet away from a wall and lean against it with the knees slightly bend. Keep your heels flat on the floor and feel the stretch in the calf muscles. Hold for a count of 10. Do 3 repetation.

(II) Stand about 4 feet away from a wall with your toes slightly turned in, legs together and lean against it, keeping your feet flat on the ground. Hold for a count of 10 repeat the stretch 3 times.

Q.176. Write the basic differences between ankle and knee injuries.

Ans. Following points should be kept in mind for ankle and knee injuries respectively.

(a) Ankle Injuries :-

— Ankle joint is basically unstable and likely to suffer with injuries.

— Unless very unstable, a third degree injury can be treated conservatively.

— With a third degree injury, a delayed primary repair can be performed if necessary.

— Reconstructive procedures are usually successful.

— Taping produces good support and recovery process will be quite fast.

(b) Knee Injuries :-

— This joint in comparison to ankle, is further unstable joint.

— A third degree ligament injury of knee always requires surgery.

— An immediate primary repair must be performed if injury needs so.

— In comparison to ankle joint, taping does not give much benefit.

— Reconstructive procedures are not a surety of success.

Q.177. After an ankle injury, what points should be observed before allowing athlete to participate in games and sports ?

Ans. Look at the following points :

— There is not even slightest chance from the examination that a fracture might be present.

— There should be no evidence of ligament instability.

— The athlete should be able to run forward; backward;

hop; run and cut; run in figure of eights at normal speed without any limp or pain.

Note : If the above can be accomplished, the athlete is permitted to return to participation. However, protective taping should be applied to support the injured structures. Immediately after the game, the ankle should be re-evaluated and treated as indicated.

Q.178. Will you write stepwise points for ankle injury rehabilitation ?

Ans. RICE is the cornerstone of injury at initial stage.

— Cold whirl pool may also be beneficial.

— in cold whirl pool Achilles stretching may by done but remember if pain is there, stop stretching.

— Alternate icing and slow walking are helpful.

— Contrast bath may be of use.

— Isometric peroneal exercises are also suggested.

— Eversion, dorsiflexion and planter flexion may be done gently with the help of another athlete. There should be no jerk while performing these movements.

— The athlete balances on one leg with eyes closed, i.e. ankle proprioception exercise.

— Movements like toe-curls, marble pick-up, alphabet writing with the foot are beneficial.

— For upper body bicycling is a good exercise to maintain physical fitness.

— It is advisable to go for Pool Running if facilities are available.

— Ice and elevation after rehabilitation session further helps in recovery process.

— Supportive taping has proved to be of great help.

Q.179. For strengthening the muscles around ankle joint what type of rehabilitation can be suggested ?

Ans. Best simple exercises are to make alphabets. Isotonic exercises with the help of sand bags are also practised.

— Hopping or bouncing a ball simultaneously.

— By using a balance :-By balancing on a tilt board improves balance and proprioception. It may be done as training exercise, but is particularly useful in the later stages of ankle rehabilitation.

— Jogging.

— Running rapidly in a place.
— Jumping ropes should be practised when complete recovery takes place.
— Hopping upstairs and in figure eight form further strengthen the ankle joint.

Q.180. What is Bursitis ? Explain bursitis of Heel.

Ans. Inflammation of Bursa is known as bursitis. It is a small sac containing fluid, which forms between two moving surfaces or tissues to provide friction free movements. A bursa sometimes forms under the heel, and it thus becomes inflamed. The symptoms are like those of heel bruising. Mostly inflammation occurs in the bursa at the back of the heel which separates the bone from the insertion of Achilles tendon. This may happen because tendon is prevented from moving normally, either by a direct strain, or by ill-fitting shoes. The back of the heel becomes tender to touch but there is no pain when the tendon is contracted.

Example : Standing on toes.

Q.181. How to help such patients ?

Ans. It may be treated by putting shock absorbing cushioning, injections and electrotherapy. Remember : alongwith these supports, rest is also needed.

Q.182. What is heel spur ?

Ans. When a tissue is repeatedly strained at its attachment into a bone, it may cause inflammation and finally set up a reaction of new bone growth. This can happen to planter fascia, where if joins the heel, and the new bone can be seen on X-rays as small bone outgrowth on the front of the underside of the heel. It may eventually be necessary to have the tiny bone removed surgically. But initially in the first instance, treatment aims at relieving the repeated pressure on the planter fascia which has caused the problem. If the heel is sore, heel pads should be used, while the arch and mid foot should be supported by a soft cushioned support or insole. Iodine therapy is also found to be useful.

Q.183. What do you understand by epiphysitis of Heel ?

Ans. Before discussing it we should understand that the heel bone is formed in parts which join together as child grows older. If for any reason the blood supply to the bone is poor, the back edge of the calcanium may fail to join the greater part of the heel properly. The usual cause is repetitive jarring. It may happen because the child has been running too much or jumping, on hard floors as in gymnastics. Pain is felt down the sides of the back of the heel. Any pressure on the feel, such as running, jumping, hurts. The problem usually happens to children between the ages of twelve to sixteen. It needs rest from any painful activities. The cushioned heel supports will reduce jarring during walking. If the child continues sport, the pain may persist for many months, whereas if rest is given to the part it usually clears within a few weeks. Pain free activities, such as swimming and cycling, can safely be continued during the rest time.

Q.184. What is Metatarsalgia ?

Ans. This is a term to describe pain in the forefoot, between the metatarsal heads. This pain may be associated with, or caused by, structural defects such as an excessively high arch. Treatment aims to correct the defects and improve overall foot function. This is done usually by exercises to improve the balanced working of the muscles in the foot, and by the foot supports to improve the mechanical alignment of the joints.

Q.185. What do you understand by Morton's metatarsalgia ?

Ans. In such cases there is severe localized pain, which occurs only occasionally, between two metatarsal heads in the forefoot. By rubbing, the foot pain may be relieved. The main cause of pain is a swelling in the nerve which lies between the two bones. This results in the nerve occasionally 'catching' and being compressed between the bones, causing a kicflicke pain in area. If the swelling or neuroma is big enough, it will feel tender if one presses the area between fingers from above and below the foot. If the condition is not severe, it may be helped by a pad placed directly, behind the affected metatarsal bone, which stops the bone rubbing over the enlarged part of the nerve. However, if the condition is very bad, giving frequent episodes of pain, it is usually necessary to have the swelling removed by an operation.

Q.186. What do you understand by the condition 'Sesamoidites' ?

Ans. Inflammation of sesamoid bone is called 'Sesamoidites'. Typical sign of this disease is pain under the ball of the foot, behind the big toe. It may be caused by damage to one of the foot, behind the big toe. It may be caused by damage to one of the sesamoids, the tiny extra bone lying in the tendon under the first metatarsal head. The bone can be broken by direct force, especially if it happens when the toes are bent back or it may be bruised by persistent jarring, possibly associated with a change into footwear or foot movements. Treatment in the first instance is aimed at reducing pressure over the bones with padding. Second phase of treatment is by improving the efficiency of the small muscles of the foot, especially those which act on the big toe. If the damage is great and the pain is severe, the only answer is to have the sesamoid removed surgically.

Q.187. Please explain the condition "Hallux Rigidus".

Ans. This condition is generally found in adolescents where there may be stiffness in the big toe joint. It is a gradual process which may be due to the late result of an injury to the big toe. The commonest symptom is that the joint may become painful when stressed either by forceful bending movements, like those involved in sprinting, hopping, or landing from a jump, or by badly fitting shoes. Unusually the pain is relieved/subsides by rest and if a soft support in the inner arch is given. As in all cases of pain of the forefoot, it is important to avoid high heeled shoes which lift the body weight towards the toes. Similarly, one should choose sports shoes having good sole thickness. If the problem of hallux rigidus rigidus becomes long-standing and causes a lot of pain, surgery may be necessary to trim down the bones and relieve pressure in the joint.

Q.188. What do you understand by 'Hallux Valgus' ?

Ans. In this condition, the big toe is pulled towards the second toe, causing the big toe joining with the first metatarsal to form an angled protrusion on the inner side of the foot. The condition is caused by excessive pull inwards from the tendons acting on the toe. Shoes with pointed toes can contribute to the problem. The deformity may become severe, but it is not necessarily very painful. If it does cause pain, pads are used around the protruding bone. In this way, one may prevent friction from shoes over it. To try to rebalance the weight bearing load underfoot support may be tried. If the joint becomes very painful, and especially if the second toe is crushed by the side way, drift of the big toe, an operation is needed to remove the protruding part of the bone and straighten the joint.

Q.189. Will you explain the 'Hammer Toes' ?

Ans. This condition essentially has shortened tendons. This condition may be associated with a high arch, or because of tight shoes, they can pull the toes into a deformity in which they are bent up in the middle, so that the ends of the toes are pressed downwards into the ground. The condition may be, painless. If so, one should ignore it. Keep in mind that the individual should not wear shoes which rub over the joints of the toes. If needed, one can place a circle of padding around the bent joints. To prevent friction it is advisable to use an arch support to relieve excessive weight bearing pressure over the ball of the foot. Even if the pain is too much, surgery is the answer.

Q.190. Can you describe in brief the most common injury - 'Ankle Sprain' ?

Ans. This classic injury is one of the inversion and internal rotation which results in sprain of the lateral ligament complex. In acute injury with local pain and swelling the treatment is by strapping. Of course the formula of RICE is of cornerstone value. If the lesion is very severe after two to three weeks when it resolves; more problematical is the less acute ankle sprain which is often ignored because of the paucity of signs. The only gross physical sign being limitation of movement although careful inspection from behind shows filling of the sulcus on either side of the Achilles tendon due to posterior bulging of the joint. It in such cases immobilization is not done, they may go into a condition of chronic sprained ankle.

Q.191. What is the footballer's ankle ?

Ans. It is not an osteo-arthrosis of the ankle joint; during the surgical examination. It is observed that there is no damage to the hyaline cartilage. However, numerous small capsular tears cause marginal osteophytes which may impinge on the neck of the talus during' dead ball kicking'. This may also lead to discomfort on shooting and later on a dull pain of continuous type develops.

Q.192. How can you diagnose a 'Footballer's Ankle' ?

Ans. The common signs and symptoms may be : Tenderness which is found over the anterior (and sometimes posterior) joint line and X-ray may show the small spicules of bones. A somewhat similar condition involves fracture or degenerative changes in the posterior part of the talus and a small spur may develop. A separate or trigonum may also be subjected to repeated minor trauma. Lateral and anteroposterior X-ray will help in differentiating it among the other conditions.

Q.193. Give the tabular comparative picture of signs and symptoms of ligament injury ?

Ans.	Ist Degree Sprain	2nd Degree Sprain	3rd Degree Sprain
Synonym	Mild Sprain	Moderate Sprain	Severe Sprain
Etiology	Direct or indirect Trauma to joint	Same	Severe direct or indirect Trauma to joint
Symptoms	Pain, mild disability	Pain, moderate	Pain, Severe disability
Signs	Mild point tenderness; no abnormal motion; little or no swelling	Pint tenderness, moderate loss of function slight to moderate abnormal motion: swelling; localized hermorrhage	Loss of Function; marked abnormal motion; possible deformity; X-rays: stress films demonstration abnormal motion
Complication	Tendency to recurrence aggravation	Tendency to recurrence, aggravation; Persistent instability; traumatic arthritis	Persistent instability; traumatic arthritis
Pathology	Minor tearing ligment	Partial tear of ligament	Complete tear of ligament

Q.194. So, What can be the line of treatment ?

Ans. In early stages kicking should be reduced and short wave diathermy given. Surgery is needed when the spicules have become prominent or fractured, and when loose bodies are present.

Q.195. What is Sever's Disease ?

Ans. This disease usually occurs in boys of about 9-10 years of age. It is due to mild traction; pain and tenderness which is localized at the insertion of Achilles tendon. Sometimes there is an increased pain and fragmentation of the apophysis.

Q.196. What is the possible treatment in such conditions ?

Ans. A self-limiting condition where rest is most important treatment. After a blow to the heel, as in soccer, a localized heel haematoma can simulate Sever's disease, and occasionally an infection of the calcanium may develop. When the heel is quite tender and swollen a precautionary E.S.R. should be done. Bursitis just above the insertion of the Achilles tendon may also result from ill-fitting footwear and has to be differentiated from this condition.

Apart from fractures and Sever's disease, calcaneal pain may be due to a localized infection or calcaneal spur (in plantar fascitis). Acute plantar fascitis may have a rheumatological (Reiter's sydrome) or infective (e.g. gonorrhoea) basis and the appropriate tests should be made.

Q.197. How does the condition of 'painful tarsus' develop ?

Ans. Especially, among children, pain in mid tarsal region is rare; one cause is Kohler's disease (osteochontritis of the navicular bone). The bony muscle of the navicular becomes dense and fragmented. A comparable condition occasionally develops in middle aged women (Brailsford's disease). In young adults, especially if arch is high, a ridge of bone sometimes develops on the adjacent dorsal surfaces of the medial cuniform and the first metatarsal ('the overbone'). This interferes with kicking and may have to be exercised. Sometimes a hard ganglion on the dorsum of the foot is confused with this condition. It also requires removal.

Q.198. What is evulsion injury ? How will you treat it ?

Ans. Forced inversion of the foot may cause an evulsion injury of the fifth metatarsal base. In children the styloid epiphysis feels tender.

Strapping and early mobility are encouraged. However, normal inversion which stretches the peroneus brevis during walking sometimes exacerbates the pain and thus a plaster is required for 2 weeks.

Q.199. What is 'march fracture'? How can it be managed ?

Ans. The stress fracture of metatarsal is known as march fracture. It commonly develops among soldiers who have to walk for hours together. In young athletes, especially after prolonged road work, the foot becomes painful and a tender lump may be felt just midshaft of the metatarsal bone.

The common site of involvement is 2nd metatarsal. In clear sciagram a fine crack may be seen, later mass of callus forms.

Management : Rest from sports and alternate exercise programme. The symptoms usually subside within 3 to 4 weeks. Correct attention to good sole on the running shoes, while tight training on grass surface may prevent its recurrence.

Q.200. What do you understand by the pronated foot disorders ?

Ans. Due to excessive running with this disorder mostly the athletes suffer. The pronoted foot disrupts the normal path of weight-bearing and causes exaggerated internal rotation of the leg. Flattening of longitudinal arch with tenderness of the planter fascia, medial ankle ligament and posterior tibial tendon, occurs. Spasm follows in the peroneal muscles and the interosseous ligament becomes stretched. Finally, the forefoot spreads out and the metatarsal heads become painful. In the mildly pronated foot there is 40-60 of calcaneous valgus, a severe deformity of 120 may sometimes also be found.

Q.201. How can it be treated ?

Ans. Ice massage, cold whirlpool and galvanic muscle stimulation or transcutaneous nerve stimulation are used.

Anti-inflammatory agents are given. Arch supports or orthotics devices supplied by a pediatrist can be used. Some exercises help to control pronation. Toe rises and Achilles tendon stretching exercises strengthen the calf muscles; the toes should be exercised by picking up small marbles or stones. Lastly, the player should be encouraged to walk with a slight toe-in-gait and an exaggerated spring in pushing off.

Q.202. What are dorsiflexion and planterflexion strains ?

Ans. They can be described in two different groups :

(a) Dorsiflexion Strain. Dorsiflexion strain can happen if one jumps from a height and land flat footed, with the knee bent and forcing the weight forward over the ankles. A moderate strain pushes the talus between the lower ends of tibia and fibula causing stress on ligament between the two bones. A more severe injury may cause the ligament to break. A very severe injury may break the ligament and cause a crack on the top of the talus or the lower end of the front of the tibia.

(b) Planterflexion Strain. Planterflexion strain is the least common type of ankle injury, but it can occur, for example if one catches the front of the foot while running. A moderate strain will simply overstretch the front of the ankle. A severe strain, combined with compression force, may cause a crack in the back of the lower end of tibia, when talus is driven against it.

Q.203. Why do people use the words 'shin soreness' or 'shin splints'? What do these interpretations mean ?

Ans. These are vague expressions, capable of multiple interpretations. They generally describe pain over the front and sides of the leg, especially the lower inner side. The pain may be just a nagging ache, usually associated with running. It may start gradually, but developed into a noticeable pain over a space of time. It is often difficult to remember how the pain started, as it comes on insidiously. It is usually caused by running, or even walking for unaccustomed long distances, but is sometimes triggered by an accident such as a kick or direct blow to the leg, developing after the initial brusing and pain have subsided. Generally it develops due to sudden overloading player with event having same biomechanics.

Q.204. What do you mean by 'snapping hip' ?

Ans. It is caused by long standing bursitis over the greater trochanter. It is more common in young girls. When this condition is not allowed to heel, the bursa becomes thick, and obstructs the tendon which should ride over it. This causes a snapping sound each time the tendon goes over the thickest part of the bursa. If it is painful, surgery may be needed to cure the problem. Quite often, the condition causes only the notice, but no pain, and in such type of cases there is nothing to worry about it.

Q.205. Explain in brief the condition 'Ankylosing Spondylitis'.

Ans. Out of the inflammatory joint condition which can cause intermittent, unexplained pain, one particularly tends to affect his sacro-iliac region. This is a progressive disease causing stiffness and gradual loss of function. It usually starts in the back and spreads up the spine, but may also affect the other joints like shoulders, elbows, hips and even it can cause the pain and tightness of planter fascia under the soles of the feet. The disease generally affects the teenage boys, so the pain may be mistakenly related to over-exercising on the previous day.

Q.206. How to diagnose and treat this condition ?

Ans. It can be diagnosed on the basis of history of pain, X-rays and blood tests. After diagnosing, it should be managed with appropriate drugs to relieve pain. The most important factor in controlling the disease is to maintain good power and flexibility in the trunk, while avoiding activities which tend to increase pain. Back exercises may be done; regularly to keep the back mobile. The pain of the disease is intermittent and arbitrary, so athlete should not try to play game during an episode of pain. The more sporting activities are maintained without pain the more better results it gives in the long run. Swimming is considered as a very useful activity for maintaining power and movement in spine and limbs, without overloading the joints.

Q.207. What is 'Morton's foot'? What problems does it create for the athlete ?

Ans. Though it is not an injury yet it is the condition which develops because second metatarsal is longer than the first so that a disproportionate amount of weight is borne on this head. The characteristic finding is a heavy, tender callus on the sole of the foot over the second metatarsal head and absence of callus over the first metatarsal head. Pain may not have been present until the athlete becomes active in running with the whole of his body weight being thrown forward on to the ball of his foot.

This may be treated by placing a self pad in the shoe under the head of first metatarsal so that the pressure is removed from the second metatarsal head.

Q.208. After injury what changes take place in soft tissues ?

Ans. The following changes may occur :

Synovial swelling;

Local chemicals are released which affect pathological changes (histamine, serotonin, bradykinin and various polypeptides).

Recent research has shown the role of prostaglandins. They are involved in pain platinisation and increased vascular permeability, thus causing persistent oedema and late fibrosis. Prostaglandins also increase collagen biosynthesis and may be responsible for excessive fibrin formation after injury.

Q.209. So, what role do anti-inflammatory agents have to play ?

Ans. Anti-inflammatory agents appear to accelerate the rate of recovery in sports injuries when given early. This is important for individuals who are keen to regain match fitness as rapidly as possible. The availability of safe simple therapy compatible with this aim is important to this group.

Thus anti-inflammatory agents have a part to play in the immediate treatment of a soft-tissue injury, supplementing other more traditional methods of rest, strapping and plaster of paris immobilization. The relative paucity of side effects in fit persons over a short course of 5 to 7 days makes one of the non-steroidal anti-inflammatory agents the drug of choice.

Q.210. What is the role of Hyaluronidase in soft-tissue injury ?

Ans. It is useful in acute soft tissue injuries especially when hydrocortisone or other steroids have been given lically for instance in a case of tenosynovitis of the wrist. However, the use of oral enzyme preparation is hindered by their vulnerability to gastric acidity. Although many tablets are enteric coated, their role in soft tissue injury is still not clear but, in one double blind trial of chymotrypsin plus trypsin in ankle sprain no benefit was found over placebo.

In local application of heparinoid substance, methyl salicylate liminent (oil of winter green), to some extent by turpentine oil cooling sprays also have a soothing effect on the skin. But there is little convincing evidence to support their efficacy in treatment of soft tissue injuries and most of them are of historical importance only.

Q.211. What are snapping tendons ? What is the ultimate remedy for it ?

Ans. The following examples can be given for snapping tendons:

In hip, a facial band may slip over the greater trochanter;

Snapping shoulder may be caused by the long head of biceps

displacing in the sulcus or by the supraspinatus syndrome;

In scapula, it may be due to an exostosis on the thoracic cage or the body of the scapula itself;

Snapping knee may be due to an exostosis on the medial aspect of the tibia which impinges on the pes anserinus during flexion and extension movements;

Knee feels locked and a small bruise may appear on the inner aspect of the knee.

For all these problems, surgery is the last resort.

Q.212. Explain, how Mysositis ossificans develops.

Ans. Generally it occurs following a musculo-skeletal injury. Such type of injuries are more common in the thigh, elbow, shoulder and ankle.

Pathologically, it forms due to ossification of a heamatoma when there has been periosteal avulsion. It is believed that the periosteal calls proliferate within the blood clot and ossify it. During the acute stage muscle may be warmed and tender. Any manipulative therapy such as deep friction massage, only adds to the problem.
On X-ray, new bone formation at 4-6 weeks as a faint cloud of ossification may be seen. This tissue gradually becomes denser until if finally assumes the radiological appearance of mature bone by 3-6 months.

Q.213. Is it possible to treat such problems ?

Ans. During the acute phase, the injured area is treated by rest which is most important. It is generally provided by using Plaster of Paris for 2-4 week; no heat or manipulations are suggested at this stage. Remobilization should only commence after pain and tenderness have subsided, and extreme care is taken not to provoke further bleeding or swelling. The maturity of new bone can be assessed by Z-rays or bone scan using a radio-active isotope. If the bone is mature and causing symptoms by pressure, nerve entrapment or friction, it can be excised. In most of the cases no surgical treatment is needed.

Q.214. What is Bruised heel ?

Ans. This complaint is common among hurdlers and long triple jumpers. Repeated heavy landings on the heels cause rupture of the fibrous septa between the skin and calcaneus so that protective fatty layer becomes dissipated, and local pain and tenderness are found.

Q.215. How can it be managed ?

Ans. There is a need to give heel support. Heel pad consists of a thick soft sponge-rubber, It works as a good heel support. However, a moulded heel cup may also be used; this cup is designed to compress the lateral aspects of the heel and prevent displacement of the soft-tissue.

Q.216. What is the sprain of the spring ligament and how can it be managed ?

Ans. Sprain of the planter calcanio-navivcular ligament may follow unaccustomed running over uneven surfaces with soft shoes. The clinical picture is similar to that of planter fascities but the tenderness is more anterior and medial side. A moulded felt insole and intrinsic foot exercises with ultrasound are required.

Q.217. Sketch the pathophysiology of overuse syndrome leading to a stress fracture.

Ans. From the following representation, it can be understood easily :-

Too much and forceful repetition of a movement.
Increase Muscular Forces + Increase rate of Remodelling
Resorption and Rarefaction
Microfractures
Periosteal and/or Endosteal Response ('Stress Fracture')
Linear Fracture ('Stress Fracture')
Displaced Fracture.

Q.218. What can be the etiology of Plantar Fascitis ?

Ans. One of the most incapacitating and prolonged effect overuse syndromes, is inflammation of the planter fascia. This malady occurs from the repetitive stretching of the planter fascia between its origin at the anterior planter rim of the calcaneous and its insertion into the metatarsal heads. The athlete usually incurs the injury from marked increase in training duration or frequency. Hill running and speed work are often responsible for irritation or the inflammation because of increased traction to the fascia in these activities.

Q.219. What are the common signs and symptoms of planter fascitis ?

Ans. The following are the common signs and symptoms of planter fascitis :

(a) Pain in medial arch or heel or both. It may also be present at planter surface of calcaneum. Sometimes both feet may give same symptoms.
(b) Patient prefers to walk on lateral side of foot as he avoids pain which is due to inflamed planter fascia.
(c) Tenderness on deep palpation towards medial edge of fascia or at the anterior edge of calcaneum.
(d) Walking on toes may elicit the pain.
(e) X-ray may show ossification changes.

Q.220. What is Achillis Tendinitis ?

Ans. It is a common and recurring problem. The etiology is a combination of short achillis tendon and repeated forcible traction such as from running or jumping. As with the most overuse syndromes it initially is most pronounced after exercise. In more advanced cases, it often produces pain and stiffness early in the morning hours. The location of the pain in vast majority of cases is around the tendon itself at the level of ,malleoli, Occasionally it may be as proximal as the musculo-tendineous junction or distal as its insertion on the posterior calcaneum.

Q.221. What are the signs and symptoms of Aachillis Tendinitis ?

Ans. Tendinitis can be diagnosed on palpation between thump and finger.

- In dorsiplanter flexion crepitus may be felt.
- In severe cases, pain increases even on walking.
- On X-ray cancaneal spur may or may not be there.
- Swelling on posterior side of malledoli may be seen.

Q.222. What do you understand by Anterior Leg Pain ?

Ans. It is also a common overused syndrome generally seen among unconditioned athlete or the athlete not conditioned for new sports. 'Coaches may accuse shoes, track surfaces or other situations as the cause of anterior leg pain. But these relationships are of minor importance. The etiology usually is increased training intensities to athletes. The origin of the pathophysiology seems to be traction at the origin of anterior compartment muscles especially at the edge of tibia.

The athlete complains of diffuse linear pain along the anterior or medial edge or the midshaft of distal one third of tibia. Occasionally they can reproduce the pain by forced contraction of the dorsiflexors of the foot. On examination an area of diffuse tenderness may be observed along the origin of either the anterior or posterior tubialis muscles.

Q.223. On an average what is the percentage of incidences of Stress Fracture on different bones ?

Ans. The stress fractures can occur on any bone to which sufficient repetitive stress is applied, but more common sites include.

- — Tibia-50 percent;
- — Metatarsals-18 percent;
- — Fibula-12 percent;
- — Femur-6 percent;
- — Other sites less than 1 percent each.

Q.224. What are the common signs and symptoms of Stress Fracture ?

Ans. The following common signs and symptoms may be found in a case of stress fracture:

- — Sharp, persistent, progressive pain or,
- — a deep persistent dull ache located over a bone,
- — Increased pain on impact (heel strike),
- — Point tenderness over a bony surface,
- — rarely bony irregularity of callus may be felt,
- — tuning fork test is positive,
- — clear sciagram sometimes reveals diagnosis.

Q.225. Describe in brief the Osgood-schlatter's Disease ?

Ans. This condition is nothing but traction apophysitis of the tibial tubercle. It is a malady confined mostly to the young athlete. The large forces of the extensor mechanism of the leg are magnified by the patellar mechanism, and repetitive forces transmitted to the insertion of the infrapatellar tendon at the immature tibial tubercle. When continued for a longer duration of time, this results in a traction apophysitis. Sports involving repeated flexions and forced extension of the knee are the inciting factors.

Q.226. What are the common signs and symptoms of Osgood-Schlatter's Disease ?

Ans. The following may be common signs and symptoms of this disease :

- — Pain and tenderness directly over prominence of the involved tibial tubercle.
- — Pain is enhanced with forceful leg extension or due to direct pressure on tibial tubercle.
- — Tenderness and occasional swelling over the involved tubercle.
- — Tubercle may be enlarged in size.
- — Pain on deep knee bend may also be there.

Q.227. What is the principle used for treating overuse injuries ?

Ans. Reduce the inflammation by :

- Rest or alteration of activity;
- Physical modalities;
- Medication.

Q.228. What types of alternate exercise may be used ?

Ans. For running sports-

- running at deep end of swimming pool;
- cycling with heel adjusted to pedal;
- rowing, weight by uninvolved limbs.

Q.229. Name the common therapeutic modalities.

Ans. In cases of overuse syndromes, the basic purpose of using these modalities is to promote healing by decreasing pain, swelling, spasm, enhanced blood flow etc.

- Cryotherapy;
- Cold whirlpool;
- Contrast-therapy;
- Therapeutic heat-hot packs, diathermy etc.
- Electrical currents (electrogalvanic stimulation) and ultrasound;
- Good stretching, and off season conditioning;
- Taping, splints, braces, and orthotics.

Q.230. What do you understand by tenosynovitis of the ankle ? Explain it by giving example of footballer.

Ans. Repeated kicking in soccer can produce a tenosynovitis chiefly affecting the dorsiflexors of the toes. It responds to local steroids and strapping for 3-7 days. Often in professional footballers. There are numerous capsular osteophytis which may cause ankle pain due to impingement or fracture. This pain may be misdiagnosed as tenosynovitis of the ankle.

Q.231. Write about the sprain of the tibialis posterior and peronei. How will you manage this injury ?

Ans. Any contact sport with sudden body checking may cause strain of the above tendons and swelling, bruising is localized to the affected tendon sheaths.

The best treatment is firm strapping or a plaster for two

weeks. Sometimes excessive scarring results in nerve entrapment. Surgical release may be needed under these circumstances. It is also worth noting that an ankle haemarthrosis may escape through a torn ligament and into the personal sheath.

Q.232. What happens when there is displacement of the peroneal tendons ?

Ans. The tendons are displaced from their normal position on the posterior surface of the lateral malleolus and lie obliquely over the lateral third of the distal surface of fibula; since the fulcrum of pull is lost, the mechanical efficiency is also impaired. This is not an uncommon injury in contact sport-soccer. The diagnosis can easily be made by making audible clicks as they sublux. They are easily felt on surface of lateral malleolus.

CHAPTER FIVE
REHABILITATION IN SPORTS

Q.1. What is Sports Physiotherapy ? Explain it in brief.

Ans. Sports physiotherapy is a specialized branch of Physical medicine and Rehabilitation, mainly concerned with the prevention treatment and rehabilitation of the athletes.

Sports Physiotherapy employs Kinesiological principles not only for the prevention of the injuries, but also helps to achieve the targets and goals in a particular game.

If injuries at all occur, this specially helps them in getting treated, and the injured athletes are properly, scientifically rehabilitated.

To achieve all above, highly specialised techniques of exercises and various electrotherapy measures are of equal importance provided they are used judiciously, optimally and timely.

Q.2. What is functional adaptation ?

Ans. Adaptation of the connective tissue to the physical exercises is called functional 'adaptation'.

It can be further explained in the following manner :

(a) an insufficient adaptation may result on account of minor stimulus or loss of stimulus of tissue,

(b) an extreme, i.e., pathological reaction of tissue may be caused on account of stimulus.

The effects of physical exercises, especially of training, have been cleared up as concerning muscular tissue. The adaptation of skeletal system, especially of bone tissue has only been explored in recent years.

The different time of adaptation between muscular tissue and cartilage and bone tissue is of great importance, for the strength of stimulus concerning physical exercises.

Q.3. How do skeletal tissues adapt to activity ?

Ans. Muscles show reaction on physical exercises within weeks by an increase of muscle force while cartilage and bone needs some years before being adapted to high loads of physical exercises.

The formative stimulus for bone is pressure, for cartilage

extension and smooth joint play. These kinds of stimuli are necessary for formation and growth of bone and cartilage.

Q.4. What do you understand by manipulative therapy ?

Ans. Manipulated therapy is based on the concepts of joint play and joint dyfunction. Joint play is the normal range of involuntary movement of which a joint is capable. Without normal joint play, pain is experienced. Manipulation restores normal joint play by taking a joint's movement to its limits, thus correcting the joints dyfunction. It must be practiced by trained, experienced therapist or physicians. Contra-indications for manipulative treatment include bone or joint disease or inflammation, healing ligament sprains or muscle strains, disc injuries and vertebral fracturer. The muscle spasm accompanying joint dyfunction can be treated by conventional therapies, but manipulative therapy can often correct the cause of the problem.

Q.5. How does the body react to the activity ?

Ans. Mostly reactions of tissue enable sportsmen to do more physical exercises on a high level with more load bearing. These signs of functional adaptation of physical exercises are :

(i) Activity hypertrophy of bone which should be gradual.
(ii) Morphological adaptation of structures of bone and joints on physical exercises.
(iii) A better formation of none in the form of osteophytes at origin of muscles, tendons and ligaments insertion.

For further explanation, example of vertebrae may be quoted here. After ten years of physical exercises including weight bearing, they will be less high and have a larger base. We measure the vertebrae of sportsmen, will have a larger fundamental basis and will not be as high as they are without a regular physical exercise.

Q.6. Why is it important to increase the load gradually ?

Ans. The reactions mentioned above enable sportsmen to do more physical exercises without injuries as stress fracture of the tibia and slipping of intervertebral disc. It is absolutely necessary to increase stimulus of physical exercises step by step and for a long time, preferably in a duration of five years.

That is why it is always necessary to do physical exercises for many years before having training for championship.

Q.7. What is morphological adaptation of hones, joints etc. ?

Ans. Many minerals are brought into tissue at pressure line. Where, there is no pressure, a loss of minerals takes place. A great strength of bone is reached with minerals deposition. A long time of physical exercises is necessary for the transformation of bone. This is the best prevention for bone injuries and diseases (e.g. osteomalacia).

Osteophytes increase at the place of bone where there is the origin of muscles, tendons and ligaments. This feature proves the process of adaptation.

It is also well known that bone needs at least 5 years for these reactions of bone tissue to take place.

Q.8. What do you understand by "Pathological adaptation"?

Ans. It may result when there is too high a load of physical exercises upon an individual's fitness. It may be characterized by

(i) External high movement in joints with extremely large osteophytes.

(ii) Bone transformation to sclerosis of bone or loss of bone structure up to a stress fracture.

If there is the first sign of these reactions, physical exercises have to be reduced for some time and are to be performed at a lower level with charge in biomechanics of the part.

Q.9. Why is physical activity important ?

Ans. It is necessary due to the following reasons :

— Bones will be weak if they are not used by physical exercises.

— Bones will become strong if physical exercises were done in agreement with individual fitness.

— Bones will be damaged (osteomalacia) if there is too high a demand concerning physical exercises and no agreement with the efficiency of the individual.

Therefore, physical exercises are important for the health of sportsmen and general people as well.

Q.10. What type of pastoral deformities can be corrected ?

Ans. Postural deformities usually occur due to the

(i) fault of attitude,
(ii) fault of position,
(iii) fault of form,
  (a) Scoliosis
  (b) Kyphosis

Among these, the first two factors caused postural deformities can be easily corrected. Therefore, physical exercises are necessary especially for young boys and girls. Compared with a tree, a young tree can be easily corrected for proper growth and so a healthy strong tree will be the ultimate result, whereas an old curved tree will never get a correct form.

Q.11. Explain with details the word 'Traction' ?

Ans. Cervical and lumbar traction is used to treat non-inframmatary musculo skeletal conditions, muscle spasm and pain. Its effects are decresed muscle spasm, increased blood flow and length of fibrotic tissue, encouragement of range of motion and relief of nerve pressure. Traction is frequently combined with moist heat packs and can be applied continuously or intermittently. Continuous traction is said to enlarge the intervertebral space and to reduce compressive for irritative press on nerve routes. Treatment with continuous traction begin with 15 to 20 pounds of pressure for 30 minutes daily. Intermittent traction uses a gradually increasing sbaich alternating with periods of relaxation. Intermittent traction is more easily tolerated than continuous traction because it is less likely to cause overstretching and resultant muscle spasm. Treatment may build up to 5 to 15 pounds with 5 to 10 interruptions per minute.

Q.12. What are the different forms of vertebral column ? Explain.

Ans. Following are the different forms of vertebral column:

(a) normal,
(b) flat back,

(c) total kyphosis,
(d) thoracic kyphosis and cervical and lumbar lordosis,
(e) scoliosis.

These different forms of vertebral column are not to be regarded as postural deformities. But if nothing is done during growth to diminish the abnormal forms, postural deformities will be the result. Stability and movement are necessary so that the vertebral column can perform the function desired by the individual.

On account of this function, intervertebral discs are provided between the different vertebrae. As the discs are not provided with a circulatory system after the age of four years, a constant change between pressure and extension is necessary in order to keep the intervertebral disc in a healthy condition. These principles have to be regarded in performance of physical exercises and daily work as well. Asymmetrical pressure on the intervertebral discs should be avoided.

Q.13. Explain the word "Kyphosis-lordosis"

Ans. There is at first a Kyphosis without any change as to the form of vertebrae. It is only a matter of attitude. At this early stage, a complete correction will be possible by means of physical exercises. By the treatment of Kyphosis, lordosis will automatically decrease.

As soon as Kyphosis is due to a change of form, it is to be regarded as a postural deformity. Physical exercises will be able to diminish symptoms, e.g. back pain, but they will never be able to cure the deformity.

Thoracic kyphosis is followed by an extreme lordosis in the cervical and lumber part of the vertebral column. Therefore, back pain will be especially localised therein.

Q.14. To prevent injury to the back. How you will perform lower back stretch and lumbar stretch with perfection?

Ans. **Lower back stretch**

— Sit on an exercise mat or soft surface with your hands by your sides.
— Lie down flat and then slowly bring your legs over your head until your toes are touching the floor behind you. Hold for a count of 5 and then slowly bring them back over your head.

Lumbar Stretch

Lie on the ground and raise yours upper body supporting your weight with your hands palms flat on the ground as shown. Keeping your arms straight stretch gently upwards, raising your head and chin. Repeat 3 times.

Q.15. What is Scoliosis ? Explain in detail.

Ans. There exist three forms of scoliosis :

C-Scoliosis,

S-Scoliosis-Double scoliosis,

S-Scoliosis-Triple scoliosis,

There must also be a difference between scoliosis as an attitude and scoliosis with changes of the form of the vertebra. Scoliosis with changes of form of vertebra are to be regarded as postural deformities. Especially during growth there is a great danger for increase of scoliosis if it already exists.

By X-ray of an ilium with demonstration of the epiphytes of ilium, it may be decided whether growth of the vertebral column has come to an end or not. As soon as the epiphytes comes into osteosynthesis with the ilium, growth will finish so the danger of progress of scoliosis will be lost.

Q.16. Can you suggest a few common physical exercises for the correction of these defects ?

Ans. As soon as feasible, take exercises to correct attitude in childhood. In case of kyphosis there must be a special muscular training of:

— stretching of front muscle of chest,
— erector spine muscle including oblique abdomens muscles,
— muscles of the back,
— stretching erector spine muscle and strengthening gluteus maximus muscle at lower level. In case of scoliosis, the following fundamental principles are to be observed.
— muscles on the side of concavity are to be stretched.
— muscles on the side of convexity are to be strengthened.

But these exercises can only help to a limited extent.

Q.17. Explain in brief the trunk rotations and trunk truns.

Ans. I. Stand with feet shoulder or width apart and knees slightly bent, with fingers interlacked behind your head, bend from the waist and touch the right knee with the right elbow. Rotate the trunk to the left to touch the left knee and back to the starting position.

II. Trunk Turns: Stand with feet apart and knees slightly bent. Raise your arms to shoulder height and close your hands. Turn from the waist to one side as far as you can go. Hold for a count of 5 and then turn to the other side. Keep your legs and hips still and turn only the upper body.

Q.18. How will perform side bends and chest flings.

Ans. **Side bends :** Stand up straight with hands by your side and knees slightly bent. Slowly raise one arm high above your head, easing the other arm down your leg. Pull your arm over your head as far as it will go while pushing down on your thigh. Return to the starting position and repeat on the other side. Do 3 repetitions on each side.

Chest Flings : Stand up straight with feet shoulder width apart elbows bent at shoulder height and finger tips touching. Filing your arms out gently backwards at shoulder height and then return to the original position. Repeat 10 times.

Q.19. What is your opinion regarding use of electrotherapy for sports injuries ?

Ans. The effect of electrotherapy for treating sports injuries is not well known. On the one hand nearly all injuries of athletes are treated with electrotherapy without a complete examination of sportsmen, while, on the other hand, the advantages for treatment of sports injuries without electrotherapy were not taken into consideration. Therefore, a critical assessment of electrotherapy for treatment of athletic injuries is necessary.

Sports injuries are to be regarded from the patho-physiological point of view and the symptoms as well. A difference must be made of the findings and symptoms resulting due to the acute and chronic lesions.

Q.20. Will you give brief account of injuries and their management by electrotherapy ?

Ans. Acute injuries, e.g. contusion, strains, incomplete or complete dislocation of joints, irritation at insertions of muscles and tendons are characterised by acute symptoms. Pain and swelling within the injured tissue along with increased capillary blood flow to the place concerned. Thus temperature increases.

The chronic stage of injuries is characterised by diminished blood circulation, increased tension and atrophy of muscles.

On account of the difference between an acute and chronic stage of sports injuries, different methods of electrotherapy must be used. During the acute stage of injury, short wave diathermy, which increases temperature within the tissue, even in the deeper parts of the body, is contraindicated.

Q.21. Write the general principles in treatment of fracture and stress fractures ?

Ans. 1. Principles of Treatment (Aims of treatment)

(i) Complete recovery,

(ii) Recovery as soon as possible,

(iii) Recovery without risk,

diagnoses as soon as possible, Clinical examination; X-ray examination.

3. Final treatment from the very beginning, e.g., operation or plaster bandage or functional treatment.
4. Physical therapy as soon as possible, e.g., isometric muscle contraction.
5. Methods of physical therapy depends upon adaptation and complete osteosynthesis.
6. Movement of joints and contraction of muscles should be done as soon as possible.
7. No risk for fractured bone is allowed by early movement.
8. Physical therapy is to be performed on order of the doctor of medicine only.
9. No massage is allowed within localization of fracture especially elbow joint, where danger of mystics ossification should always be kept in mind.
10. Medical treatment should be done until complete recovery and rehabilitation is achieved.

Q.22. What do you understand by the world "Rehabilitation"?

Ans. Recovery of injured or ill persons upto the best possible degree of physical, mental and professional fitness.

Rehabilitation in sports means recovery of injured or ill sportsmen upto fitness (physical fitness) for training and competition by specialized coaches and medical doctors of sports medicine (Helga Schmidt, Prof. of Sports Medicine from G.D.R.-a talk).

Q.23. Write the contents of Rehabilitation ?

Ans. Rehabilitation is necessary :

— to keep morphological and functional adaptation to physical exercise.

— to regain physical fitness.

— to avoid atrophy of the injured side by exercises with the non-injured side-arms or legs.

— to avoid uncontrolled physical exercises of sportsmen on account of pleasure in physical exercises.

— to guarantee a high level of physical fitness and make sportsmen ready for systematic training.

Q.24. How one should approach for rehabilitation of an athlete ?

Ans. Rehabilitation of an athlete should always include the following aspects :-

— Strength of stimulus,

— Frequency of stimulus,

— Frequency of movement,

— interval must be adapted to individual medical findings and to regain physical fitness.

Importance of regular medical examination for developing physical fitness should not be overlooked.

Q.25. What does this medical examination mean ? Explain it in the light of "Knee Joint" ?

Ans. It means clinical examination, i.e. joints, muscles, detailed ligaments of the knee joint i.e. lateral and medical collateral ligaments and cruciate ligaments etc.

If the clinical examination detects something then it ought to be treated as soon as possible by either functional treatment or treatment with plaster bandage or operative treatment.

All these aspects depend upon the special findings detected during examination.

Care should be taken not to damage injured ligaments.

By clinical examination and X-ray it has to be decided whether there is a strain, a sprain, a rupture of the ligament or even a rupture of several ligaments, any fracture or dislocation of the joint.

Q.26. How to rehabilitate a case of meniscus damage ? Explain with suitable examples.

Ans. It depends upon the findings during operation whether there is' a meniscus with :

(i) a simple longitudinal rupture which may be removed easily,

(ii) a rupture in the posterior part which sometimes is difficult to be removed and bleeding may occur during operation,

(iii) a damage of the cartilage of joint surfaces combined with the rupture of the meniscus.

(I) First case :

First day after operation: beginning with isometric muscle exercises in bed.

4th day : beginning with movement of leg in bed.

8th day : getting up, patient begins to take steps.

Exercises out of bed : Strengthening of quadriceps muscle.

After two weeks : Swimming with stretched knee joints if possible.

Special training in competition discipline begins when complete strength of quadriceps muscle has been regained.

(II) Second Case :

First day after operation, beginning with isometric muscle training, movement of leg and knee joint according to liquid in joint capsule.

Getting up avoided before all the liquid in capsule of knee joint is absorbed.

(III) Third case :

Rest in bed for at least 8 weeks with extension of the leg.

NOTE : There may be slight variation in the treatment line, depending upon the liking of an operating surgeon.

Q.27. What is the line of treatment in a case of ruptured achilles tendon ?

Ans. It may be treated in the following manner :

Ruptures of achilles tendon are to be operated within the first 6 hours after injury in order to get the best results. If no operation is done then it will result in a weak gastrochemius and soleus muscles.

Rupture of achilles and its management :

1 day : isometric muscle exercise in plaster bandage and exercises with non-injured leg.

(a) After 3-4 weeks : Plaster bandage may be made show and movement of knee joint started gradually.

(b) After 5-6 weeks : taking off plaster bandage and movement of foot, without extreme dorsal flexion (only upto an angle of 90 0).

(c) After 8 weeks : Out of bed and walking with a high heel shoe.

(d) After 10-12 weeks : Walking-normal range and more dorsal flexion may be tried.

(e) 3-6 months : Competitive sports are allowed.

Keep in mind that there are no fixed timings for increasing physical exercises during rehabilitation programme.

Q.28. How to assess the level of physical activity in a particular rehabilitation programme ?

Ans. Concerning an increase of physical exercises depends upon the :-

— individual medical findings after injury,
— morphological changes seen during operation,
— reactions of tissue during rehabilitation,
— increase of muscle strength during rehabilitation.

Q.29. What basic points to be kept in mind in relation to hematoma.

Ans. (1) Diagnosis should be prompt, with aspiration, if necessary, to make a final determination.

(2) The volume of contained blood should be reduced by aspiration. Hyaluronidase, pressure, cold first and then heat, and closely controlled activity.

(3) Re-injury should be prevented by protection against trauma or against excessive activity.

(4) Resorption should be encouraged by exposing the

hematoma to a larger surface area of circulation by improving the local circulation and by maintaining the general circulation. Excessive scar formation assification or calcification can be prevented by the preceding measures.

Q.30. What do you understand by word "Cryotherapy" ?

Ans. When applied to the injured part, ice or cold pack results in the cooling of that part, by the transfer of heat energy from the part to the water or ice. Cold has been found to be very effective modality in treating athletic injuries. Ice has advantage over cold water as it takes latent heat for its melting, so injured part gets quick cooling effect.

Q.31. What are its common indications and contra-indications ?

Ans. This may be used in any soft tissue injury, i.e. sprains, strains and contusions. It relieves pain and muscle spasm, controls the oedema formation and also produces temporary anaesthetic effect.

It should not be used in cases of circulatory disorders and coronary heart disease, i.e. Raynaud's daises. External haemorrhage and cold allergy also contra-indicate for cryotherapy. There may be skin blisters or even frost bite if not applied carefully. Patients need an extra care.

Q.32. Give in brief the management of hematoma ?

Ans. 1. RICE.

(i) Prevention of further bleeding
(ii) Evacuation of the blood
(iii) Encouragement of absorption of the blood,
(iv) Protection of the part until healing takes place.

Q.33. What are the common physiological effects of cold ?

Ans. It can have the following effects :

(a) Reduction in swelling and inflammation.
(b) Reduction in pain through an anaesthetic effect.
(c) Decrease in muscle spasm by reduction in nerve conduction and muscle spindle excitability.
(d) Reduction in the metabolic and oxygen needs of the injured tissues limiting the extent of the initial injury.

Q.34. What are the common methods used in Cryotherapy?

Ans. Following methods are commonly employed :

(a) Ice Massage : Keep ice in a polythene bag and rub the skin in circular or to and fro movements. A very minimal pressure should only be applied. It may be applied at a time for 5 to 10 minutes and repeat it number of times in a day. Repetition depends upon type and severity of injury.

(b) Immersion : Here, as per need, temperature of water is kept between 0 to 10. It is better to use the solution of 50% ice and 50% water. The part may either be immersed for a single ten minute duration or a series of shorter immersions comprising total of 10 minutes.

(c) Ice packs : Here crushed ice is used and kept in a double layered plastic bag or towel bag. Treatment is usually given for 20 minutes at a time. It should be repeated many times a day. For ice cube massage and ice pack techniques, it is better to spread a thin layer of vegetable oil over the area to be treated to minimize the possibility of ice burn especially when treating at cold climatic conditions.

(d) Evaporative cooling : Ethyl Chloride spray gives effect by heat exchange process due to rapid evaporation and results in reflex muscle relaxation.

Remember, time, type and duration of cryotherapy depends upon :

Site of injury,

Type of injury,

Severity of injury

Structure involved, and

Type of effect to be obtained.

Q.35. What do you understand by Cryotherapy and compression ?

Ans. Ice plus cold compression wrap which may be in any form-cotton and bandage; crepe bandage and crushed ice or through a machine.

Q.36. What are the treatment techniques of Cryokinetics ? Also write its physiological effects.

Ans. (a) Method : After applying cold to the injured part, begin an exercise programme appropriate to that particular injury. When pain is felt the exercise is to be stopped. The same process is repeated many times.

(b) Effects : The injured part is allowed to be numbed by the effect of the cold, and then put through a range of movement and controlled exercise. It enhances the healing process by stimulating the circulation, while at the same time preventing inhibitory neural responses and allowing the surrounding tissues and muscles to early activity.

Q.37. Give an example and method of its application ?

Ans. Suppose there is a mild second degree inversion sprain involving the lateral ligament of ankle. One should follow this treatment programme :

(a) Ice : Ice application; compression; gentle range of motion or exercises provided there is no pain or uncomfortable feeling.

(b) 2nd day onwards : Ice for 10 to 20 minutes; then athlete attempts a normal heel to toe walking gait. If this can be achieved without a limp, the athlete should continue until pain is felt. Repeat it five times. Perform the same routine with eversion exercises, toe raises and if possible other couple of days hopping also, Always conclude the exercise session with Ice.

Q.38. What is cold spray therapy technique ?

Ans. In the technique of "Spray and stretch" ethyl chloride is used. But so far in India, it has not received the wide popularity. But it has definitely a place in athletic injuries, especially during a match on the field when athlete wants immediate response.

Method :

(a) The muscle to be sprayed should be stretched to the point of discomfort.

(b) The container is held approximately eighteen inches (45 cms) from the skin.

(c) The jet stream should meet the body's surface at an angle, not perpendicularly.

(d) The stream should meet the trigger point or origin of the muscle to the reference area or insertion of the muscle.

(e) The speed of moving the part is generally kept at 10 centimetres per second.
(f) There should be no frosting of the skin if technique is properly applied.

Q.39. What are the mechanisms and physiological effects of cold spray ?

Ans. Any muscle spasm produces pain regardless of the cause. In order to relieve the spasm and achieve normal resting muscle length, the cycle producing the muscle pain, spasm pain should be blocked. It is through the effectiveness of cold spray in relieving muscle spasm due to the cold respecters, conducting the sensation more rapidly than the pain impulses. This is also known as gate theory. Thus results in the muscle-pain impulses being blocked and the muscle spasm is being relieved. In this way, it restores the normal patterns, so long as the muscle is stretched during the application of cold spray. Whatever the exact mechanism might be, the counter irritation of cold applied in a specific way, together with stretching of muscles, produces a reversal of muscle spasm in many cases, especially when dealing with trigger points.

This procedure may also be used for non-specific muscle spasm.

Example. When an athlete is subconsciously protecting an injured limb by contracting a particular muscle, this can produce an intense pain in that limb with the athlete's being aware of this cause. Spraying along the muscle from origin to insertion, together with gentle stretching of the involved muscle, may produce immediate and complete relief from the discomfort of the muscle spasm.

Q.40. Is there any advantage in applying alternating cold and heat?

Ans. Yes, this procedure is found useful in aiding recovery for the post-acute phase, particularly after sprains of extremities (contrast bath).

Q.41. How is it advantageous to the athlete ?

Ans. By its use there is an increase of circulation to the injured areas, thus aiding healing, reducing inflammation and improving range of motion.

Q.42. What is the procedure of contrast bath ?

Ans. For applying alternate hot and cold, two containers are partially filled-one with ice slush and one with lukewarm water (33.9° C to 36.7° C). The application starts from cold side and ends at cold. The ratio may be decided by sports physician. It may be three minutes to half a minute in warm water or

— Two minutes to 10 seconds in warm water or,
One minute to 10 seconds in warm water.

The procedure may be continued for 15 to 20 minutes in the same frequency. In the fatigue and overuse lesions of the limbs, it gives excellent results when started and ended with not immersion. In these cases, the ratio of hot and cold immersion usually recommended is 4 and 1 minute. If the part to be treated is such that it cannot be immersed in the containers, then the alternate towels or packs may also be used to give contrast bath.

Q.43. How does the liquid paraffin help in treatment of athletic injuries ?

Ans. It is particularly needed for enhancing circulation and providing relief from pain. The cutaneous respecters are shut off from all stimuli except the warmth of the paraffin and the insulation (layers of hardened paraffin) prevents the heat loss. As the melted wax solidifies, the energy release i.e., latent heat of solidification is conducted to the tissues. The paraffin wax is commonly used in the post-traumatic lesions of the hands and feet.

Q.44. For applying paraffin on body, what should be its temperature ?

Ans. The ideal range is 40° C to 48° C.

Q.45. Will you explain the word "paraffin painting" ?

Ans. In this procedure, a brush is dipped into a melted paraffin wax and with this plain-brush, paraffin is applied on the skin of the part. This procedure is repeated six to twelve times to form a thick layer. Now medicated liquid paraffin is allowed to dry. After this, the part treated must be wrapped in a plastic sheet and a towel in order to retain the heat. The duration is kept between 15 to 20 minutes.

Q.46. What is "paraffin dip and soak method" ?

Ans. Here the part is immersed and soaked in paraffin wax to form the thick layer of the wax. Usually this is repeated many times. Duration is the same i.e. 15-20 minutes. Exercise following paraffin wax bath gives good results.

Q.47. Is there any contra-indication for the paraffin wax treatment ?

Ans. Yes, the paraffin wax therapy should not be given in the open wounds or haemorrhagic conditions, skin diseases, and over the areas of defective sensations and impaired arterial blood supply.

Q.48. What is Joule's law ?

Ans. Joule's law is concerned with heating the body tissues by high frequency electrical currents. According to this law, the heat producer is directly proportional to the :

1. Square of the current strength ;
2. Resistance of the conductor, and
3. Time for which the current flows.

Q.49. What are the implications of Joule's law ?

Ans. When the high frequencey electrical currents are used for heating deep body tissues; regulation of treatment is done by :

(i) power output,

(ii) the different types of body tissues after the different resistance and so heat in them is produced proportionately.

(iii) treatment time.

Q.50. What are general principles to be kept in mind while using electrotherapeutic devices ?

Ans. Following points should be kept in mind :

1. The type, severity and antomicalsite of injury.
2. The indications and contra-indications of the modality to be used.
3. The individual treatment time and its frequency and the operational procedures of the modality.

(a) warm up.

(b) safety procedures.

(c) positioning of the athletes.

(d) instruction the athlete.

Q.51. Write the indications, contra-indications and effects of Hydrocollator packs or hot moist packs ?

Ans. (a) Contra-indications : Anything causing an impairment of deficiency in skin thermal sensation and thermo-regulatory control and arterial insufficiency.

(b) Indications : All soft-tissue injuries, psyches contusions, muscle strains and localized muscle spasm in sub-acute and chronic lesions.

(c) Therapeutic effects : Analgesic; reduction of muscle spasm; increase in surface circulation (cutaneous and sub-cutaneous both).

Q.52. What is the procedure of applying hot moist packs ?

Ans.

1. First the temperature of the unit must be set at approximately 65° C, then remove the packs from the unit and permit the excess water to drain off.
2. Place a few folds of a towel to avoid an excessive amount of heat from reaching the skin.
3. Duration of the treatment is usually kept between 20 to 30 minutes. Immediately after the treatment, the part should not be exposed to cold.

Q.53. What do you understand by Diathermay ? How does it function and affect the treatment ?

Ans. It produces effects in tissues mainly by increasing local temperature due to direct heating and general temperature through reflexes associated with temperature receptors. There is an increase in blood flow and tissue metabolism. The increased blood supply brings more oxygen and nutrients to the tissues and takes away the metabolities. Tear tissue may yield more easily when stretched, and tension within a musculo-tendinous unit may decrease, possibly as a result of decreased sensitivity of the muscle spindle to stretch.

Theoretically, Diathermy may be sub-divided into three on account of the relative wavelengths of the wireless waves that they set up :

Long wave,
Short wave, and
Microwave Diathermy.

Long wave diathermy was extensively used in the past. But now-a-days, in the treatment of athletic injuries, short wave and microwave diathermy are more commonly used to heat the deeper tissues. Microwave is more local and comparatively less penetrating while shortwave produces a generalized heating effect.

Q.54. What is short wave diathermy ?

Ans. It is a form of heat that makes use of a high frequency alternating electric current to heat the deeper tissues. The frequency commonly used for the treatment purpose is around 27 million. Such a high frequency does not stimulate motor or sensory nerves and result in conversive heating e.g., the electric current is converted into heat within the deeper tissues without burning the intervening ones. The does should be administered by the athlete's subjective feeling of warmth since the different body tissues in individuals may vary in dia-electric constant.

Q.55. Write the indications and contra-indications of short wave diathermy ?

Ans. Patient should be thoroughly evaluated before starting short wave diathermy treatment. Signs of defective blood supply and sensations to be noted and the nature of the treatment well explained to the patient.

Indications : Strains of the musculo-tendinous unit during post-acute stage. Capsulitis, tendinitis, rheumatoid and osteo-arthritis, frozen shoulder etc.

Contra-indications : Non-draining infections, loss of skin sensation, areas with ongoing haemorrhrage, pregnancy, acute inflammation, arterial insufficiency, venous thrombosis, neoplasms, cardiac pace-makers, turberculosis of the joints etc.

It should not be used over clothing, dressing, adhesive, casts, metal implants, crews etc. Before applying short wave diathermy skin sensation should be tested. It should also not be used on metal table. Lack of thorough evaluation, carelessness on the part of the therapist and patient as well may all lead to the burns, scalds, shocks, precipitation of gangrene, chill and faintness.

Q.56. Summarize the effects of short wave diathermy in brief ?

Ans. (i) Short wave diathermy, in various conditions, leads to an early resolution of inflammation.

(ii) This relieve pain because of its sedative and counter irritant effect on the sensory nerve endings. Pain may also be relieved because of the elimination of the waste product of the metabolism.

(iii) It also induces muscle relaxation.

(iv) Certain traumatic and bacterial infections respond well to short wave diathermy, because of the increased blood supply made available in the body tissues.

Q.57. What is the exact procedure of applying short wave ?

Ans Short wave diathermy may be given either through the condenser field method in which the electrostatic field is utilised, placing the electrodes in various arrangements like "Coplaner" through and through Monopolar etc., or by means of cable method using an induction coil. With this either a magnetic field developed at the centre of the cable may be used or the electric field between the ends of the cable may be utilised.

Method of application should be selected and the electrodes arranged according to the structure to be treated. A double layered towel is placed between the electrodes or the cable and area to the treated. Treatment time may vary from 10 to 30 minutes depending upon the lesions i.e. sub-acute or chronic.

Q.58. Explain what do you understand by micro wave diathermy ?

Ans. Microwave diathermy uses electromagnetic waves where frequency of machine may vary from 900 MHz. Heat is produced by absorption of radiation and conduction in tissues. Tissues with a high blood or water content, such as muscles, are best treated with micro-wave energy. Penetration of micro wave diathermy is more than infra-red rays but less than short wave diathermy. Commonly used frequency for the treatment purpose is 2450 mega cycles/second with a wavelenght of 12.25 cm. Now a days, the MW radiations having a frequency of 900 cycles/second is claimed to have deeper effects.

Q.59. What are the indications and contra-indications of this therapy ?

Ans. **Indications :**

(i) Same as of short wave diathermy, but more effective in fluid content lesions.

(ii) It has selective use on trigger points.

(iii) If the skin lesions contra-indicate hydrocollator usage then micro-wave therapy may be used.

(iv) The overheating of fat as with short wave diathermy does not occur with microwave diathermy. The overheating provided by microwave diathermy makes its use preferable over shortwave diathermy.

Contra-indications :

(i) Same as short wave diathermy.

(ii) Eyes and testicles should not be irradiated to microwave diathermay.

(iii) X-ray exposures, malignant growths, pulmonary tuberculosis are also contra-indicated.

Q.60. What are the effects of micro wave diathermy ?

Ans. Same as of short wave, i.e. vasodilatation with increased blood flow making more O2 and nutrients available to the tissues and removing the waste products and reduction of muscle-spasm. A burned or cylinder heating pattern produces deeper and more localized tissue heating.

Q.61. What do you understand by "ultrasound therapy" ?

Ans. It is a form of treatment with sound waves. Ultra sound waves are the sound waves that human ear cannot detect and therefore the name "ultrasound" is given. Normally human ear can detect the sound waves with frequencies between 30 and 20,000 cycles per second but not those of higher frequencies. For treatment purposes, the sound waves with a frequency of about 1 million cycles per second is commonly employed. These waves may be pulsed or interrupted to reduce the heating effects. The pulsed type ultrasound produces mechanical effects.

Q.62. How are the Ultra-sonic waves produced ?

Ans. Ultra-sonic waves are produced with the help of a crystal. It is the oscillation of crystal that sets the motor in motion and produces the ultrasonic waves.

Q.63. Write the indications and contra-indications of ultra-sound use ?

Ans. **Indications :**

Most effective in localized lesions. Post-acute soft tissue traumas (sprain, strain, contusions, tendinitis, bursitis and fibrositis); Neuromata; joint contracture; scarring etc.

Contra-indications :

(i) An actively haemorrhaging contusion.

(ii) Area of iirnited vascularity (it may not be able to meet the metabolic demands), thrombus formation, theoplasms, glands, C.N.S., heart, ears and eyes; epiphyses of growing bones; reproductive organs, and in an area of anaesthesis, acute sepsis. This should not be given in the acute inflammatory lesions. Only after 48 to 72 hours of the injury, this treatment can be started. There should not be any increase of pain during the treatment session.

Q.64. How does it influence the local part ?

Ans. (i) It is mostly due to local heat which is produced at the tissue interfaces such as fats and muscles, and at the periosteum where the waves encounter a different medium.

(ii) Other effects may be mechanical due to diffusion of ions across the cell membrane under the influence of ultra sound waves and so fluid interchange is accelerated and absorption promoted.

(iii) Changes in the biochemistry of tendon and joint capsule, collagens and other items, may also be accounted for the increase in extensibility sometimes found during treatment.

Q.65. What is the exact treatment techniques of ultrasonic waves?

Ans. Direct contact technique is most frequently used.

(i) It is used generally on flat or smooth surfaces. Coupling medium, i.e. liquid paraffin or gel is used so as to transmit the sound waves from the transducer into the body area. The treatment head should be held at right angle to the skin surface and it should always be kept moving with small circular or longitudinal strokes at a speed of about 1 inch per second. Overlap each previous stroke by half.

(ii) Duration of the treatment ranges from five to eight

minutes. Week, Intensity may be adjusted during operation of machine.

(iii) Intensities - Low intensity 0.1 to 0.8 watt per square centimetre of treatment head or five to eight total watts should be given in the early sub-acute stage. Medium intensity 0.8 to 1.5 watt per square centimetres or eight of fifteen total watta may be used in the late sub-acute stage. High intensity 1.5 to 3 watts per square centimeter or over fifteen total watts may be given in the chronic lesions.

Q.66. What is under water technique of ultra-sound therapy?

Ans. Ultra-sound may also be given underwater especially for uneven surfaces or where body areas are highly sensitive to pressure.

Method : Place the body part to be treated under water and hold the treatment head one half to one inch from the surface. Keep it moving in a similar manner. The transducer should be held parallel to the skin.

Q.67. What can be the misuse and dangers of ultra-sound therapy ?

Ans. The following may result :

Burn, and Damage to equipment.

(i) Burn may occur due to great intensity of ultrasound energy. For example, during treatment if the treatment head is allowed to remain stationary, so that the effect is confined to a small area.

(ii) If there is incomplete contact between the treatment heat and the tissue, it may lead to the over concentration of the energy at the area of contact. This may cause overheating of the ultrasound head, which subsequently burns the patient.

(iii) If the energy is applied to the crystal with the treatment head held in air, waves pass to and fro between air and crystal because the air is a poor transmitter of these waves. This leads to the setting up of the long standing waves and may increase the vibration of the crystal to be shattered.

(iv) Over bony surface : As the surface reflects the waves which pass to and fro between the bone and the treatment head, the energy is concentrated in a limited area and may give rise to a burn.

Q.68. What do you understand by Iontophoresis ?

Ans. It is a method of treatment by which ionized medication is introduced through the skin by means of an electric current or by Ultra-sound. Mostly, an ionized solution of dexamethasone in combination with a 4% viscous xylocaine preparation is used.

Q.69. Mention indications and contra-indication of Iontophoresis ?

Ans. Indications : Post-acute soft-tissue trauma such as contusions, tendinitis and strains.

Contra-indications : Same as ultra-sound and the drug being used

Q.70. What is the exact technique of using this method ?

Ans. The directing pad is first soaked in 1-2% solution of the salt that is to be introduced. This pad is kept directly on the tender area and the current is applied for approximately five minutes. The number of joins introduced into the tissues depends upon the intensity of the current and duration of the treatment. If a larger area is to be covered, the medication is applied on larger affected area, and ultrasound is used in does of 1.5 watts per square centimetre for five to ten minutes at a time.

Q.71. What is phonophoresis ?

Ans. It is the technique by which molecules of medication are driven through the skin by means of ultra-sound. Usually hydrocortisones are used. These preparations reach upto six, centimetres in depth.

Q.72. Will you mention indications and contra-indications of this method ?

Ans. Indications : Post acute soft tissue trauma (tendinitis, strains, contusions and painful areas).

Contra-indications : Same as in drugs used and ultrasound therapy. Note,10% hydrocortisone cream is frequently used. It may also be used with xylocaine.

Q.73. What are the common effects of this therapy ? Explain the method of application in brief.

Ans. Effects are the same as those of ultra-sound and drugs used.

Both the lectrodes are on the same muscle or muscle groups. For example, on quadriceps muscles, the active electrode is placed over the motor point of the thigh, while the dispersive electrode is placed over the proximal portion of the femoral nerve. An intermittent surging current of five secodns on and five seconds off may be used. The intensity of the current can be increased as per toleration. The length of time for instance can be one minute off and one minute on .

Q.74. Can ultrasound and electrical muscle stimulation be used together ?

Ans. Yes, especially when there is a risk of development of adhesions within the healing tissues.

Q.75. Will you mention this procedure by giving suitable example ?

Ans. Yes, take example of severe quadriceps muscles strain.

1. Three days of injury : Cryotherapy (gentle stretching with ice).
2. Fourth and fifth days after the injury : Ultra-sound (at 1.0 watt per square centimetre) plus electrical stimulation (pulsed and set at rate of seven to eight, intensity set at six to seven). Generally a high number of contractions at a low intensity is preferred.
3. Two treatments per day of five minutes duration each, may be given.
4. Sixth day onwards ultrasound (1.5 watts per square centimetre for five minutes) plus electrical stimulation (pulsed and set at six with intensity set at seven is given. At this stage of treatment, the rate of contractions begins to decrease and intensity is increased. Continue this procedure for fifteen minutes, then gradually modify the setting until the rate reaches four and the intensity ten.

Q.76. What is electrical muscle stimulation ?

Asn. Here, electrotherapy modalityused is either a direct or an alternating current or a combination of the two. The current may be altered in a variety of ways :

(a) Interrupted-Thecurrent is turned off and on at regular intervals.

(b) Surging-The magnitude is slowly increased or decreased.

(c) Modulation-The magnitude of the wave form is altered.

Q.77. Write common indications and contra-indications alongwith therapeutic effects ?

Ans. Therapeutic effects : During atrophy of a muscle, enzymatic and structural changes occur. Modern muscles stinulation techniques help prevent many of these changes.

Indications :

1. Prepheral nerve lesions involving the musculotendinous unit.
2. Electrical muscle stimulation may help prevent, as well as treat the muscular atrophy which occurs when limb is immobilized.
3. In muclse re-education programmes.
4. In reducing swelling and pain around a join, and for treating localized trigger points and spasm.

Contra-indications :

Doubtful use where premanently interrupted nerve pathway is treated. Also the lesions of more than two years' standing are hardly to derive any benefit.

Q.78. What are the methods of giving this type of treatment?

Ans. Two methods commonly employed are mentioned here.

(i) Unipolar Approach : Here electrodes are of unequal size and used when treating small muscles or trigger points. The active electrode is placed over the motor point of the muscle to the treated, and the dispersive or indifferent electrode is placed at a point distant to the area, being stimulated (usually on the same side under the extremity).

2. Biopolar Method : In this method both the electrodes are of equal size and are used to exercise muscle groups or a large muscle on the same aspect of the body.

Q.79. How do Transcutaneous Electrical Nerve Stimulation affect the human body ?

Ans. Varioud theories are put forward to prove its usefulness.

(a) Gate control theory : This theory of pain was used to explain the effectiveness of its pain control. It has been found that if larger diameter afferent never fibres are electrically stimulated, pain perception decreases, perhaps by the inhibition of pain conduction through a small fibre at the dorsal horn level of the spinal cord.

It is also thought that the activation of inhibitory substantial gelationosis cells will close the gate to transmission of pain sensation.

(b) It is also though that chronic pain may depend upon neuroreverberating circuits and that TENS break these circuits by activating the descending pain inhibiting pathways, thus decreasing the amount of pain experienced.

(c) It has recently become apparent that the endorphins and enkephalines, the pain inhibiting chemicals are released by the body in certain situations. These are found in increased quantities, both during and after TENS treatment, and this also explains the effectiveness of TENS.

Q.80. What is the method of giving the treatment by TENS?

Ans. 1. Operation of the machine (Setting the controls). The current amplitude should be such that the athlete perceives a comfortable sensation, and there should be no muscle twitching or contractions. No discomfort should be experienced by the patient during the treatment session.

placement of electrodes : It needs good knowledge of anatomy, dermatome and trigger points. Generally one electrode is placed near or directly onto the site of discomfort or onto an area served by the peripheral nerve. The second electrode is placed more proximally, either along that dermatome or on a trigger point area.

Improvement may be felt by an athlete within first 5 minutes, usually treatment is continued for 20 minutes. Effect lasts for hours together. If no effect is produced, one should see if electrodes are placed at proper site or not.

Q.81. What is neuroprobe ?

Ans. Based on Acupuncture therapy, best results are usually obtained through a comprehensive programme that includes stimulation of acupuncture points, both local and auricular, as well as appropriate use of other modalities and exercises where indicated.

Q.82. What are infra-red rays ? Explain in brief.

Ans. Infra-red rays are the electromagnetic waves having wave lengths between 4,000000 A -7,700 A unit. The infra red rays are usually emitted from any hot object, i.e., Sun, electric heater etc.

(i) Non-luminous and

(ii) Luminous generators.

The infra-red rays are the invisible rays. Luminous generators also produce the visible rays alongwith the infra-red rays of shorter wavelengths, so they have a greater penetration whereas the non-luminous generators mainly produce the pure infra red rays of the longer wave lengths and so they have a less penetrating effect.

Q.83. What are the indications of infra red rays in the treatment of injuries ?

Ans. Infra red rays work by reducing the muscle spasm, increasing the vascularity of the tissues and by analgesic effect, so these rays can be used in the soft tissue injuries when the initial inflammation subsides.

Q.84. What effects are produced by infra red rays ? Explain how they are produced ?

Ans. Mainly the effects produced by the infra-red rays are :

— relief of pain,

— muscle relaxation,

— increased blood supply,

— elimination of waste products.

Relief of pain :

(a) When heating with I.R.R. is mild, there is a sedative effect on the supeerficial sensory nerve endings.

(b) Strong heating irritates the superficial sensory nerve

endings causing counter irritation to them.

(c) Pain may be due to the accumulation of waste products in the tissues. Ray therise in temperature, there is an increased flow of blood through them and thus removing the waste products.

Muscle relaxation is brought about by the relief of pain and also due to the direct effect of heating rays into the tissues.

Relief of muscle spasm which is generally associated with injury of inflammation.

Greater range of movements can be achieved after heating of the tissues due to the relief of pain.

Increased blood supply :

In superficial wounds and infection, a good blood supply is essential for healing to take place. In infections the increased number of white blood cells and the oxidations of fluid are of assistance in killing the bacteria.

Resolution of inflammation is also sometimes desired with I.R.R. through vaso-dilatation. This will increase the supply of oxygen and food stuffs available to the tissues and accelerate the removal of waste products. This helps to bring about the resolution of inflammation.

Elimination of waste products is accelerated by increased activity of sweat glands from extensive irradiation throughout the body.

Q.85. We have discussed so much of heating devices but what does actually "Electrotherapy" mean ?

Ans. It is the treatment by electricity which is utilised for heating, stinilating the various tissues and structures.

Q.86. Please mention the misuse Electrotherapy ?

Ans. Unqualified and careless operator may create the following problems for a patient :

1. Burns, i.e., heat burns, chemical burns etc.
2. Electric shock.
3. Precipitation of gangrene.
4. Headache.
5. Constipation.
6. Faintness.
7. Chill, and
8. Injuries to the eyes.

Q.87. Please explain each point in detail ?

Ans.

1. Burn : Irradiation can cause superficial heat burn. A red patch can be seen on the skin, which may be converted into a blister. It can be caused due to great intensity of irradiation. Defective skin sensation and impairedblood flow may also result in burms. Usually burn results by touching the lamp by mistake when it is hot.
2. Electric shock can occur due to touching of some exposed part of the electric wire.
3. Precipitation of gangrene : It can be caused by irradiation with rays to an area with defective arterial blood supply.
4. Head-ache : It occurs due to irradiation of the neck area of the head. Also due to lot of sweating, i.e. fluid loss, it is sometimes reported (dehydration in summer).
5. Constipation : This may occur if the water lost by sweating is not replaced by increased fluid intake.
6. Faintness : Extensive irradiation is accompanied by a fall of blood pressure which may result in faintness due to lack of blood supply to the brain. It can also occur if the patient rises suddenly from lying position after an extensive exposure.
7. Chill: There occurs a rise in body temperature nearly 2° F due to extensive irradiation and if the patient goes out immediately after such a treatment.
8. Harmful to the eyes : Exposure of eyes to rays may predispose to cataract.

Q.88. What do you understand by Ultra Violet Rays ?

Ans. These are the electromagnetic waves with wavelengths between 3900A to 136A unit. For treatment purposes, the UVR with wavelengths between 3900-1849 A are only used. The UVR are absorbed in the skin.

1. UVR with wavelength between 2900 A to 1849 A are absorbed in superficial epidermis.
2. UVR Wavelength between 3300 A to 2900 A are absorbed in deep epidermis, and
3. UVR Wavelength between 3900 A to 3300 A are absorbed in the blood of superficial capillary loops of dermis.

Q.89. Explain, how ultra violet rays are produced ?

Ans. When an object is heated to a very high temperature, it produces rays with wavelengths of a type to be perceived by the human eye, including ultraviolet rays. The chief artificial sources of ultraviolet radiations are electric arcs between electrodes of metal end of carbon and mercury in quartz. These rays penetrate tissues to a very limited extent like infra red rays. The human skin allows these rays to penetrate upto two millimetres only. There are many factors associated with ultraviolet (production, transference and recipient) to make the exact prescription and dosage of this radiation.

Q.90. What are the contra-indications for use the of ultraviolet rays ?

Ans. If an athlete is taking drugs like tetracyclines, steroids, tranquilizers, it should not be given as it increases the sensitivity to the rays. Certain diseases like T.B. eczema also contra-indicate therapeutic use of ultraviolet rays. Eyes should be covered or special goggles should be used while receiving treatment. It is also contra-indicated to a person receiving deep X-ray therapy.

Q.91. What are the common uses of ultra violet rays ?

Ans.

1. Indolent wounds and certain skin conditions such as psoriasis, acne, alopecia and some superficial circulatory defects, benefit is derived due to the visitational bringing more blood supply to the skin. More oxygen and food stuffs are the available and the nutrition of the tissues is improved.
2. Destruction of bacteria : It is used in bacterial infections such as boils, infected wounds, adenitis and acne. The increased blood supply increases the number or white blood cells and antibodies in the area. There is exudation of fluid into the tissue from the dilated capillaries. These changes reinforce body's normal defence mechanism for destroying bacteria.
3. Acceleration of healing process : UVR irradiation to damaged cells of epidermis stimulates the growth of new tissues through the liberation of repair hormone.
4. To prevent spread of infection in boils and acne : It is due to the increased blood supply or nutrition to

the skin. There is increased number of W.B.C's and pigmentation.

5. Used in acne frequently affecting the face. In acne, there is thickening of epidermis resulting in the blockage of sebum. Peeling off results by exposure leading to the free drainage of the sebum.
6. Also used in chronic inflammatory lesions and in after effects of trauma. A third degree ultra violet rays irradiation gives counter-irritation to the superficial sensory nerve endings. So relief of pain occurs.

Q.92. What are its misuses ?

Ans. If used by unqualified person or due to carelessness it may reult in the following problems :

1. Conjunctivitis,
2. Vomiting, a high temperature and collapse by overdose (very rare).
3. Electric shock,
4. Burn.

1. Conjunctivitis :

Conjunctivitis is caused following exposure of ultraviolet rays to the eyes. There may be pain or photophobia (inability to expose the eyes tot the light) or Lacrimation (outflow of tears) from both eyes.

2. Overdose :

There may be erythemia with red and painful skin.

3. Electric shock :

It is a painful stimulation of sensory nerves and may be caused by :

(i) If there is some fault in apparatus.

(ii) If the patient touches an exposed part of the circuit.

4. Burn :

Tissue is destroyed and a burn appears as a sport surrounded by reddened area. This may result when the hot part of a lamp is touched.

Care :

(i) It should be kept dry and avoid infection as far as possible.

(ii) Burn be protected with dry sterile gauze.

Q.93. What is Heliotherapy ? Write its important uses.

Ans. It is the irradiation of the body tissues the natural sunlight rays. The effects produced are those of infra-red and ultraviolet rays.

Q.94. Please explain in detail the uses of faradic currents?

Ans. It is an unevenly alternating current. The duration of stimuli is of 0.1-1 millisecond and they are repeated 50-100 times per second.

Uses :

1. To increase the power and bulk of the muscles.
2. To reduce the oedema of tissues.
3. For loosening adhesions.
4. Re-education of muscle action.
5. Exercise for a paralysed muscle.

1. When a muscle contracts as a result of electric stimulation, it leads to increased metabolic rate and the increased demand for oxygen and food-stuffs, which further result in the increased output of waste products. The notabilities cause dilatation of capillaries and arterioles further leading to an increased blood supply of the muscle. As the muscle contracts and relaxes during stimulation, there occurs a pumping action on the lymphatics lying within. Thus there is an increased lymphatic return. If a muscle contracts a sufficient number of times against resistance there occurs an increase in the bulk of the muscle fibres and the muscle is strengthened.
2. To reduce the oedema of the limbs : Here the current is applied to the limb under pressure so that there is an increase in venous and lymphatic drainage. There is need of contraction for many muscles so that they cover the motor points of the main muscle groups. The limb is supported in elevation so that the gravity assists the flow of venous and lymphatics. Elastic crepe bandage is used further to help it.
   The bandage increases the pressure on the blood vessels where the muscle contracts and it recoils on muscle relaxation. The treatment lasts for 20 minutes with frequent rest to avoid fatigue.
3. For loosening adhesions : For this aim, faradism is given under tension. The limb is fixed in fully extended position so that the muscles involved are in a stretched position. The intensity of the current is increased

until a contraction is obtained. The increased tension in the muscles leads to stretch the adhesions.

4. Re-education of muscle's action : When there is a pressure to contract a muscle, i.e., in a flat foot the intrinsic muscles of the foot are not long used due to pain, faradic may be used to produce contractions and so help to restore the sense of movement.
5. Exercises for a paralysed muscle : In neuro-paralysis of a muscle, there occurs loss of voluntary power. By stimulating with faradism below the site of lesion, impulses pass to the muscles causing them to contract, so keep the paralysed muscles in good condition again till the muscles are innervated.

Q.95. What do you understand by exercise therapy to an injured athlete ?

Ans. Exercise therapy is a means of accelerating the individual's recovery from injuries or weakness that have altered the individual's normal way of life.

Q.96. What are the techniques of exercise therapy ? Explain them.

Ans. Basically all exercises or the movements are done either actively or passively.

1. Active movements.

Active movements are those which are performed by the individual according to the choice.

They may be further classified into voluntary and involuntary types.

(I) Voluntary : Voluntary movements are performed by the voluntary action of the muscles opposite to some external force, i.e., force of gravity, resistance etc. Voluntary movements may be further sub-divided into the following :

a. assisted,

b. free,

c. resisted.

(ii) Involuntary : It is the motor response to sensory stimulus, and is not under our conscious control.

2. Passive movements :

Passive movements are performed by the application of some external force during muscular inactivity. They are either.

a. Relaxed : within limit of pain and very gentle movement.
b. Forced : within limit of passive stretching of tight structure, or
c. Manipulation : Forced movement performed by a surgeon when the patient is relaxed under anaesthesia. They are given to break the adhesions.

Q.97. What are the aims of exercise therapy ?

Ans. There are following three aims of exercise therapy :

1. To promote activity whenever and wherever it is possible to minimise effects of inactivity.
2. To correct the inefficiency of specific muscles or muscle groups and regain normal range of joint movement without delay to achieve efficient functional movement.
3. To encourage the individual to use the ability he has regained in the performance of normal functional activities and so accelerates his rehabilitation.

So, briefly summarizing, the maintenance and increase in the muscle power, joint mobility and co-ordination are the important functions of the exercise when done therapeutically.

Q.98. Explain the details traumatic myositrics osification.

Ans. During stage I, or the inflammatory phase of myositis ossification traumatic, the involved extremity should be protected from further injury. Immobilization is usually helpful, and limitation of motion at adjacent joints is usually beneficial. No active exercise should be given to the involved area during this stage. Use of ice and compression to aid in limiting the extent of the hematoma.

During stage II, or the proliferative stage, It is usually helpful to begin quadriceps setting exercises for the thigh, or, in case of myositis ossification traumatica involving the arm, hand grip and upper extremely, "setting" exercises are helpful. Active range of motion exercises are allowed as pain and soreness subside, but no attempt is made to forcibly increase motion.

During stage III, or the repair stage, it is usually possible to begin light resistive exercises through the available range of motion. Joint motion should be monitored daily and if there is a decrease in motion or return of symptoms the exercise must be reduced or completely ommitted. If the response to light resistive exercise is favorable, then gradually progress to the normal progressive resistive exercise routine, as outlined for rehabilitation elsewhere. In patients with myosities ossificans, these exercises must be carefully controlled. Pain in the involved muscle indicates overload. The exercises should be pain free.

Q.99. What do you understand by "Assessment to the individual's condition" ?

Ans. It means the following :

— What does the patient need to do ?

— What can the patient do ?

— What is the patient unable to do ?

Q.100. What is a normal posture ?

Ans. Posture is the attitude assumed by the body to maintain stability. Here we mean the alignment of the head, neck, shoulders, trunk, pelvis and limbs.

Q.101. What do you understand by wind mill ?

Ans.

1. Stand up straight with arms hanging by your sides. Swing your right arm forwards and up and round behind you in circle. Repeat 5 times.
2. Repeat the exercise with the left arm 5 times. If wished, you can then do the exercise again with both arms.

Q.102. Though in brief, you have already mentioned couple of postural defects. For better understanding enlist the common defects and explain them in brief ?

Ans.

1. Lordosis,
2. Kyphosis,
3. Scoliosis,
4. Knock-knee, and
5. Flat-foot.

In the early stage of postural defect, we find some degrees of alteration in the length of soft structures, e.g., muscles and ligaments. It leads to the contraction on one side and stretching to the other side. At this side the treatment can be of great value. In chronic cases the body changes may be there.

Q.103. Explain the various types of shoulder stretch.

Ans. (A) Above the head shoulder stretch-Stand up straight and raise your arms above your head, clasping your hands together. Pull them down behind you and hold for a few seconds. Repeat 5 times.

(B) Shoulder stretch - Reach down your back behind you with one hand and up with the other. Try to bring the two hands together and then pull hard in the opposite direction.

(C) Bent arm shoulder stretch - Bend your right arm back over your head and right shoulder. Hold the elbow with your left hand and then gently pull it towards your left shoulder. Repeat the exercise on the other side.

Q.104. What are the common causes of postural defects ?

Ans. Chronic muscle strain, fibrositis or muscular rheumatism may lead to chronic changes, besides this there may be other causes also.

1. Any form of nervous disturbances or imbalances.
2. Unilateral lung disease.
3. Paresis or paralysis of the muscles and/or their poor development.
4. Shortening of any of lower limbs, and
5. Idiopathic (unknown cause).

Q.105. Does the weakness of certain muscles lead to such defects ?

Ans. Yes, the weakness of the following muscles is responsible for the following postural defects:

1. Toe flexors (brevis and limbricales).
2. Middle and lower trapezius.
3. Upper back erector spinae.
4. Lower back, anterior abdominals.
5. Anterior muscles of neck.

Q.106. Does the position of certain postural defects have some relation with right or left handed subjects ?

Ans. In right handed individuals the following are found weak:

— Right hip abductors,
— Right hip external rotators, and
— Left tibialis posterior.

In left handed individuals the following are found weak.

— Left hip abductors
— Left hip external rotators, and
— Right tibialis posteriors.

Q.107. Write in brief the etiology and pathological changes in kyphosis.

Ans. Causes and incidence :

Common in females or in heavier type of individuals :

1. Habitual poor posture.
2. Nasal obstruction causing a flat chest.
3. Weakness of longitudinal back muscles.
4. Mental or physical fatigue.
5. Rickets.
6. Failure of development of normal curves of spine.

In such type of case, the back is rounded and the chest remains flattened. The shoulders are round and the scapulae are being too forward on the chest wall.

Following pathological changes may also be seen :

1. Pectoralis muscles become shortened leading to kyphosis.
2. Longitudinal backmuscles are over-stretched and weakened especially the rhomboids and middle part of trapezius.
3. The posterior leigments of the vertebral column are lengthened and those on the anterior aspect are shortened.
4. Bones in late stage, i.e. the vertebrae become wedge shaped.

Q.108. Explain in detail, how you will correct kyphosis.

Ans. Health education may be imparted to the people on the following aspects :

1. To correct the deformity and habitual posture, and re-educate the postural sense.
2. To stretch any tightened structure (especially muscle).
3. To strengthen the muscles concerned in postural control so that they can maintain the correct position.

4. To improve respiration-most important in kyphosis and scoliosis conditions.

Q.109. So what can be initial line of treatment ?

Ans. At initial stage, two points are to be kept in mind and practised :

1. Massage : Deep friction will be given to all affected muscles leading to kyphosis.
2. Relaxation : As the muscles are in tension, so it is most important to relax them in lying position. In kyphosis, the tense muscles are pectoralis group. So the patient should be asked to stretch the shoulder as much as possible.

Q.110. Suggest basic exercise for neck stretches.

Ans.
1. Stand up straight and lift your head to look upward.
2. Bring your head slowly forwards until your chin is resting lightly on your chest.
3. Raise your head and turn it slowly to one side. Hold the position for a few seconds.
4. Roll your head round to the other side, keeping your chin down. Hold for a few seconds. Repeat the exercise 5 times to stretch and loosen your neck.

Q.111. How to achieve postural correction and how to stand? Discuss it.

Ans. **(A) Strengthening Exercises :**

1. Arm bending and stretching forward and outward : Start from pelvis, since the position of the pelvis governs the posture. Shoulder girdle must be in alignment with pelvis. The position of the head and neck needs attention by giving movement to cervical spine and not merely to the occipito-atlantic joint. Full size mirrors are proved to be invaluable aids.
2. Lying on the abdomen and head raising causes strengthening of erector spinae muscles.
3. Head backbending will give support to neck muscle.
4. For transverse back musckes, standing arm parting movements.
5. The and nominals be strengthened by abdominal exercises. Hollowing of the lumber spine must be corrected by sleeping on hard bed in supine position for an hour daily.

6. Back raising in knee sitting position.

(B) Balance Exercises :

— Marching with a weight on the head.

— Marching with a stick held behind the head and arms, and

— Balanced walking.

(C) Mobility exercises :

If there is any stiffness of the spine or shoulder, then swinging movements, head and trunk rolling, active side bending and rotation may be practised.

(D) Breathing exercises :

These are needed to stretch the pectorals, expand the chest as much as possible and to increase the range of respiration. Emphasis must be given on inspiratory movements.

(E) Postural treatment by free exercises :

Many physical therapists believe by their long practical experience that the above mentioned free exercises are really good. It is more satisfactory to treat these cases by free exercises rather than resisted exercises. It is also felt that the posture of the body as a whole needs attention, rather than any single muscle group which is of limited value only.

Q.112. Explain the basic points of triceps stretch.

Ans.

1. Stand up straight and raise your right arm with the fingertips resting on the right shoulder.
2. With your left hand, push against the right elbow.
3. Try to lower your fingers down your back as you do so. Hold for a count of 8 and then repeat on the other side.

Q.113. What is the etiology of Flat-foot ?

Ans. It is common in women than in men. The condition is usually bilateral. It is generally painless.

Causes :

1. Paresis of the muscles which support the arches of the foot.
2. Shortening of the tendon-tibialis anterior.
3. Increase in body weight or much standing as in the professionals like nurse, policemen, surgeon, physical education teacher etc.

Q.114. What parhological changes may be observed in flat-footed person ?

Ans. First muscular changes occur followed by ligaments, leading to the displacement of hones.

1. Stretching of the ligaments on the inner side of the foot-the inferiorcalcaneo navicular ligament; the internal lateral ligement of the ankle; the small ligaments and planter fascia on the medial side of the sole-all need attention.
2. Shortening of those on the outer side, i.e., external lateral ligament of the ankle.
3. Stretching in severe cases : Atrophy occurs in tibialis anterior and posterior, the intrincis muscles of foot specially of the interossen group.
4. Spasm : later structural shortening of the peronei from over action of these muscles.
5. Shortening of the achillis tendon with contraction of the calf muscles

Q.115. What are the common signs and symptoms of flat-foot ?

Ans. Following complaints can be made by the patient :-

1. Sensation of weakness and strain on the inner side of the foot.
2. In severe cases, pain is a prominent symptom.
3. Mobility-inversion is limited. Extension and flexion at the ankle may also be incomplete. The movements of the toes are often limited.
4. Loss of spring effect in walking. The gait is awkward and unmerciful. The patient brings down the heels heavily and walks with the feet turned out.
5. Circulatory symptoms such as coldness or increased perspiration of the feet may also be present.

Q.116. What is isometric ankle wrestling.

Ans. Sit and place one ankle over the other (half way through, switch ankles). Exert an out ward force with both ankles that your feet are firmly pressing against each other. Hold for 10 seconds release, and repeat 10 times.

As your ankles become stronger and less painful or stiff allow them to move in and out against each other as you exert the outward force. Make each full movement last 10 full seconds. Repeat 10 times.

Q.117. What are the basic principles to be kept in mind during treatment ?

Ans. The following five principles need to be given attention :-

1. To restore the arches as far as possible.
2. To strengthen the muscles concerned.
3. To re-educate the patient in their correct use.
4. To re-educate the patient in walking.
5. To mobilize the joints of foot, if necessary.

Q.118. How will electric modality, if used, help such cases ?

Ans. Faradic foot baths is an important aspect of the treatment in flat foot cases. It is given not only to strengthen the muscles but also to regain the feeling of movements. The foot is stimulated longitudinally and transversely. Specific stimulation may be given to lumbricales and interossei. The posterior tibialis muscle and tibialis anterior may also be stimulated.

Q.119. What type of exercises will help in the treatment of such cases ?

Ans. The following exercises may be given in sitting and standing position :-

1. Heel raising and lowering either with both feet together or alternatively.
2. Sitting with feet crossed, resting on outer borders.
3. Drawing the sole of one foot up the shin of the opposite leg. Foot must be kept dorsi-flexed.
4. Legs crossed over knee. The flexion and extension-this may also be done with the feet in dorsi-flexion, the heels resting on the ground.
5. Pick up objects with toes, e.g.,towel or marble pieces.
6. Sitting toe separating.
7. Abduction of the toes, if possible.
8. Pressing the toes on the ground, the metatarsal heads not being raised. This is an exercise useful to lumbricales muscles. Patient tries to shorten the foot, keeping the toes pressed down throughout the movement.
9. Walking on the inclined board.
10. Standing on the edge of plinth, toes over the edge. Flexion and extension of the toes of both feet.

Q.120. What type of foot-wear should be used in flat foot condition ? Also mention if massage plays any role in this condition.

Ans. A leather shoe with a crooked and elongated heel, i.e., about quarter of an inch thickness pad along the inner side of the shoe provides the best footwear. If the foot is painful, then massage may be given to improve blood circulation and removing fatigue products or inflammatory exudates from the muscles.

1. Effleurange should be given to the whole leg to promote drainage-the leg should be well supported over pillows and foot end kept elevated.
2. Finger kneading and effleurage be given to the dorsum of the foot and malleolar region.
3. Effleurage, stroking, kneading and friction may also be applied to the sole if patient can tolerate these.
4. Wax baths, hot soaking and contrast bath may sometimes also help to relieve pain.

Q.121. Classify the manipulations used in massage ?

Ans. The manipulations are mainly classified into four types :-

1. Stroking manipulations,
2. Pressure manipulations,
3. Percussion manipulations,
4. Shaking manipulations.

Q.122. Explain what Massage is ?

Ans. Massage is a scientific art and manipulation. This is one of the oldest techniques used for heating different parts of body. Hypocrites, the father of Medicine used to manipulate his patients for treatment.

Q.123. What are the effects of massage ?

Ans. The massage, in general, may include the following effects:-

1. It shortens the period of recovery.
2. This also leads to local and general relaxation, through its effects on the superficial sensory nerve endings.
3. It causes venous and lymphatic return by alternate pressure and relaxation and thus improves the muscles circulation. The notabilities are removed from the part relieving the pain.

4. By stretching and softening effect on fibrous and subcutaneous tissues, adhesions are prevented and broken if already existed.
5. Massage does have psychological effect. The patient feel being given an individual attention which may be of value in relieving the symptoms associated with mental tension.

Q.124. Describe in brief the "Effleurage Manipulation" ?

Ans. It is a stroking manipulation which is always performed from the distil to the proximal part of limbs and should end at the nearest lymphatic glands. The distal end should always be kept elevated. All the aspects of the limb must be treated by the physiotherapist. Both the hands may be used together or the right and the left hand alternately. The pressure of the upward stroke must be firmly applied and the downward stroke must be very light, just to maintain the continuity of the mainpulation.

Q.125. What are the effects and uses of effleurage ?

Ans. (a) It exerts a mechanical pressure on the soft walled veins, pressing the blood towards the heart. In this way, venous congestion is removed and it is used in the early stages of sprains and dislocations.

(b) It also increases the circulation of the skin and thus improves its nutrition. The skin becomes soft and supple and the tone of the skin is improved.

(c) It mechanically exerts pressure on the lymph moving it towards the lymphatic glands. So it reduces oedema through reduction of lymph stasis. It is used in cases of swollen limbs due to lymphg stasis.

Q.126. What are its contra-indications ?

Ans. The effleurage should not be given in the following conditions :-

1. Gross oedema : When there is danger of breaking of stretched skin.
2. Early infantile paralysis : Where the weak muscles might be unduly stretched.
3. Varicose veins and severe thrombo phlebitis.

Q.127. Explain "Stroking" ?

Ans. This is also a superficial manipulation. For stroking to be effective to a patient first support and hold the limbs as in effleurage. After this stroke can be followed in any direction. The movement can be performed briskly to stimulate a part or, slowly to obtain sedative effect. Fingers and thumbs can be used for stroking small areas such as the face, the palm of the hands, the dorsum of the foot.

Q.128. What are the effects and uses of "stroking" ?

Ans.
1. The main effect of stroking is one on the peripheral nervous system. It is given firmly on the back with finger tips to stimulate the peripheral nervous system. Generally it is used in the cases of debility and depression.
2. It may be done briskly and rhythmically with a perfectly relaxed hand on the region of the stomach to stimulate the organ.
3. Same techniques performed over small intestine and colon region, reduce intestinal stasis.
4. When it is done briskly down the length of limb with the finger tips, it causes a stimulation of the peripheral nervous system and is valuable in the treatment of anaemia and debility.
5. Brisk stroking of the scalp through hair stimulates its glandular activity, producing more sebum and thus promotes better growth of hair. It is used in case of falling hair.

Q.129. What advantages can be had by using slow deep stroking method ?

Ans. It has proved useful in the following conditions :-
1. When it is done on back from accept to sacrum by one hand following other, it produces a feeling of relaxation. It may be used in Hypertension cases.
2. In limbs, it helps to produce relaxation and, is used in recent injuries when the muscles are in protective spasm.
3. When applied to the thumb or finger tips, over the eyebrows pain is reduced in cases of frontal headache.
4. It is also used in reducing tension associated with upper motor neurone lesions.

Q.130. Classify the Pressure Manipulation ?

Ans. Pressure manipulation is divided into three types :-

a. Kneading,

b. Petrissage and

c. Frictions.

Kneading type of pressure manipulation may further be sub-divided into the following :-

(i) Squeezing,

(ii) Stationary,

(iii) Circular, and

(iv) Ironing.

Q.131. Describe in brief the Squeezing kneading ?

Ans. The muscles are gently squeezed, lifted and released in a rhytmic manner. In treading the larger surface, one or both hands are used.

Effects and uses : This promotes the blood circulation which is sufficient to maintain the nutrition of the muscles and prevents their disuse atrophy :

1. It is used in lower Motor Neuron Lesions.
2. It is used for recent injuries where there is pain and muscle spasm persisting.
3. It is used in the cases of gross oedema of the limb.
4. This may also be used in the cases of flatulence and destinations by the experiences of operators only.

Q.132. Explain Stationary Kneading ?

Ans. In this type of massage, the muscles are pressed against the underlying bone. It is performed with fingers of thumb on small areas such as face, palm of the hands and sole of the foot.

Q.133. Write in brief about "Circular Kneading" ?

Ans. Circular kneading is performed with one or both hands working alternately. In this manipulation, the whole length of the limb must be covered. The soft tissues are pressed against, the underlying bone in a circular manner. The soft surface of palm of hand and fingers must be used. Care must be taken to avoid bony prominences. Pressure should be deep and the muscles should be moved on the bone.

Q.134. What are its effects and uses ?

Ans. They can be mentioned in the following points :-

1. It promotes better blood supply to the muscles thus increasing their nutrition. It is commonly used in the cases of muscular weakness.
2. In cases of twitching or cramp in the muscles, it is done slowly along the length of the limb to get a sedative effect.
3. By giving brisk light kneading on the back, a general stimulation of the muscles can be produced.
4. Kneading is frequently used on the abdomen. It produces a more active flow of blood to the organs and the cells, further stimulating their activity and thus the digestion and the absorption are promoted.
5. By kneading of the limbs, the circulation and nutrition of the bone is also improved by pressure against the bone, the blood supply of the periosteum is stimulated from which the bone receives its nourishment.
6. Abdominal kneading may be used in cases of chronic constipation, squeezing and kneading are done with hands. Deep pressure is exerted on the organs followed by relaxation. The portal circulation is accelerated and there is better supply of bile which acts as a natural purgative and stimulates peristalsis.

This method should not be used in the following conditions:

1. In hypotenuse cases,
2. Very hairy surfaces,
3. In severe abdominal distension,
4. In early stages of recent injuries.

Q.135. What is "Ironing Kneading"?

Ans. This form of kneading is performed chieflyon the back and gluiteal muscles. In this, one hand re-inforces the pressure of the other hand, and the body weight may also be used to get the maximum depth to move the thick structures on the underlying bone.

Q.136. What are its benefits ?

Ans. Its use has advantages in following conditions :

1. This is used largely in cases of chronic lumbago : Low back-ache, and sacroiliac strains.
2. It produces heat and helps in relieving the waste

products from the muscles and therefore making them more mobile.

Q.137. What is percussion manipulation ?

Ans. This type of manipulation is further divided into four forms. :

1. Hacking,
2. Clapping,
3. Beating, and
4. Pounding.

All percussion movements have a penetrating effect and stimulate deep seated structures.

Q.138. Describe the "Hacking" in brief, with its effects and uses.

Ans. Hacking : To perform this movement the arms are adducted, elbows flexed with extended wrists. The movement consists of promotion and supination of the forearm. In this the ulnar border of the little finger supplemented with other fingers strike the part. The little finger is the first to strike the part and divergent, convergent and longitudinal movements are made.

In patients with habituated constipation, smooth hacking on the abdomen increase peristalists.

Most commonly used over the back after long immobilisation.

It also stimulates the spinal nerves when given highly and briskly down the spine from occiput to the sacrum and helps in depression, debility, and anaemic conditions. This can also be used to tone up the muscular and vascular systems and so produces a feeling of well being.

Q.139. Describe in brief the clapping manipulation ?

Ans. It is a movement of alternate flexion and extension of the wrist joints in which the hand should be completely relaxed. The fingers remain lightly in contact with the skin and the wrists are alternately raised and lowered alongwith small range elbow movements. In this, the fingers should be adducted and the palm cupped. This can be used over the back limbs and chest.

Effects and uses :

Applied chiefly for the skin and the contents of the thorax.

When it is applied on thorax it causes gentle shaking which leads to

(a) Increase in activity of the cells of the lung tissue and bronchi, increasing their resistance powers.

(b) There is more active circulation throughout the lungs, leading to increased interchange of gases in the lung capillaries.

(c) Mucus is loosened and expectoration gently facilitated. It is used much in cases of chronic lung diseases especially in bronchitis and bronchiectasis.

Q.140. What is "Beating" ?

Ans. It is a heavy movement usually performed with right hand. This is quite similar to clapping, but is performed with a loosely clenched hand. The dorsal aspect of the fingers and the base of the hand come in contact with the part treated, arms lifted-up and falling heavily to produce the manipulation. This produces definite shaking of liver cells and so secretions are stimulated and more supply of bile occurs. It is used in cases of sluggish. Liver and chronic constipation patients.

Q.141. What is "Pounding" ?

Ans. It is a heavy form of percussion. It is quite similar to hacking and is performed with a loosely clenched fixed hand striking the part with the ulnar border of the hand. Few therapists perform it keeping the fingers over the part to be treated, and heels of the hands are heavily raised and lowered. This is also used on liver for chronic constipation and sluggish functions.

Q.142. Describe the types of shaking manipulations and their uses.

Ans. Shaking manipulations are divided into two types :-

1. Vibration, and
2. Shaking.

1. **Vibration :** There are fine forms of tremors conveyed through hands or finger tips. They may be performed with one hand or both as required. They may be used to treat the joints, stomach or any abdominal organ. The movement is one of very fair tremble shaking of the tissues by the slightest possible flexion

and extension of the wrist joints or with the fingers from carpophlangeal joints.

2. **Shaking :** This is a movement of coarse, rhythmic vibrations perormed with all perfectly relaxed hand. This is performed by holding the part with one or both hands moving it from side to side, up and down or in and out. They may be performed on small intestine, colon, stomach or limbs.

CHAPTER SIX
HYGIENE & ATHLETE

Q.1. What do you understand by the word 'Hygiene' ?

Ans. Hygiene concerns with the mode of living that is adopted by an individual to adjust himself with his environment and vice versa, in order to preserve and promote the health of body and mind.

Q.2. What is Personal Hygiene ?

Ans. Personal Hygiene deals with routine activities of body care and maintenance, and the mental attitude forwards the healthy habits with the aim of achieving the higher status of health. This is one's own responsibility and so, it is personal.

Q.3. Explain Environmental Hygiene.

Ans. Environmental hygiene is the alteration and adjustment of environment according to our needs in order to promote and maintain the health. But, the environment is not constructed by any one individual. It is created by nature and affected by the activities of group of individuals and the whole community. Therefore, it is the responsibility of the groups, who have to play their roles at different levels for the promotion and maintenance of favourable atmosphere.

Mode of living is governed by the habits which are learnt and developed by the practice and then becomes a part of life and character.

Q.4. Mention the general aspects of Hygiene for an athlete.

Ans. They can be divided into the following groups :

(i) Good and bad habits of eating and drinking etc. :
 Balanced diet
 Alcohol
 Smoking
 Costly and cheaper foods.

(ii) proper maintenance of posture as
 Role of fatigue
 Optimum exercise

Need of sleep and rest
Need to control the weight.

(iii) Care of body parts, bath and cleanliness :
Hair
Mouth and teeth
Eyes and ears
Skin
Hands
Feet
External genitals

(iv) Miscellaneous :
Clothing
Mental hygiene
Sex education.

Q.5. What are the basic principles which a player should observe while eating and drinking ?

Ans. One should form regular habits of eating and drinking. Only wholesome food should be taken for the preservation of health and also for better health. Meals should be taken after sufficient intervals and at fixed hours. The quantity and quality should be compatible with one's type of work. Eating should be avoided when too much fatigued. It is a bad babit to overload the stomach. Water should be sparingly taken alongwith meals, but should be taken freely between principal meals. Too much of water during meals will dilute the effect of digestive juices.

Q.6. How does alcohol affect the human body ?

Ans. It is a food and a narcotic, but its food value is very limited. It can replace an equivalent amount of carbohydrates or fats and economise proteins. But it can definitely be neither stored in the body, nor utilized for repair. Although on certain occasions, if used in small doses, it may aid digestion or induce sleep to some extent. It has a devitalizing action upon the tissues. The feeling of exhilaration that follows after taking a mild dose of alcohol is due to depression of higher nerve centres that normally provide inhibition. Symptoms of delirium, trembling and mental distress are thought to be due to vitamin starvation and the toxic affects of alcohol, especially when consumed in large amounts for longer periods. This is because of damage to the brain cells which do not have power to regenerate.

Q.7. Mention the effects of alcohol on various systems.

Ans. It effects the following systems :

— It acts as a narcotic on the central nervous system.

— Heart rate is increased.

— Cutaneous Blood Vessels are dilated leading to loss of heat.

Drunkards are found dead on roadside in extreme cold weather. It is due to loss of heat in drunkards.

— The functions of special sense-organs like eyes and ears are impaired. A drunkard may talk and give reply to questions but he forgets what has been just talked.

— Very large amount of alcohol brings about paralysis of respiratory centres.

— In the case of digestive process, peristaltic action may be lessened and flow of saliva and also the gastric juice is increased with the difference that this is lower in pepsin contents but higher in hydrochloric acid contents than normal-a change liable to be harmful to persons suffering from peptic ulcer.

— One general effect of excessive intake of alcohol is that normal restraint in conduct may be lost involving the risk of promiscuity, and of contracting such diseases as gonorrhoea, syphilis or AIDS.

— There is a lowered resistance to respiratory and septic infections and shortening of normal expectation of life.

Q.8. Why is the knowledge of Hygiene necessary for sportsmen ?

Ans. Sportsmen are also human beings and in no way can escape the requirements of general hygiene, rather it is more important for the them. It should be understood that no one is a sportsman since birth. Most of the sports are learnt after certain period of life in schools and colleges and till that time the habits affecting health have already been established. Some adopt sports as professionals and others take it casually just for the maintenance of the fitness. Like other occupations, sports has also its own problems and hazards. The professions have to adjust their way of life in their fields through the development of proper health habits. There are various health problems arising due to careless attitude and lack of knowledge about hygiene in the field of sports also. As far as communicable diseases are concerned sportsmen are more exposed to them because when they go from place to place for competitions, their routine about food, rest and sleep is affected. In India, during most of ordinary tournaments, the rooms and places which they get for accommodation are not according to the requirements; the food they get during their journey may not be hygienic. They also have to face the lack of washing and bathing facilities. All these aspects have detrimental effect on their health.

I don't say that India sportsmen are always at disadvantage if they themselves are not particular about their own health. Only at the national and international level sports competitions, they get favourable sanitary lodging and boarding, particularly when the competitions are held in a very big way like Common-wealth games, Asian or Olympics etc.

Q.9. What do you understand by 'Hygiene for sportsmen' ?

Ans. Hygiene for sportsmen may be considered under the following headings :

— Hygiene in daily life, i.e., general aspects of hygiene.
— Hygiene while playing.
— Hygiene in competition.
— Hygiene in travel.

Certain common points to be remembered for hygiene during and after playing:

— Water may be sprayed over the ground to avoid unnecessary dust.
— Nails should be cut properly to avoid injury in contact games.
— The dress and socks should not be used for more than one session without washing. All the dress material should be preferably cotton especially in hot humid climate (Bombay, Calcutta, Kerala, Madras etc.)

— Special care should be taken about the dressing of genital organs. Tight synthetic undergarments favour the collection of sweat and cause injury to the skin by friction. It will be difficult to control fungal infections in such cases.

— Shoes should be given time to dry up after each session of playing. It is advisable to have at least two pairs of sports shoes. Avoid shoes with plastic lining and too much of other synthetic materials.

— One should take bath invariably after playing exhausting games but keeping in mind that temperature of water should not be very low than that of body temperature. Warm water bath gives relaxation after exhaustive work-outs. Common towels should never be used.

— Individual slippers may be used for common bath rooms to avoid spread of skin infection to the feet.

— Don't use dirty hands for drinking water directly from the tap. Water container and some tumblers should be kept by the side of play ground.

— One should not play if one feels tired or one's resting pulse rate is higher than the normal rate.

Q.10. Explain the term 'Hygiene of Competition'.

Ans. Following points may be kept in mind :

— Avoid excitement.

— Proper amount of water and electrolyte should be used to replace sweating.

— Do not play with full stomach, i.e. immediately after meals.

— Do not play in conditions of fever and injuries.

Full protective devices should be used according to the requirement of game.

Q.11. Harpies among athletes writes its management ?

Ans. Soap and water cleansing or use of germicidal agents.

Topical drying agents for viral blisters,

Benzoyl peroxide 5-10%

Tincture of benzin

Camphor agent (champho-phenique)

Zinc solution, 4%

Antiviral agents for early lesions.

Q.12. What points of Hygiene should be kept in mind while travelling ?

Ans. One must observe the following points :

- It is essential to take care about hygiene of food, water and general clealiness during journey.
- Loose eating from unregistered shops should be avoided.
- One should have one's own arrangement of drinking water.
- One should make a point to avoid unnecessary tiredness during journey. (Do not travel when reservation of berth is not there.)

It is a well accepted fact that the changing of old practice is more difficult than to develop new ones. Some basic scientific knowledge, motivation and proper guidance is essential to achieve voluntary participation for the development of favourable habits. Some common problems faced by sportsmen due to unhygienic habits are :

- The problems of indigestion and constipation,
- Skin diseases of various types,
- Over anxiety or awakening problems, and
- Drugs abuse etc.

Q.13. Give brief management of acne and pimples in young athlete ?

Ans. Astringent lotion.

Benzoyl peroxide 5-10% applied twice daily to inflammatory lesions.

Topical Retain-A Gal or cream applied to black head acne at bedtive.

Parenteral Antibiotics:

Tetracycline 500 mg. twice a day for 6 weeks, then 500 mg/day taken on empty stomach. or

Erythromycin 500 mg twice a day for 6 weeks, then 500 mg/day

Topical antibiotic lotions or creams twice a day.

Elindae a is also quite effective as reported.

Q.14. What do you understand by 'Hygiene : Health and Sports' ?

Ans. Hygiene is that branch of medicine which aims at

maintaining the state of health. To attain this goal, two courses should be followed. The first consists of avoiding and applying all those rules which tend to increase the robustness of the organism in such a way as to render it more resistant to the action of harmful external factors. The second consists of studying and neutralising the exigences morbid factors of all kinds (physical, chemical, biological etc.) which may have a negative action on the state of health.

Within the framework of Sports medicine, Hygiene concerns all measures liable to safeguard the health of the athlete in the environment in which he carries out his activity and fights against easily diffused illness and harmful agents; lastly, attention is also paid to the rules of living such as sexual activity, pleasure seeking habits, etc.

Q.15. What do you understand by personal hygiene of sportsmen ?

Ans. Hygiene of a person is essential in order to avoid contagious diseases especially of the parasitic type. It should be borne in mind that the fact of living as a group vastly facilitates the transmission of such illnesses, and that accordingly the rules of personal hygiene should be much more sever than in the case of an individual. It has already been stressed as to how essential it is to avoid any promiscuity of clothing. It is advisable that every sportsman be educated in this that he should take utmost care regarding personal washing, taking repeated baths preferably showers, and using disinfecatants and soaps. Steps should be taken to isolate those athletes who may be bearers of parasites of the skin and its annexes (hair of the head and pubis) until such time a suitable cure has been effected.

Infestation by lice (Pediculus louse)causes a reaction of the skin, which becomes red and highly irritable. On the infested Zone, the typical small parasites (about 1-2 mm long) grey-brown in colour, together with their eggs laid at the base of the hair of the head or the pubis may be noted. The cure for this condition consists in shaving the hair and in using anti-parasitic powders having a basis of mercury derivatives and DDT. Prophylaxis is necessary in the utmost personal hygiene especially in groups. by avoiding the possiblity for contagions.

Q.16. How you will manage fungal infections among athelete.

Ans. Dry lesions.

— Soap and water cleansing
— Topical keratolytic agents (acene soap)
— Topical antifungal agents applied twice a day for atleast 1 month (eg-Tinactin, 2% Micatin,)
— Wet Lesions
— Soap and water cleansing
— Wet dressing (Domeboro Solution)
— Topical antifungal agents,
— Phonetics dyes or antifungal creams or lotions.

Q.17. Mention the point for avoiding contact dermatitics ?

Ans. — Avoiddance of contactant.
— Acute wet dressings twice or thrice a day.
— Topical corticosteriod lotions, gels or creams.
— Chronic topical conticosteroid ointment or cream.

Q.18. Can you explain the role of coffee or tea on the health of sportsmen ?

Ans. It may be allowed in small quantities, that is to say, two to three cups per day on an average. In fact, it has a tonic action on the organism; but if abused especially in hypersensitive subjects, it may cause psychic hyper-excitability and hyper-sensitivity of the cardio-circulatory and digestive systems. Though, rarely these drinks may also cause appearance of intermittent extra systole, palpitations of the heart, gastric hyperacidity, etc..

Q.19. Is smoking a bad hygienic practice ?

Ans. Smoking should be extremely forbidden. In fact, it is the opinion of all experts competent in this field that smoking harms the organisms through various mechanisms, both on account of the substances it contains (nicotine and its derivatives) and its physical state (smoke, carbonmonixide or dispersion in the air of carbonoised corpuscles).

Q.20. Mention in brief the role of sex among players.

Ans. It is well to clarify the repercussions which may be produced by natural sexual activity and by spontaneous nocturnal emission. The former, provided it takes place without artifices, excesses, or psychic commitment in periods of not excessive athletic and physical commitment at sufficient intervals, does not raise any problems of antagonism on the energetic plane.

In this connection, we would like to undramatic the erotic attention raised in certain individuals precisely as a result of the obligation to respect an abstinence which, in such cases, in shown to be more harmful than useful.

It should, however, be considered that, without attaching excessive importance to the problem, sports activity itself tends to unfocus the athletes' attention on sexual activity.

It is necessary to explain that nocturnal emission is a purely mechanical and natural phenomenon which has no negative effect on the physical state of the subject or on his athletic performance. Always remember, that a complex of culpability is not created in the athlete on account of such phenomenon, which would have the effect of convincing him of having been the victim of an impairment of his athletic capabilities.

In this case, a negative effect is obtained which has consequent depressing effect on the youngman's moral aspect and athletic performance.

By respecting such general hygienic advice, and above all by avoiding the excesses either of abstinence or of a sexual hyperactivity, the problem of sexual hygiene in athletes may be considered as solved. In addition, the chances of getting contagious diseases should not be underestimated.

Q.21. Why is there an urgent neet of 'Tetanus Immunization'?

Ans. In Indian conditions every player in the field or during contact sports is likely to get injury on skin or wound contaminated with horse manure or cowdung. Since ground is polluted with the above mentioned articles which are potential sources of tetanus infection, It is suggested to have immunization against tetanus.

Q.22. Mention the Immunization schedule of 'Tetanus Toxoid'.

Ans. Injections may be taken in the following order :
1st dose : Injection of Tetanus Toxiod 0.5ml I/M
2nd dose : Repeat it after 6 weeks.
3rd dose : Have the booster dose after 6 months.
The immunity effect lasts for 10 years.

Q.23. How to handle the blisters ?

Ans. They are the result of unaccustomed training alongwith use of new rigid equipment. They are produced due to skin stresses. Management of small blisters is possible by a small felt pad or adhesive dressing, but larger blister may be punctured by sterile needle and then dressed . Surgical spirit or mercurochrome can be used to dry up weeping surfaces and harden skin.

Boots, shoes, rackets etc. should be checked for friction areas, often minor ridges in the soles may lead to blistering. These faults can be rectified with soft padding.

Q.24. How can you manage the condition of ingrowing of toe nails?

Ans. Daily inspection is to be carried out and the demonstration is to be made, how to cut toe nails and the details must be explained how the smallest of sharp points from an incorrectly cut nails could lead to eventual infection. Toe nail should always be cut horizontally and not allowed to become jagged.

Treatment : Ingrowing toe nails can be treated by padding between the toes (such as cotton wool) to separate the great and second toe when the lesion is on the opposing surface. Antibiotics do not help and once a granuloma has developed it require excision either by trimming of the nail or partial or complete nail ovulation.

Q.25. What is the most common skin infection of Indian players ?

Ans. Players are prone to fungal infections between the toes (athlete's foot) and in the groin. These infections are transmitted in communal baths, and therefore showers, if available, should be preferred. Our athletes have the habit of exchanging under clothes and towels. These are the root causes which lead to the transmission of the disease.

Antifungal cream containing undecylenic acid, miconazole and clotrimazole are usually used. Sometimes the long term administration of grisofulvin in needed. In resistance cases gention violet may prove better.

To eliminate infection from a sports arena, strict attention to personal hygiene, showers and the regular washing of equipment (stocking, shorts etc.) must be observed.

Q.26. Can common cold prove harmful for an athlete ?

Ans. The common cold impairs efficiency in that the congestion of the nasopharangeal mucosa restricts the hyperventilation of effort. By virute of increased ventilation, the risk of incurring a descending infection of the respiratory tract is increased and bronchitis may occur. While in most instances an athlete is able to compete when he has a cold, his performance may fall short of his best. Nasal discongestants are often useful. Swimmers, however, should be advised against taking part unless the event is of vital importance. During somersault turns in water may wash, infected material from the nose to the nasopharynx into the accessory nasal sinuses or via the Eustachian tubes into the middle ears. The same thing may also happen with divers who in their routine include 'feet first' entries, the body entering in water with high velocity.

Q.27. What is otitis media and otitis externa ?

Ans. Otitis Media (push in ear) does not offer the same danger of complications due to use of antibiotics. Pain is the initial symptom accompanied by malaise and fever. Antibiotics-local and general, after cleaning the ear with analgesics, if pain is severe, should be give. The infection may settle without perforation of ear drum.

When perforation occurs, after cleaning, ten volumes hydrogen peroxide on wool swab sticks, or syringing gently with boric acid may be effective. The question may be asked about future swimming and diving. According to Philip Garson even if the drum is perforated, swimming may be allowed provided the infection is cleared, pus is absent and cotton plug is used to avoid entrance of water in the ear.

Some swimmers use nose clips in order to prevent sinusitis

and middle ear infections. These certainly do appear to prevent nasal catarrh. Most swimmers exhale through the nose when pushing off under water on their backs. This action prevents the entry of water through nose.

Otitis Externa can be very painful, it may be acute and associated with pyrexia, deafness, and oedema over the mastoid process. Antibiotic alongwith local application of glycerine and ichthyal on gauze may be effective.

Q.28. Explain health education steps in relation to the gastro-entritis.

Ans. It is a very common problem especially with foreign competitors. Even in its mild form, it affects the performance of players to a great extent. Following points should always be kept in mind :

(a) Adequate Health Education : Orientation of all team members, coaches, trainers and officials as to possible causes and effects of traveller's diarrhoea. An outline of preventive measures should be given to these people whenever they accompany them.

(b) Personal hygiene of especially washing and personal toilet.

(c) Use of bottled water for everything except bathing.

(d) Dietary restrictions : No food is to be consumed except at dining table (specific dining halls).

(e) Supervision of food services : Including preparations, serving and dishwashing by medical doctor.

(f) Avoidance of excessive fatigue : Especially on arrival at competitive site.

(g) Isolation of active infected cases and carriers.

One must always remember the following sings and symptoms of the disease :

(a) Mild : Simple diarrhoea without Abdominal cramps; Nausea; vomiting and fever which leads to impairment of capacity to train or compete.

(b) Severs : Diarrhoea with one or more of the following: Adbominalcramps; Nausea; Vomiting; Fever; significant impairment of capacity to train or compete.

Q.29. Describe in brief the pediculosis pubis.

Ans. Pediculosis pubis is caused by the crab. Infestation by this parasite has risen sharply in the population as a whole. Typically, it invades only the pubic hair, but it may involve the eyelashes, beard, moustache, and axillary hair. P.Pubis is not present in the hair. Pubic lice are usually transmitted by sexual contact. There is pruritis and the movement of the louse can be felt. Treatment consists of application of lindane (Kwell) or gamma benzene hydrochloride to all areas after a soap and water bath and thorough drying. In hairy individuals, this application should include the thighs, trunk, as well as axillae and pubic areas. When a shampoo product is used it is removed after 10 minutes: a lotion production is washed off after 12 hours. Clothing and bedding used before treatment should be disinfected by machine.

Q.30. Among adoloscent athletes 'Acne Vulgaris' is a big nuisance. Suggest treatment for it ?

Ans. Face should not be rubbed after sweating because it makes the problem more complicated.

— Astringent lotions should be used.
— Benzoyl peroxide 5-10% be applied twice daily to inflammatory lesions.
— Topical Retin-A gel or cream be applied to blackhead once a bet time.
— Parenteral antibiotics : Tetracycline 500 mg-thrice a day x one week, Erythromycin 250 mg-four times a day x two weeks
— Topical antibiotic lotions or creams twice a day.
— Ultraviolet rays exposure proved to be beneficial (While exposing care of eyes should be taken).
— Certain vitamin like A-D capsule may give some relief though it may have psychological effect only.

Q.31. Mention in brief the treatment of impetigo.

Ans. Alongwith consultation of doctor the following treatment may be taken :

- Soap and water cleaning.
- Erythromycin 250 mg four times a day for a week or more.
- Topical microbial or antibiotic application.

Q.32. When athlete suffers from 'Herpes Simplex' - a viral infection, can we help him ?

Ans. Athlete can be helped by the following :

— Soap and water cleaning or use of germicidal agents.
— Topical drying agents for viral blisters :
 * Benzoyl peroxide 5-10%
 * Tincture of benzoin
 * Camphor agent
 * Zinc solution 4%
 * Anti-viral agents for early lesions; if available.

Heavy exercise of involved area should be avoided. Athlete should be prohibited to take part in contact and competitive sports.

Q.33. Write the treatment for Warts and Molluscum contagiosum ?

Ans. The treatment mentioned below has been found to be effective:

40% salicylic acid daily for 3-4 months.

— Topical Retin-A cream or gel twice a day for 4 months.

— Topical destructive agents; Caustic acids, Cryotherapy, Electrodesiccation.

Q.34. Fungal infections are very common (especially on athlete's foot) among players. What should they do to avoid these infections ?

Ans. (A) Treatment for dry lesions : Soap and water cleaning.
— Topical keratolytic agents (soap if available).
— Topical antifungal agents, applied twice a day at least for one month.

(B) Treatment for wet lesions : Soap and water cleaning.
— Wet dressing.
— Topical anti-fungal agents.
— Phenolic dyes or anti-fungal creams or lotions.

Three weeks of Griseofulvin proves to be effective for cure.

NOTE: The skin diseases observed in athletes are common dermatological problems related specifically to the individual skin type hereditary factors, age, sex, environment and the sports activity. Anticipation, early recognition, and treatment of these skin diseases usually permit the athlete to continue participation without disability or reduced performance.

Q.35. Why are Blisters of foot developed and how will you managed them ?

Ans. The problems encountered by bare foot runners or with improve soles or with spikes, even wearing of socks with wrinkles can cause this painful condition which pathologically is due to any source of chronic friction and leads to a formation of fluid between the layers of the skin, that is epidermis and dermis, initially called 'Hot Sports'. It can be prevented by wearing properly cushioned shoes and putting extra cushions or felt pads at the sports which are tender. The application of vaseline on feet and hot fomentations after every session can prevent this condition.

Blisters formed should be treated immediately by pricking them with sterilized needle to prevent super added infection and applying antiseptic bandage.

Q.36. Describe the problem of Corns and Collosities among athletes.

Ans. Another condition commonly seen in distance runners due to constant running with ill-cushioned shoes or congenital deformities of the feet. Collosities are thickening of superficial layers of skin while corn is thickening of all layers of skin Common sites are the head of first metatarsal and the side of fifth metatarsal. On the dorsum surface of the feet at the phalanges of the 2nd, 3rd and 4th toe, and the heel. Neglected collosities can turn into thickening of tendons and bones, this is sesomoditis.

Collosities can be prevented by good lubrication and massage of feet making the skin supple and elastic. The shoe should be comfortable and well-snug. Excess of callus can be removed with a file or sand paper, while application of petroleum jelly will keep the callus soft and maintain elasticity of the skin.

On the other hand, corns are painful, tender and harder than collosities Corns can be softened by application of salicyclic acid and keeping felt pads. Corns are deep-rooted, and even after surgical excision, there are fair chances of recurrence.

Q.37. How to manage Athlete's Foot (Tenia Pedis) ?

Ans. Fungus infection is like an epidemic amongst athletes and goodpersonal hygiene can prevent this virulent infection from spreading. General rules of personal hygiene, wearing of clean socks at every training session keeping the webs of toes dry and use of fungicidal powders can prevent this condition, but common shower rooms, towels and toilets spread this condition in the community of sportsmen.

Q.38. What do you understand by Traumatic Arthritis ?

Ans. It is the degenerative condition of distance runners involving calcaneal and talus bone. Athletes complain of pain and stiffness in the morning hours and tenderness is elicited while foot is rotated. Weight bearing is painful. Diagnosis is by radiological confirmation. Condition is an overuse injury and can be controlled by running on grassy surface and use of anti-arthritic drugs, electrotherapy etc.

Q.39. What points should be kept in mind by Marathon runner in relation to care of their feet ?

Ans. Following points should be kept in mind :

1. Training shoes should be comfortable, well snug, heavy sole with adequate box having proper width and height. Shoe should be with good cushioning under the heel and also protecting the achilles tendon while extra cushioning be provided at the pressure points.
2. Laces of the shoes should be worn in ladder pattern convention, cross lacing is to be avoided. It causes friction on the extensor tendons on the dorsum of the feet.
3. Thick cotton socks should be used by runners and the wrinkles before wearing shoes should be removed. Nylon socks should be discouraged.
4. Biomechanical evaluation of the feet should be done to assess the congenital problems, viz, flat feet, dropped transverse arches, hammer toes and high arched feet. Necessary orthotics, matatarsal bars and felt pads should be used to have an even balance of the feet.
5. Collosities, sesmoid bones and corns should not be ignored and any thickening of the skin taking place at any pressure point in the feet should be immediately taken care of.

6. After a long distance run, contrast bath with massage of feet should be a regular feature.
7. Runners not using socks should use a good lubrication of vaseline or petroleum jelly.
8. Nails should be trimmed regularly and cut horizontally.
9. Proper cleaning of the webs of toes after every practice session is to prevent fungus infestation of toes.
10. To maintain the arches, the following exercises should becarried out :
(a) Tip-toe jumping;
(b) Walking on straight line with weight on the outer border of feet;
(c) Pigeon toe walking, i.e. to walk on toes turned in placing one foot across the other;
(d) Sit on chair and roll up a towel with toes, until fatigued; and
(e) Pick up marbles with toes until muscles are fatigued.
11. Foot wear should be according to the surface; length of the spikes, according to the training ground and any shoe worn out or trodden over from inside, which can be a source of friction, should be immediately changed.

Q.40. Why is there the need of 'Pediatric Sports Medicine' ?

Ans. Participation in organised athletic competition is a reasonably well established feature of childhood and youth throughout the world. The extent of participation by young people in sports is partly hightighted by the notably swimming, gymnastics etc. Hence a consideration of injuries athletes offer a potentially significant contribution to the developmental literature.

Q.41. These days a trend is developing-An athlete ,marries another athlete. Is there any advantage ?

Ans. These types of marriages tend to produce a relatively high percentage of athletically gifted children. In addition to genetic effect, there is the very important influence growing up in a family where sports have a very high priority and where everyone participates in some type of sports activity.

Q.42. Has growing population any influence in bringing out better records ?

Ans. Now the population one arth is more than 5 billion. It is not only creating a bigger base from which more outstanding athletes may appear but it inevitably brings about a greater genetic mix and bringing more people together for more times to create the situations inwhich sports competitions develop.

Q.43. Write the effect of cold on athlete ?

Ans. In a cold environment muscle viscosity increases, and joints stiffen, impairing performance considerably. With minimal clothing, as in running or swimming costume, energy stores must be used at an increased rate available for running or swimming. Swimmers in marathon events frequently have to give up the event because of hypothermia.

Though it is rare in India, yet it should be remembered that the combination of cold air temperature and highwind velocity will include hypothermia and frost-bite rapidly in the person who is not well protected.

Q.44. In relation to development, does training give advantaget to growing children for muscle development ?

Ans. Quite often, many people are of the opinion that larger size and/or 'optimal' growth or the delayed maturation of young athletes is related to the regular training and competition. Regular training has no apparent effect on stature. It is, however, a significant factor influencing the growth and integrity of specific tissues such as bone, muscle and fat. Activity enhances skeletal mineralization and density and stimulates bone growth in width. Regular physical activity results in muscular hypertrophy, an increase in contractile proteins and enhanced oxidative enzyme activity. Some evidence indicates a significant increase in the DNA content of muscle tissue in growing animals above that expected with normal growth suggesting perhaps that training during growth may be a significant factor determining adult levels of DNA in muscle tissue.

Physical activity is important in regulation and maintaining body weight. Regular activity in growing children generally results in an increase in lean body mass and a corresponding decrease in body fat, quite frequently without any appreciable change in body weight.

Q.45. How do exercises effect health of children ?

Ans. Young athletes as well as non-athletes of both sexes grow. The experience of athletic training and competition does not harm physical growth and development of the youngsters. The young, trained athlete has generally a lesser percentage of body weight as fat. Maturity relationships are not consistent across sports. Male athletes more often, than not, tend to be advanced maturationally as compared with non-athletes. On the other hand, female athletes tend to be delayed in maturity, except for swimmers. Maturity associated variation in size and body composition is thus a significant factor in comparing athletes and non-athletes, especially during the circumpuberal years.

Q.46. What are the optimum ages for starting sports training and competition ?

Ans. Here* is the list of some popular sports activity and suggested ages.

Games	**Age in years.**
Hockey	10 years
Basket ball	13
Boxing	15
Cycling	14
Football	10
Gymnastics	9
Handball	11
Track and field	11
Rowing	10
Swimming	8
Table tennis	8
Tennis	10
Volleyball	11
Weight lifting	15
Wrestling	12
Water polo	12

*American college of sports Medicine.

Q.47. What is the need and importance of cardiac evaluation of a young athlete ?

Ans. Mostly heart beat of young athlete can be readily evaluated by the primary physician. Evaluations of blood pressure above accepted norms for age should be evaluated and the individual who wishes to participate in high intensity sports should have a maximum exercise stress test. More complete rhythm disorders necessitate consultation with cardiologist familiar with heart diseases in young. One should allow the young individuals to achieve maximum exertion and, whenever possible allow participation rather than arbitrarily impose restrictions that might predispose to all of problems attended with 'cardiac crippling.' It is likely that psychological harm due to limitations of activities overweight the risk of leniency in permitting participation. We, therefore, advise a consultation with cardiologist familiar with problems of children and adolescents prior to making a decision to exclude a boy or girl from athletic competition.

Q.48. What happens in Adaplation to endurance Training ?

Ans. Formation of a stereotypes motor programme in the slow Twitch Fibers (STF) Extension of the energy stores i.e. glycogen in muscle and liver, Triglyceride in muscle. Increase in aerobic glucose utilization and increase participation of fats in energy metabolism. Increase utilization of gluconeogenetic metabolic paths. Elevated activity of oxidative key enzymes in the STF. Breaking down of about half of the body fat deposits. Increase in capillaries net work. Adaptation in oxygen uptake increase in VO_2 max.

Q.49. Explain why there are sporadic instances of 'Sudden death' in sports among child population.

Ans. There are certain medical and environmental factors associated with unexpected sudden deaths in sports in children. Restrictions or environmental alterations to prevent sudden death associated with an individual sport have been recommended. Medical problems such as cardio-myopathies, posterior mitrai valve leaflet syndrome, and underlying congenital heart problems have been in sudden deaths related to sports. It is also necessary to emphasize the abnormalities of hypertrophic cardio myopathies, Marfan's syndrome, and the need to monitor constantly the medical, environmental, and safety factors for all sports in which our youth now actively participate.

Q.50. What age is suitable for a child to start team sports ?

Ans. For an individual child it is determined by his own pattern of development and expressed interest. Generally children begin at about 6 years age to compare themselves with others in both skill and ability. Most children begin to play sports (contact) by the time they are 10 years old. Late maturing adolescent should delay entering in contact sports until they can withstand the physical pressure of these sports.

The real question here is, does the child want to participate in team sports or do the parents want it ? We get some clues to the child's interest from: pride in warning sports uniform, collecting sports items, or talking about sports. Sports development is the same as the other areas of the child's development; the more the child is pushed, the less likely are the chances of success and the more he or she will resist. Thus, premature involvement may least to withdrawal because of boredom, pressure of failure.

Q.51 Should one let his child quit a team ?

Ans. Before a parent reacts to a child's declaration that he or she wants to quit, it is necessary to gather the facts. The first step is to talk to the child. Although commitment to play a team sport should not be taken lightly, there are acceptable reasons to allow a child to withdraw. Some valid reasons are the coach is abusive and lacks skill to coach the child, or the child is experiencing stress-related symptoms such as vomiting, headache, or depression. No benefit is derived from playing under these circumstances and continued participation may result in the occurrence of more problems.

Q.52. If a child is an extra-ordinaryathlete, should it be considered anything special ?

Ans. The athlete who has superior abilities and skills may lack the maturity to handle the prestige and pressure that come with recognition. Parents have the delicate job of helping the gifted athlete handle these pressures. They must be reminded frequently that they are loved for themselves and not for their athletic or academic accomplishments. This applies particularly to younger children who succeed in sports. Boys and girls who mature early may not be able to maintain their early levels of athletic accomplishment when their peers catch up in physical development. It is important that parents begin early to emphasize the value of the individual without success and the value of participation without regard to winning. This will help to protect the early maturing child, from pressures that might otherwise be overwhelming when later maturing children begin to equal and surpass his or her performance.

The younger who is able to achieve sports' success during adolescence has different set of potential problems. The parent's task is to help the athlete and avoid an exaggerated sense of self-importance or distorted view of the role of sports and help him or her build a healthy self-image. Frequently, the physician's task is to tell the parents that they are doing fine job.

Q.53. How can a handicapped child participates in sports activities ?

Ans. As a matter of fact, sports involvement offers psychological and physical benefits for boys and girls who have health handicaps. Some handicapped adolescents desire to participate in those sports activities which parents and sports doctors feel are inappropriate for them. In such instances, unless the activity endangers the adolescent (e.g., a hemophilic playing football), he or she should make the final decision. The sports doctor's responsibility is to help the handicapped in getting the consultation when necessary, recommend a physical programme, and acquaint the parents and adolescents with the pros and cons of participation. If the handicapped adolescent decides to participate, the parents and physician should make sure that appropriate equipment is available and used.

Q.54. Should a child having trouble with academic work be allowed to participate in sports activities ?

Ans. Yes, because everyone should be involved in regular physical activity. Sports activities may be an important vehicle of success for a young person who is not experiencing success in the class room.

Q.55. Should boys and girls play sports together ?

Ans. It is now generally accepted that boys and girls in the prepuberal years can play sports together without fear of physicalinjury or significant imbalance in the development of abilities and skills. Questions have been raised about the psychologic effect on boys who find it difficult to accept being defeated by the girls. Changing standards make this problem less important for the children, but the parents may find the problem as difficult as ever.

Q.56. Are injuries more likely to occur in certain sports than in others ?

Ans. Football is implicated in more injuries than any other sports. There are relatively high injury rates in wrestling, gymnastics, and hockey. Even in these sports, the risk of significant injury is minimal when the programmes are properly supervised. Information about the risks involved in some sports is widely available. There is certain attraction to risks for adolescents. However, there is increasing participation in a relatively high risk sports short of reckless when there is good coaching and equipment and the rules are adjusted to protect the young athletes. When children need intense physical activity, supervised activities may be preferable to reckless persuits divorced from sports and any type of supervision.

Q.57. Are sports activities too stressful for young children ?

Ans. Many feel that prepubescent children should not participate in organized sports because of stress. However, the fact that children experience some stress while participating in sports is not the major issue. The question is, does sport participating in sports is not the major issue. The question is, does sport participation create inordinate or undesirable stress ? Sports activities involve children in stressful situations, but this is a part of learning and development. Competition is a part of all phases of everyday living including sports. But unreasonable pressure to win creates an unhealthy stress and distorts a child's developing value system, but total avoidance of stress undermines learning and growth.

Recent studies have shown that the stress of performing a music solo was far greater than that created by participants in a sports contest. The biggest problem occurs when adults add their own competitive drives to their children's normal competitive instincts. The combination can prove to be too much for children and lead to overwhelming stress experienced in the home throughout the day. The solution is withdrawal of adult pressure -not the withdrawal of child from the sport.

Q.58. Should parents coach their own child ?

Ans. Both advantages and disadvantages are there if a parent is coaching a team in which his or her childplays. It is no doubt convenient; but, even gifted coaches have difficulty in coaching their own children. Many find it impossible to arrive at an attitude that is neither too critical nor too approving. Sometimes it is best to avoid the situation.

Q.59. Is it important to know the genetic background of a child player ?

Ans. The inherited characteristics from both mother and father have an effect on the ultimate body configuration of the individual. Adult height is related to mind parental height, as was pointed out by Sir Francis Galton in 1889; most of the children will attain a height in the range of the mid parent height. Similarly, the child's body shape is related to the parents shape. Weight is more difficult to correlate because it is also affected by caloric intake and energy expenditure, which are related to life style.

Q.60. Why is there a need to have separate groups of boys and girls during growth spurt ?

Ans. The average boy and girl can compete equally in any sport upto adolescence. After that, the changing levels of hormones cause considerable changes in body proportions, muscle mass and fat distribution that preclude equal competition. Changes in boys usually start two years later. Because of this, trying to use chronological age to establish team participation limits become meaningless after the athlete begins to mature. During adolescence, there can be no equal competition between the sexes or within the sexes based on chronological age. During the period of most rapid growth, the risk of injury to epiphyseal plates is the highest, as is the risk of ligament injury because of the normal joint laxity at this age. Expecting early, average and late maturers to compete equally is unreasonable; and the difference is growth and maturation should be taken into account when advising parents as to when to compete and in which sport, or whether not to compete at all.

Q.61. What is the importance of C.V.S. check among children ?

Ans. The young child should be allowed to achieve maximum exertion and, whenever possible, to participate in sports rather than have restrictions arbitrarily imposed that might predispose of all the problems accompanying 'cardiac crippling.' Psychological harm from a limitation of activities may far outweigh the risk from leniency in permitting participation. Therefore, physician should consult a cardiologist familiar with the problems of children and youth before excluding an individual from all opportunities to participate in sport activities.

Q.62. Should epileptic children participate in contact sports? Explain.

Ans. Some children or adolescents with epilepsy want to play contact sports. In general, such type of children should be encouraged for non-contact sports, but each instance must be evaluated individually. The frequency, type and time of seizures, and the degree of seizure control should be taken into account. Children and adolescents with frequent daytime seizures, patitmal seizures, or psychomotor seizures should not participate in contact sports. Children with generalized seizures may participate if their seizures are well under control. There is no evidence that repeated head impacts in football worsen seizure disorders. Boxing, with its potential forhead trauma and primary goal of producing injury, is not an appropriate 'sport' for any young person.* Swimming should be totally forgotten by the children suffering from epilepsy. It can be fatal.

Q.63. What have you to say about participation in Gymnastics and Swimming ?

Ans. There is a general agreement that child or adolescent with epilepsy should not perform athletic activities where a fall because of a seizure could result in a serious injury. Activities, thus, excluded are rope climbing, performance on the parallel bars, rings and balance beam.

Swimming may prove fatal. It should not be allowed under any condition.

Q.64. Explain in brief the participation in games and sports when involved in chronic health problem.

Ans. The over-riding goal of the physician caring for a child or adolescent with a chronic health problem should be to make it possible for these young persons to lead a life as normal as possible. Whenever a doctor is consulted by a family, the doctor should attempt to understand the nature of the family's interest in making their child participate in a particular sports activity.

All children should be encouraged to take part in typical childhood activities as well as organized athletic pursuits with peers.

Q.65. What is the role of exercise in a case of chronic lung disease ?

Ans. Training programmes using aerobic exercise improve exercise tolerance in patients with chronic lung diseases. The parameters of pulmonary function are not changed by exercise training, but ventilatory muscle endurance and resistance to fatigue improve with aerobic training. Improved ventiatory muscle endurance may be a reason for improved exercise tolerance observed in patients with chronic lung disease following exercise training. Childhood with chronic ling diseases can probably achieve the same benefit by participating in aerobic sports (e.g. tennis, hockey, cycling, swimming, running). More debilitated

*The Americal Academy of Paediatrics does not approve of boxing as an Interscholastic activity

patients may require a more structured exercise programme. Some hypoxic patients may also require supplemental oxygen to improve tolerance for exercise to the point where daily activities can be easily performed. The effects of physical training are not maintained if exercise is stopped. Thus, exercise programmes should be designed to enable patients continue the exercise in their own. Improvement of exercise tolerance by an aerobic exercise training programme may significantly improve the rehabilitation potential and quality of life for some children and adolescent with chronic lung disease. Whether or not exercise training improves survival in those with chronic lung disease is not known.

Q.66. What do you understand by 'Thermo-regulation, fluid and electrolyte' needs ?

Ans. Heavy physical activities overtax a number of body systems and regulatory mechanisms with specific metabolic, cardio-respiratory, and muscular responses. Physical exertion also stresses the thermo-regulation system, and severe losses of fluid and electrolytes may occur during strenuous activity. Thermo-regulation and losses of fluid and electrolyte become matters of paramount importance whenever the stress of increase in environmental temperature, humidity issue perimposed on metabolic load. When the environment is too hot, too cold, or too humid, subpar athletic performance and hazards for the health of the athlete may result.

Q.67. Write the importance of liquid in games and sports.

Ans. It is a proven fact that injury is more likely when the player is dehydrated. At the other extreme overhydration prior to an event may lead to discomfort and stitch. Training should be used to prepare for competition and the well trained sportsperson will have discovered long before the day of competition how much fluid he finds comfortable to drink. As relative dehydration beings immediately, it is also sensible to be prepared to drink from an early stage in any drawn out competition requiring stamina. By the time thirst is felt, it is almost certainly too late to replace the lost fluid.

Q.68. Why and how does 'Thermoregulation' take place ?

Ans. The chemical energy involved in muscle contraction, 70 to 80% is transformed into heat, with a rise in muscle temperature. Distribution by the blood stream and conduction by neighbouring tissues disperse this muscle heat throughout the body. The resulting rise of body temperature is related to the degree of increase in metabolic rate involved in muscle work. When the active muscle mass is large (as in walking or running) and exercise is intense, there can be an 8 to 10 fold increase in the resting metabolic rate. The core temperature of the body can increase 1° to 1.5° C in 20 to 30 minutes two physiological regulatory mechanism are available to human beings to prevent an excessive rise in core temperature :

(a) With an increase in blood flow to the skin more heat can be transferred from core to periphery, and

(b) With the increased production by the sweat glands, there is greater evaporation from the surface of the skin. The other factors are climate, clothings, radiant heat etc.

Q.69. What are the basic differences between adult and child in relation to thermo-regulation ?

Ans. There are some morphological and functional differences between adults and children that make the latter less efficient thermo-regulators. The basic difference is the lower sweating capacity of children resulting from the level of sweat production by their sweat glands (an unexplained mechanism that increases the ability to sweat starts operating during puberty). Another disadvantages of children in this regard is their greater heat production in exercise and their less ability to convey this heat from the muscles to the skin. Their greater relative surface area may not be important in mildly warm or cool climates; but children will be at a disadvantage in performing strenuous activities for prolonged periods in extremes of warm or more humid climates.

Q.70. What common physiological changes occur in dehydration ?

Ans. It results in a reduction of total plasma volume, stroke volume, and cardiac output; elevation of heart rate during submiximum exercise; a reduction in renal blood flow and glomerular filtration rate; depletion of liver glycogen; losses of electrolytes Na, K, Ca and Mg, and compromised thermo-regulation. Dehydration will also adversely affect performance because of reduced muscle strength, endurance time and mental activity. Prevent 'involuntary dehydration' during prolonged activities and to curtail deliberate dehydration for 'making weight'.

Q.71. How to make fluid and electrolyte replenishment ?

Ans. Fluid and electrolyte losses must be minimised in the exercising child. If these losses are not controlled, performance, physiological functions, and well-being of the athlete will suffer. A rational approach to fluid and electrolyte replacement include a number of principles :

1. The fluids used should stimulate more drinking rather than just quench the thirst.
2. Gastric emptying to the small intestine should be rapid to avoid fluid stasis and subsequent gastric distension during exercise.
3. The quantity taken should be enough to minimize fluid loss.
4. A mixed diet sufficient in amount to satisfy the energy needs of the athlete will replace all electrolyte losses.

Q.72. What have you to say about cold and commercial drinks ?

Ans. (a) Cold drinks are preferable to tepid or warm ones because they stimulate thirst and are emptied more rapidly from the stomach. The overall direct cooling effect of a cold drink is not evident, and there are no documented adverse effects from drinking cold drinks before, during and after competition provided they are not taken in excess otherwise gas may cause distension (very rare).

(b) Commercial drinks with various concentrations of sodium chloride postassium chloride, and sugar have become popular among athlete and joggers. These drinks contribute nothing special to meet the needs of the athlete but are expensive. For Indians, plain water is sufficient (with one glass of fruit juice) for exercising children who eat a balanced diet.

Q.73. Is the use of salt tablet beneficial ?

Ans. The use of salt tablets is potentially dangerous for the following reasons :

(a) The salt content in regular diets is adequate to replace the sodium and chloride lost in sweat.

(b) As aldosterone activity is increased with exercise, sodium is conserved by the kidney, and in fully acclimated individuals by the sweat glands. Thus, habitual exercisers who eat and drink normally maintain a positive sodium balance.

(c) Because sweat is hypotonic, body fluids become hypertonic during dehydration from excessive sweating. A disproportionate consumption of salts will increase the hypertonicity of the extra-cellular fluid and may further deplete the intra-cellular space by hypernatremic dehydration.

Q.74. What guidelines should be kept in mind in relation to Thermoregulation in the conduct of the Athletic Events ?

Ans. The following guidelines for preventing harmful effects of heat are intended for people who are working with athletes or helping to plan athletic events :

1. Ensure acclimatization to exercise in heat. Before this stage is reached, control the intensity and duration of activities. Remember that children acclimatize slowly, and most adverse reactions to heat happen during the first few days of the training season.
2. Schedule activities to the prevailing climate. Remember that humidity, solar radiation, and air velocity are factors to be considered in addition to environmental temperature.
3. Schedule periodic rest periods is in shade during a practice; this is important for dissipation of heat previously accumulated.
4. Identify and screen for close observation and attention to those athletes at high risk because of obesity. Poor conditioning, exercise, weight loss during exercise, or health problems. Preparation of health history and evaluation is recommended.
5. Secure full hydration prior to any practice or competition.

6. Identify athletes who loss more than 3% of body weight during practice.
7. Enforce periodic drinking above and beyond the amount required by thirst, with special attention to the athletes who have lost excessive weight.
8. Never use water restriction as a disciplinary measure.
9. Discourage deliberate dehydration in young athletes. Help enforce regulations to reduce the temptation for this practice.
10. Avoid excessive clothing, taping or padding in hot and humid climates. Ensure optimum evaporation from the skin by use of porous clothing and frequent changes from sweat saturated to dry garments. Avoid prolonged exposure of skin to direct solar radiation. A hot clothing of light colour is recommended whenever feasible.
11. Adjust the timing of practice and competition (hour of day, time of year) as needed.

Q.75. Describe the role of increasing flexibility during warming up sessions ?

Ans. Flexibility is an essential component of muscle performance. Stretching exercises develop flexibility. One method is to assume a stretched position for a given amount of time, usually 6 to 10 seconds at first and increasing to 1 minute as flexibility increases.

Another method forces the ligaments and muscles to an extended and flexed position, and the final stretched position is held for any period of time.

Many exercises are designed to develop flexibility in a specific portion of the body. The frequency of flexibility exercises is arbitrary, in general, 2 to 3 days a week for 30 minutes is sufficient.

Maximum obtainable flexibility must be re-established by warm-up exercise, immediately before any intensive activity involving muscle contraction and stretching. Warm in a predetermined routine is absolutely necessary prior to strenuous activity and after any extended rest period during a schedule contest or work-out.

Q.76. What do you understand by the word 'Athletic Trainer'?

Ans. Historically, athletic trainers have been caring for competitors since the days of 'Greek Olympics'. They were there to care for bruised and sore muscles, to rub and oil 'their charge' before competition and bathe him after, and to bandage and to take care for his injuries. The rubber was still part of the atheletic scene in the early days of modern era of sports. Many former day athletic trainers were individuals whose active athletic career ended because of accident or age, or perhaps they earned their way from locker room boy (ward body) to equipment man and then to trainer. Many become proficient in mastering or developing athletic training techniques. Through reading, on the job training, and associate with team physicians and other remedial professionals, they created the foundations of the present day profession of trained, certified athletic trainers.

Q.77. Who can be the athletic trainer in India ? What are the common functions of athletic trainer ?

Ans. A better oriented person in Sports phyisotherapy and sports medicine can look after the work of athletic trainer, provided he/she has physical education as the base. The athletic trainers (coach, PT, in India) interact with school administrators, equipment and other sports staffs, physicians (team, family, consultant), pubic school nurses, paramedical professionals, teachers, parents and athletes themselves. The athletic trainer's role has functional value in four areas of primary responsibility :

- first aid and emergency care,
- treatment and rehabilitation,
- injury prevention,
- programme administration.

Q.78. How can school nurse, compounders, ward boys be useful for school level players ?

Ans. School paramedical staff, junior or senior can encourage positive attitudes towards health and fitness among school athletes, coaches, and parents. This staff can quickly establish mutual respect with athletes and coaches. Athletes though stronger but generally have poor immune mechanism (because they hardly get exposure to ineffective or dirty environment). The expertise of paramedical staff in the health care of children can easily be expanded to include more involvement in the prevention and management of athletic injuries and the athletic/physical education programme for all school children.

Q.79. Why is the knowledge of musculo-skeletal injury necessary for school physician ?

Ans. The skeletally immature athlete has patterns of musculo-skeletal injuries that differ from these encounters in adults. A knowledge of these injuries and recognition of their occurrences is essential to the medical management of the young athlete. In addition, medical personnel need to be acquainted with the patterns of injury unique to each of the individual sports. With these basic facts, proper training, prevention and rehabilitation programme can be devised to suit the unique characteristics of skeletally immature athletes.

Q.80. What do you understand by word 'DOPING'?

Ans. The word 'doping' first appeared in an English dictionary around the beginning of the twentieth century. It was derived from the word in the Boer Language (The word 'dop' was to refer to a local hard liquor made from grapes that the Kaffirs used as a stimulant at worship). The word 'dope' was applied to the use of narcotics in race horses to improve their performance. As a result of widespread use of 'doping' in the equestrian field, saliva test for horse came into use in 1910.

The opium is also said to be the origin for word 'dope' as since ancient time it was being used by the people.

Q.81. What do you mean by word Ergogenic aid ?

Ans. This word has been applied to the substances or methods the athlete used to obtain an 'extra-edge'. This classification included nutritional, physiological, psychological, physical and chemical aids. These materials may be provided by a coach, physical and chemical aids. These materials may be provided by a coach, manager, athletic trainer, physician or parents peer pressure encourages their use.

Q.82. In few lines what message you will like to give regarding ergogenic aids, nutritional products ?

Ans. Due to international and national competitions new

ergogenic aids will be available to help produce records breaking champions. Evaluation of these products remains an ongoing process which require the sports nutritionist to keep current, keep listening and be circumspect in taking a stand. There are lot of misinformation also available all over the world surrounding ergogenic aids. It is a necessity to keep an open mind and to admit what we do not know. In long run truth is the best antidote to inaccurate claims.

Q.83. Why do athletes use alcohol for increasing performance ?

Ans. Alcohol has been used for years by competitors in three ways in sports competitions; as a tranquillizer in shooters, as a source of energy in cyclists and as a support by athletes in several categories of weight. Alcohol is a depressant and may decrease performance by prolonging reaction time and showing neuromuscular response. Recently alcohol has been used for its caloric and diuretic effects by marathoners in competition as 'gold water'. Beer is an inefficient energy source; the resultant diuresis is undesirable for distance runners and the dehydration is undesirable for any athlete.

Q.84. Why do the athlete try to use the drugs ?

Ans. Some athletes will do anything of any new idea-to improve their normal physiologic performance. They may be superstitious, impressionable, faddish gullible or extremely susceptible to suggestion. They are unwilling to accept scientific evidence that some drugs or other agents are dangerous, will not improve performance, and have potential for creating a serious health hazards and the feeling of guilt.

A question frequently asked by athletes competing at the international level is, "If these materials are not going to improve my performance, why are you bothering me to test for drugs." Athletes are tested to protect and preserve their health. Athletes should be educated and not penalized. They should be warned of the dangers of taking drugs and taught that any claims for improved performance are far outweighed by the danger of these substances.

Q.85. Comment on the 'Drugs misuse by Adolescent Athletes' ?

Ans. Athletes have used many substances to augment their athletic performance. These substances have been referred to an ergogenic aids, and as the athlete's ability carry them closer to international competitions or professional athletics, their use seems to increase. Athletes may believe that benefits to be accured include an increase in strength and endurance, a delay in the onset of fatigue, an increased ability to concentrate and a decreased sensitivity to pain. Banning the use of ergogenic aids, as is done in international Olympic Competitions and enforcing this ban by urine testing may be a practical, albeit expensive approach to this problem in international amateur competition. The main problem is that this method cannot be used in the usual high school or college athletic programme. There is a need not only to educate the athletes about the hazards of most of these ergogenic agents but also about their relative ineffectiveness in achieving 'the illegal edge'.

The substances described have little or no ergogenic capacity, and even if they did, the danger associated with many of them far outweight the advantage of being given them to an athlete. Using these drugs for this purpose is cheating and a violation of the ethics of fairplay in sports, the use of alleged ergogenic aids by the adolescent athlete is a possibility that should be considered by sports physician whenever he performs either a routine health maintenance examination or a pre-participation physical examination on the adolescent athlete. This subject should be routinely mentioned by the physician, and the risks, and alleged benefits fully discussed.

Q.86. What have you to say about the 'Local anaesthetic agents' used as ergogenic ?

Ans. Athletics who get local injuries treated with an injection of a local anaesthetic may be tempted to return to the game since they are no longer in pain. Obviously, this decision could lead to further and more serious injury to that part of the body. These drugs can produce cardiac arrhythmias and in large doses produce convulsions and death. Idiosynoratic sudden deaths have been reported, but these may have been caused by overdose or intravenous injections. The physician should be aware that the resuscitation and other emergency drugs should be available at Health Centre if at all such drugs are to be used.

Q.87. Does Marijuana possess positive effect ?

Ans. There would be little to suggest that this drug is an ergogenic aid. One recent study has shown no difference between smoking marijuana and a placibo in measurements of vital capacity, expiratory flow rate and hand grip strength. This drug may affect skeletal muscles, reaction time and coordination. Further studies on athletics are needed to comment on this drug.

Q.88. Do anti-inflammatory drugs have any role ?

Ans. DMSO (dimethyl sulfoxide) is widely available as counter preparations in pharmacies throughout the western countries, and it is widely used by athletes of all ages because of its alleged anti-inflammatory properties. Athletes rub it on injured area in the belief that the inflammation (and therefore the pain and discomfort) will be relieved sooner than by the traditional conservative methods such as rest, heat or cold. The pungent odour of the breath within minutes of its being applied to the skin makes double blind placebo-controlled studies difficult. However, one recent study compared the effectiveness against elbow tendinitis of standard 70% solution with a 5 percent DMSO placebo, and no benefit could be ascertained.

Q.89. Why are there increasing number of overuse syndromes in young athletes ?

Ans. To excel in sports today the young athlete is forced to train longer, harder and that too early in life. Swimmers and gymnasts in junior high school can spend three to six hours a day in the pool or gym. Runners in high school may average in excess of 30 to 40 miles a week. Cyclists may cover over 200 miles a week during training rides. Beginners in sports, although not training at these intensities, are also subjecting their bodies to the rigours of trained throughout the year as they migrate from sport to sport.

The reward for this regimen is an increased level of fitness, better performances, faster times, and satisfaction in attaining goal. Hours of practising the same movements produce gradual wear on specific parts of the body. Variations in the athlete's anatomy or technique, hours of practice, and the intensity of training may combine to produce an overuse injury.

Q.90. Enlist the duties of a team physician for young athletes.

Ans. Following duties can be listed for a team physician :

1. Establish policy lines for authorities, with administration, coaches, emergency medical techniques, trainers, parents, students and physicians for competitive sports.
   a. Evaluation of playing field and equipment.
   b. Evaluation of injuries or illness and system of care for proper management and follow-up care.
   c. Evaluation for conditioning and training programme.
   b. Establishing criteria for disqualifying conditions for participation in competitive sports and returning to participation after illness or injury.
2. Set up transportation and referral system for these injuries needing special care.
3. Educate the parents, coaches, and students about the risk factors in each sport and establish their areas of responsibilities.
4. Be aware of many needs of adolescents and offer them an entry to the health care system for problems other than related to sports such as drug abuse, venereal disease, malnutrition, anaemia, chronic illness and behaviour problems.
5. Review all history and physical assessment done by other physicians and re-evaluate the participants if any doubt arise from the assessment.
6. Record a history and do a physical examination for those athletes without a primary physician.
7. Set up other rehabilitation procedures for injuries.
8. Set up a record keeping system for injuries.
9. Evaluate the coaching techniques that might contribute to injuries.
10. Learn the rules of the games and evaluate adherence

of officials to these rules.

11. Know the general factors that contribute to injuries in order of their importance.

a. Conditioning,
b. Coaching techniques,
c. Rules and regulations,
d. Equipments,
e. Physical and medical evaluation.

12. Know the most important elements in the medical examination.

a. The annual, history between each sport with questions about previous injuries or illness, operations, hospitalizations, and use of medicines.
b. An examination should be done at least every two years that concentrates on the systems most frequently affected by strenuous exercise.
c. Concentrate on problems of cardio-vascular system abdomen musculo-skeletal system, secondary sex characteristics, and review of sports history.

13. Handouts available on conditioning and training, stretching, and general risk factors are to be given to each athlete.

Q.91. Mention the names of important drugs used as ergogenic aid ?

Ans. Though there is a big list of drugs but a few important generally used drugs are-Amphetamines, Anabolic steroids, Barbiturates; Hallucinogens, Local anaesthetics, Metabolic inhibitors, Narcotic analgesics, Peripheral vasodilators, Tranquilizers etc.

Q.92. Mention important actions of each drug ?

Ans. (a) Anabolic Steroids : Described separately

(b) Amphetamines : C.N.S. stimulant, which promotes alertness and false confidence, stimulates action of the naturally occurring catecholamines on heart, arterioles, nerves and metabolic reactions.

(c) Metabolic Inhibitors : Interferes with normal metabolic reactions.

(d) Barbiturates : Central nervous system depressant, most commonly used to lessen pain or produce sleep.

(e) Local anaesthetics : Peripheral nerve depressant

which relieves pain and can prevent muscle swelling and spasm.

(f) Hallucinogens : CNS activator or inhibitor depending on person and area of CNS predominatly influenced. Creates bizarre effects, for normal though processes are charged and reality avoided.

(g) Narcotic analgesics : CNS depressant, that produces stupour, insensibility or sleep. Use can lead to dependence and addiction.

(h) Peripheral vasodilators : Dilate peripheral arterioles and coronary arteries to presumably supply more blood to working muscle.

(i) Tranquilizers : To calm or sedate. Used to enhance recovery from fatigue.

Q.93. What are the common methods of super compensation or 'Carbohydrate loading' ?

Ans. Generally the following methods are employed :

(a) Endurance athlete who consume a high carbohydrate diet for 3 to 4 days after several days on a normal mixed diet may increase their glycogen stores from the normal 15 grams to around 25gm/kg of muscle. During the period of high carbohydrate diet, no exhausting exercise should be performed.

(b) In it, muscles that are to be loaded are first exhausted of their glycogen stores through exercise, the individual then follows a high carbohydrate diet for a few days. This helps in almost doubling the glycogen stores. In this method also, no exhausting exercise should be performed during the time period of high carbohydrate diet.

(c) This method needs exercise and the special diet. Exercise is used to induce muscle glycogen depletion. The individual then follows a diet very low in carbohydrates but high in protein and fats for 3 days, after this high carbohydrate diet is followed for additional 3 days.

Exhausting exercise may be performed during the period of the diet that is high in fat and protein but not during high carbohydrate diet. This method has shown to increase the glycogen stores (in the depleted muscles) to the level approaching 50gm/kg. In body, on an average as much as 700 grams of stored glycogen, or 2800 Kcal of ready energy may be stored by this method.

Q.94. What do you understand by lean Body Mass (fat free weight)?

Ans. When the weight of the body fat is subtracted from the total body weight, the remaining weight is referred to as fat free weight, or lean body mass. The FFW reflects mainly the skeletal muscle mass, but it also includes the weight of other tissues and organs such as bone and skin. The muscle mass makes about 40 to 50 percent of fat free weight. The average fat free weight of a young male is about 85 percent of their total body weight. The females may have 70 to 75 percent of their total body weight.

Q.95. How far is this statement correct, "Exercise burns relatively few calories and, therefore, makes an insignificant contribution to changing energy balance" ?

Ans. With one example everything will be clear :

(a) An individual of 170 pounds decides to substitute 1 hour of tennis for one hour of watch in T.V.

(b) Kcal burned while playing tennis per hour (requires 0.045 calories/minute/pound=170x0.60=459.)

(c) Kcal that would have been spent watching T.V. (burns 0.008 calories/minute/pound=170x0.008x60=81).

If such an individual plays tennis four times per week for 6 months, 39,3123 extra calories would be burnt which is equivalent to just over 11 pounds of fat. So without reducing caloric intake one can gradually reduce the weight.

Q.96. What are your comments about " An increase in physical activity will automatically result in an increase in amount of food eaten" ?

Ans. Results of various research work done on this aspect indicate light and medium work result in a decrease in caloric intake and in body weight, and that heavy and hard work result in an increase in caloric intake but the but the body weight remains constant.

Q.97. Are Sauna or steam baths effective in losing weight?

Ans. One may lose weight through sweating. The way to lose weight by Sauna is temporary. The fluid will be quickly replaced and the weight will return to its original level. So, there is no permanent loss of weight. No doubt sauna is used for relaxation.

Q.98. How is the heart muscle different from others ? Explain the effect of exercise on it.

Ans. Heart and exercise :

1. Heart is a combination of 2 muscular pumps to supply blood to lings and to general circulation.
2. Individual cardiac fibres are interconnected so they function normally as one fibre.
3. Cardiac muscles have the property of Autorythmicity (the ability to self generate nervous impulse.)
4. During exercise two major changes take place :
   (a) Cardiac output,
   (b) Redistribution of blood flow.

Q.99. What is congestive heat failure ?

Ans. The heart fails when the muscle is so damaged by the infarction that it can no longer pump the enough blood for the needs of the body. This can occur any time after an infarction, but it is usually manifest between the 3rd and 7th, days after the heart attack. These patients may develop pulmonary oedema with trophy pink sputum. They consequently may have difficulty in breathing. These may also be evidence of generalized swelling in the body.

Q.100. Give tabular comparison of angina and heart-attack? (my-cardial infarction).

Ans.

Condition	Common precipitants	Duration	Frequent Manifestations (singular or in combination)	Treatment.
Dugrina	Physical stiess Emotional Stress Laege Meals	8-10mins.	Substenal pain Epigastric pain-radiating pain to jaw or aems. Pressure in chest. Shortness of breath Nausea Sweating.	1. Rest. 2. Nitroghyoine 3. Medical Follow-up
Daete Hyocardial Infaction	Not necessarely related to start may occure at rest	Louger than 30 minuts	Substernal pain Cuushing chest pain. Heaviness in chest. Inregularilty of heartbeat Radiation of pain to jaw arms, epigasturim Felling plert is failt or light headed.	1. Reassurance. 2. Marieta vital vigus 3. Send to ED as soon as possible Alert hospital of patient is status & estimated time of arrival

Q.101 . Can you explain the difference in 02 requirements during rest and exercise ?

Ans. It can be made clear by looking at this table :

Component of the oxygen transport at rest/exercise

Conditions	VO_2 ml/min		St.Vol. ml/beat		Heart rate/ min.		$A\text{-}VO_2$ diff. ml/llr.
(A) Untrained							
Rest	300	=	75	x	82	x	48.8
Max.	3110	=	112	x	200	x	138.0
(B) Trained							
Rest	300	=	105	x	58	x	49.3
Max.Ex.	3440	=	126	x	192	x	140.5
(C) Endurance at							
The rate	5570	=	189	x	190	x	155

Q.102. What are the effects of training ?

Ans. Effects of training can be divided into the following groups :

(A) At rest :

(1) Change in the heart size (Echocardiography).

(2) Slowing of heart rate/increase in stoke volume.

(3) Change in Blood Volume/Hb-concentration.

Before exercise	After exercise	Increase%
5.25 litres	6.58 ltr.	25%
805 gm.	995 gms.	24%

(4) Changes in Capillary Density in Heart/Lung/Muscle.

(5) Lowering of blood pressure.

(6) Lowering of cholesterol and triglycrides.

(B) At Sub Maximal Exercise : So that it can work more efficiently with less strain/problem.

(1) VO_2 uptake (less glycogen and more FFA use)

(2) Lactic Acid (as anarobic threshold)

(3) Muscle glycogen use.

(4) Cardiac output (S.VOl., Heart rate)

(5) Cardiac rate

(6) Blood flow rate (A-VO_2 difference).

(C) During Max. exercise :

(1) Aerobic power Vo_2 max. (more CO_2 and more extraction of O_2)

(2) Lactic acid conc. (Glycolytic enzyme acting heart rate)

(3) Cardiac output (Storke Volume Heart Rate Cardiac Hypertrophy)

(4) Blood flow to muscle ($-VO_2$ difference)

(5) No change even lowering of max. exercise heart rate.

Heart can work more vigorously and for longer duration so that total work done in increased as a result of training.

Q.103. Mention, what common instruments you will use for measuring strength ?

Ans. Commonly used instruments can be divided into two groups :

(A) Isotonic strength :- With weight (bench squat, pull-up, push-ups, dip test, leg lift, bench press and others).

(B) Isometric strength :- Dynamometers ant Tensiometer (Grip, leg and back, hand-dynamometers).

Q.104. What instruments are used for assessing Flexibility?

Ans. Goniometer, scales (for measuring distances, static flexibility-possible, dynamic flexibility-not possible).

Q.105. Mention the selected tests for assessing endurance?

Ans. (a) Local muscular endurance by various forms of ergometer,

(b) Cardio vascular endurance :

In field

(a) 12 minutes Cooper's run/walk test.

(b) A particular distance -time to be recorded

(c) A particular time-distance to be recorded.

In lab

(a) Harvard step test.

(b) Bicycle Ergometer-constant and increasing load.

(c) Treadmill.

Q.106. How to test the aerobic/anaerobic power ?

Ans. For it, specific instruments/equipments are needed :

(a) aerobic power Vo_2 max liter/min, ml/kg/min.

(b) Anerobic power 3/4
    (i) Lactic acid conc.
    (ii) ATP/CP System.

Q.107. How to assess body composition ?

Ans. (a) Under water weighing measurements.

(b) Skinfold Caliper – Lange
Harpendon

D_b = Body density (gm/wt)

W_a = Weight in air (gm)

K = Weight in air minus wt. in water divided by density of water at weighing temperature.

RV = Residual Volume.

$$Db = \frac{Wa}{K - RV}$$

$$\text{Percent fat} = \frac{4.95}{-Db} \text{ X } \frac{4.50}{} \text{ x } 100 \text{ (SIRT' FORMULA)}$$

Q.108. What for muscle biopsy is taken ?

Ans. Muscle Biopsy is taken for :
Red/white muscle fibre for
1. Size of fibre (diameter)/types,
2. Diameter of fibre,
3. Glycogen/ATP/OP conc.,
4. Enzymatic studies.

Q.109. How to assess respiratory/circulatory fitness ?

Ans. Respiratory/circulatory fitness can be assessed by :
(a) (i) Hear rate,
(ii) Blood pressure, stroke volume, cardiac output, total blood and Hb conc.
(b) Pulmonary ventilation, peak flow/air flow rate, vital capacity, breath holding times.

Q.110. What do you understand by Rehabilitation after injury?

Ans. Rehabilitation or reconditioning is a process through which the functioning of the injured athlete is restored to his full potential. It consists, of various therapeutic modalities which are utilized immediately after injury or trauma and continue till full recovery is achieved.

Q.111. How many phases are there in rehabilitation ?

Ans. There are five phases involved in the rehabilitation of the injured athletes :

1. Control of haemorrhage, hematoma formation and inflammatory reactions.
2. Absorption of hematoma or inflammatory products to minimise scarring of the injured tissues.
3. Healing and functional rehabilitation of the injured part.
4. The psychological preparation of the athlete for his return to competition.
5. The psychological preparation of the athlete for his returns to competition.

Q.112. Explain how cryotherapy is useful in rehabilitation after injury ?

Ans. The use of cold (ice therapy, cryotherapy, cryokinetics) in combination with exercise has become an accepted method of treating common athletic injuries. Grant, Bierman and Haines are the strong advocates of cryotherapy, particularly in acute musculoskeletal injuries.

Application of cold produces-four phases of sensation :

First the patient has a cold feeling which lasts for one to three minutes.

Two to seven minutes after the initiation of cryotherapy, the patient experiences a burning or aching sensation (stage 2).

In 5 to 12 minutes, local numbness of anaesthesia is achieved (stage 3).

At this point, pain and reflex impulses are inhibited.

12 to 15 minutes of ice exposure produces a reflex deep tissue vasodilation without an increase in metabolism (Stage 4).

Immediately after the injury, ice should be applied to achieve stage 3.

Once the injury phase has been stabilized, stage 3 cryotherapy should be combined with progressive slow exercises.

Immersion technique is suitable for extremities (10 to 30 minutes). Ice massage is popular for flatter areas (20 to 30 minutes). A light circular or back and forth motion is used with the application carried out circumferentially from the painful site. Take precautions of frost bite. Often and ice pack is made by putting crushed or chipped ice in a towel and attaching it to the part with tape or an elastic wrap. The athlete should be treated at least three times a day.

Many trainers believe that the phenomenon of cold vasodilation does exist and that blood can be increased through cold application and thus cold can be used throughout the rehabilitation period.

Q.113. What role has thermotherapy to play in recovery from soft tissue injuries ?

Ans. (a) Hot pack : Every training room should have moist heat pack equipment (Hydrocollator), because it is the simplest and most economical way to apply moist heat for the relief of pain and muscle spasm. The packs are contoured to fit different parts of the body. Wrapping the hot pack in a heavy turkish towel before applying it, diminishes the risk of injuring the skin. The heat penetrates 2cm. compared to the 0.1 cm. penetration of infra red heat, a 20-30 minutes treatment is sufficient.

(b) Whirlpool Bath : The whirlpool is a popular piece of equipment for giving hydrotherapy. Most athletes consider whirlpool bath a necessary part of the training room. The whirlpool has the effect of gentle massage, which helps in reducing swelling, relieves pain and relaxes muscles. The use of warm water for 30 minutes stimulates circulation, reduces inflammation and aids absorption of waste products.

In case whirlpool is not available, a hose attached to a shower connection can direct warm water to an injured part wrapped in a towel to accomplish the more or less the same purpose as a whirlpool. Warm wash should never be given to acute injury.

(c) Infra-red heat treatment : It is an efficient and easily operated therapeutic agent. It is easily applied and transported. It is applied to a local area to create a local hypermia stimulating the circulation of blood within that area. It can be applied for 20 to 30 minutes and deep heat penetration is not required.

(d) Ultrasound : An ultrasonic generator produces vibration having frequency between 700,000 and 1,000,000 cycles per second, which will penetrate as much as 6 cm into body tissues. An oil or water medium is used to conduct the waves from the generator head to the body. Properly applied by a trained person, it has been found beneficial for sprains, strains and contusions.

Q.114. How does the massage help in rehabilitation programme ?

Ans. Massage is used primarily to promote the return of flow of venous blood and lymph to the heart, thus relieving local swelling. Deep massage can break up adhesions, restoring a more complete range of motion. There are four basic techniques of massage - stroking, kneading, friction and percussion.

Q.115. Discuss in details the need and role of therapeutic exercises in injury prevention and rehabilitation.

Ans. Therapeutic exercise is defined as prescribed bodily movements used to restore specific functions in persons suffering from various physical or mental disorders.

The therapeutic objectives are : to rehabilitate the injured back to its normal function in the shortest possible time. To prevent further functional loss and atrophy to the surrounding body parts. To maintain the status-quo of the present body fitness.

Therapeutic exercise may be divided into five types passive, assisted, active, resisted and P.N.F. (Proprioceptive Neural Facilitation Techniques).

Q.116. Enlighten each exercise in detail.

Ans. Here a detailed description is given about each exercise;

(a) Passive movements are performed by the therapist or a physician; the patient, being entirely relaxed, takes no active part in the movement. The purpose of such movement is to regain the mobility in the joint by preventing the adhesion formation. Such movements are generally carried out in those cases where an active and full motion causes pain and discomfort. After ice application such movements help in reducing the oedema of injured part and helps quick recovery.

(b) Assisted movement is generally used when the injured athlete is unable to perform the free movement or to withstand any resistance. Assistance can be given by the therapist, the pulley and sling, by self-assistance or by immersion in water. Swimming pool activity is generally included for injuries of the lower extremities. It offers much versatility.

(c) Active movements are performed entirely by the patient but still under the supervision of the therapist. Active movements should be started as soon as the joints or muscles are free from pain or inflammatory products. Active exercise should be individually planned for each athlete according to his selected sport.

(d) Resisted exercises are those exercises whichare performed against some external resistance. This may be applied with the help of some weights, springs, bands, rope or manual resistance. Research has shown that resisted exercises are most potent to develop the strength of weak joints and muscles and thus play an important part in rehabilitation.

There are four types of resisted exercises :
Isotonic, Isometric, Eccentric and Isokinetic training.

Q.117. Mention the details about resisted exercises :

Ans. (a) Isotonic training involves the use of progressive resistive exercises. Weights are generally used, and the athlete moves them through a full range of motion from extension to flexion. The programme has several variable factors : repetitions, resistance and sets.

(b) Isometric exercises are becoming more and more popular in rehabilitation work. The advantage is that exercise can be used at an early stage after injury.

(c) Muscle setting tonic contraction exercise : In such an exercise the muscle remains in partial or complete contraction without changing its length. If a muscle acts to take up the slack, but does not produce motion, the action is known as static contraction. This type of exercise is similar to isometric; however. in tonic contraction, there is more play in the muscle to take up the slack without causing any appreciable motion at the joint.

(d) Eccentric strength or "negative work" is that part of the isotonic programme in which the weight is held back against the force of gravity. Eccentric movement produces lengthening contraction. The scientific literature reveals that negative exercise has little or no training evidence that negative contractions could provide much faster strength gain after surgery or bed rest than could positive contractions.

(e) Isokinetic exercises are known as a system of accommodating resistance. It allows movement at a mechanically fixed are of speed and offers a resistance force directly proportionate to the magnitude of the input throughout the range of motion. In order to achieve this control an isokinetic device is used.

Research studies have shown that isokinetic exercises have produced better results in the development of strehgth than the isometric or isotonic. However, the exercise cannot be performed without an apparatus.

Q.118. Explain, in brief, the proprioceptive Neural Facilitation Techniques (P.N.F.).

Ans. There are five basic techniques which may be used in accordance with the athletic trainer's preference and the stretch, mass movement patterns, reflexes and reversal of antagonists.

The maximal resistance is used to increase strength by increasing the number of motor units. The stretch technique in used to attain an increased muscle response as well as to initiate motion. Stretch applied to a muscle group facilitates the stretch reflex mechanism of the golgi tendon organs to produce a stronger muscle contraction.

In the mass movement pattern, the opportunity for optimal contraction of muscle groups is provided. The directions of these patterns are in spiral and diagonal motion and not in isolated planes. Some of the desired voluntary neuromuscular responses, for example, the stretch reflex is utilized to initiate the facilitated response. The last technique is the reversal of antagonist. Maximal resistance is given during isometric contraction of the antagonist as against in a rapidly alternating manner. It is used to increase the range of motion.

Q.119. How is haemorrhage or hematoma controlled ?

Ans. The basic character of the immediate inflammatory responses to injury is almost always the same regardless of the location or nature of the injurious agent. The stage is known as 'First Aid' stage and the treatment consists of the 'ICE' which stands for the application of compression and elevation of the injured part. Cold compression may be elastic bandage immersed in ice water, icebags, or towels containing finely cracked ice or sponge rubber compression bandage wrapped about the injured part which is then immersed in ice water for 30 minutes. Compression reduces haemorrhage and oedema about the joint. Effleurage massage movement, while keeping the injured limb in an elevated position also helps minimizing swelling. The patient should be treated with ice therapy for a minimum of three times a day till the danger of internal bleeding is gone. Light exercise may be combined with cryotherapy if bleeding is minimal.

Q.120. How can the Hematoma absorption be enhanced ?

Ans. The second stage involves the use of some forms of therapy to break up and absorb hematoma which has been formed. Many types of therapeutic modalities are available to aid in the promotion of blood flow to absorb the hematoma-cold whirlpool bath, steam pack, ultrasound plussed massage, massage and exercise. Sometimes the trainers use ice massage for 5 to 7 minutes, and when the part becomes, numb, exercise is helpful for stronger repair. Peapock's research on wound-healing revealed that with early controlled motion, fibro-blasts tend to orient themselves along the line of stress.

Once the inflammatory agent and/or inflammatory debris have been destroyed or removed, repair begins. Thus the size of the hematoma or amount of exudate are directly related to the total healing time.

Q.121. Explain the procedure of achieving functional rehabilitation.

Ans. Healing by tissues and functional rehabilitation : Fibroblast formation is the third phase.

Therapeutic modalities should be applied to increase blood flow to help healing. Concentration should be on exercises and particularly specific exercises. Progressive resisted exercises are not initiated until the athlete exhibits full range of motion of the injured area. This is also a stage of retraining, which requires return to the basic drills. These drills provide an excellent source for whatever active exercises may be required for rehabilitation. It also involves the restoration of the general physical capacity to high performance levels.

Q.122. What are the expected beneficial effects of training in relation to CHD ?

Ans. There are some additional benefits of physical training. One is an increase in myocardial vascularization. This may be the result of an increase of collateral vessels in the coronary artery tree or an increase in capillary/myocardial fibre ratio from capillary proliferation.

Another beneficial effect of exercise is on the other CHD risk factors. Exercise has a positive effect on lowering the blood lipids, particularly triglycerides, decreasing the percent of body fat in obesity, lowering the resting blood pressure, and indirectly helping abstinence from cigarette smoking. These combined metabolic and dynamic effects of training protect the heart against myocardial ischemia even in the presence of some degree of coronary atherosclerosis.

The greatest benefit of these protective mechanisms, however, is a primary prevention. For this reason regular, aerobic endurance exercise should be started in childhood and continue throughout life.

Q.123. How exercise helps in prevention of heart problems?

Ans.
(a) Maintain or increase myocardial oxygen supply.
(b) Decrease myocardial work and oxygen demand.
(c) Increase myocardial function.
(d) Increase electrical stability of myocardium.
(A) Maintain or increase myocardial oxygen supply-Delay progression of coronary artherosclerosis.
(a) Improve lipoprotein profile (increase HDL-C/LDL-C (ratio)
(b) Improve carbohydrate metabolisiom (increase insulin sensitivity).
(c) Decrease platelet aggregation and increase fibrinolysis (Probable)

(d) Decrease adifosity (Usually).

— Increase coronary collateral as cularization (unlikely)

— Increase coronary blood flow (myocardial perfussion) or distribution (unlikely).

(B) Decrease myocardial work and oxygen demand.

— Decrease heart rate at rest and submaximal exercise (usually)

— Decrease systolic and mean systemic arterial pressure during submaximal exercise (usually) and at rest (possible).

— Decrease cardiac output during submaximal exercise (probably)

— Decrease circulating plasma catecholamine levels (decrease sympathetic tone) at rest (probable) and at submaximal exercise (usually).

(C) Increase myocardial function.

— Increase stroke volume at rest and in submaximal and maximal exercise (likely).

— Increase ejection fraction at rest and in exercise (possible).

— Increase intrinsic myocardial contractibility (unlikely).

— Increase myocardial function resulting from decreased "after load" (probable).

— Increase myocardial hypertrophy (probable); but this may not reduce CHD risk.

(D) Increase electrical stability of myocardium.

— Decrease regional ischemia at rest or at submaximal exercise (possible).

— Decrease catecho-lamines in myocardiam at rest and at submaximal exercise (probable)

— Increase ventricular fibrillation threshold due to reduction of cyclic AMP (possible).

Q.124. How do continuous and regular exercises effect cardiac functions ?

Ans. Table showing the effects of exercise on cardiac functions

	Increase	**Improves**
Resting heart rare Arterial pressure.	Vegal tone Peripheral shunting of blood	Oxygen transport system Myocardial vascularization
Sympathetic tone	Lower function of the myocardium	Other risk factors

Q.125. How will you make selection of candidates for exercise therpay ?

Ans. The healthy subjects who are coronary prone show the best response to a regular exercise programme. Alongwith physical activity, they should receive help in modifying their other risk factors. They should have a weight reduction programme with skin fold measurements to estimate percent of body fat. They should have diet counselling, especially if hyperlipidemia is present, and their blood lipid content should be periodically evaluated. An intensive anti-smoking programme should be started. Blood pressure records before and after exercise sessions should be kept for those within hypertension. They should be encouraged to have regular medical follow-up examinations by their physicians. A change in risk taking behaviour patterns may change these persons from a high CHD risk status to lower one. The change is one of the primary objectives of a conditioning programme. Persons with clinically recognized ischemic heart disease and selected individuals with mild essential hypertension are also excellent candidates for exercise therapy.

Q.126. What are the absolute and relative contra-indications for exercise therapy ?

Ans. Contra-indication to exercise therapy. Contra-indications to an exercise programme are listed in Table 1 and 2. Certain medical problems are absolute contra-indications to physical conditioning while others are only relative.

ABSOLUTE CONTRA-INDICATIONS TO AN EXERCISE PROGRAMME

— NO EXERCISE PROGRAMME RECOMMENDED

Recent myocardial infraction.
Changing patterns of angina pectoris.
Severe vavular heart disease.
Certain arrhythmias :-
Paroxysmal ventricular tachycardia.
Untreated atrial fibrillation.
Frequent ventricular premature beats with exercise, heart block,
Congestive heart failure.
Myocarditis or cardiomyopathy within a year.

RELATIVE CONTRA-INDICATIONS TO AN EXERCISE PROGRAMME — UNDER MEDICALLY SUPERVISED REHABILITATION PROGRAMME

Myocardial infarction after 3 to 6 months.

Angina Pectoris.

Moderate to severe hypertension (B.P. greater than 160/100); massive obesity.

These later cases, however, require careful medical supervision and frequent monitoring during and after the exercise session. There are a number of reported cases of cardiovascular collapse. It is shown after the exercise session is completed. A test-retest protocol is necessary to follow the progress of these selected persons with relative contra-indications to exercise. If progress is not shown on regular testing, the exercise programme is discontinued and the medical problem revaluated. The improvement from physical reconditioning of these individuals is often rewarding.

Q.127. List the contra-indication of exercise testing, Mention once more ?

Ans. (a) Absolute contra-indications.

(b) Relative contra-indications.

(A) Absolute contra indications.

(i) Recent change in resting ECG, suggesting acute myocardial infraction.

(ii) Unstable angina.

(iii) Serious dysortythmias.

(iv) Acute pericarditis or myocarditis.

(v) Endo carditis.

(vi) Severe Aortic or mitral stenosis.

(vii) Acute pulmonary embolus or infraction.

(viii) Severe physical handicap or injury.

Q.128. Why exercise testing is needed ?

Ans. Exercise testing is an important clinical method for evaluation of cardiopulmonary function. The diagnostic accuracy of exercise testing depends on the extent of disease processes and sensitivity of monitoring methods. Present method of electrocardiographic recording provide a reasonable method for screening patients with probable inschemic heart disease.

Q.129. What are the basic concepts of stress testing ?

Ans. 1. Indications for termination of stress tests : Any test whether maximal or submaximal may need to be terminated. Conditions for terminations include hypotension, pallor, syncope, bradycardia, tarminations, ventricular premature beats, weakness and incordination. ST segment depression in itself is not usually a reason for termination.

2. S.T. : T. changes on the Electrocardiogram : The simplest method of observing myocardial ischemia is with the ECG during stress testing. A tracing with horizontal or down-sloping ST segment depression of one mm or more and of 0.08 to 0.12 seconds duration is considered significant. Persons showing such a phenomena have positive electocardiographic evidence of myocardial ischemia.

Q.130. Mention the points for sudden stoppage of exercise tast ?

Ans. (1) Absolute

(2) Relative

(1) Absolute :

— Onset of severe angina or dyspnea.

— Symptoms or evidence of acute myocardial infarction.

— Significant fall in blood pressure (–20 mm Hg)

— Severe dysrhythmia.

— Signs of pollar, cyanosis, poor skin perfusion.

— Symptoms of poor central nervous system perfussion.

(2) Relative :

— Mild chest pain.

— Marked S-T depression >-0.2 mV or S-T elevation.

— Bundle branch block.

— Less severe dysrhythemia.

— Fatigue, wheezing, leg cramps, or claudication.

Q.131. What are the common exercise-symptoms which require medical review ?

Ans. The following signs and symptoms should be subjected to medical review when they appear in any person on therapeutic exercise programme :

1. Any chest pain or pain referred to teeth, arm, ear or jaw.

2. Syncope, vertigo.
3. Irregular pulse.
4. Persistent fatigue lasting for more than one hour after exercise.
5. Nausea and/or vomiting.
6. Failure of pulse to recover in three minutes to 120 or less.
7. Change in medication dosage (hypotensive drugs, insulin, digitalis).

Q.132. Mention E.C.G. changes ?

Ans. Depression of the ischemic ST segment at its origin : Before it can be regarded as significant, the ST depression, according to some workers should exceed 0.05 mV or even 0.10 mV, especially in the presence of tachycardia. It may not be having that much importance in diagnostic value but definitely it has prognostic importance. The displacement can, if necessary, be divided into three categories of depression; 0.01-0.09 mV; 0.1-019mV; 0.2mV and above.

CHANGES IN WAVE :

An isolate T wave change during exercise is , in general, hardly specific. Continuous 24 hours E.C.G. recordings have shown that in 30% of normal subject. i.e. (those with no cardiac complaints) transitory changes in the T wave may occur, an increase in amplitude being twice as frequent is a decrease. These T wave variations are brought about by tachycardia, nervous excitation, mental activity, change of position, eating a very heavy meal, coffee, tobacco etc.

However, the appearance of a pointed and elevated T wave in V4 with three times of amplitude (or more than 0.5 mV) always indicates serious myocardial ischemia.

Q.133. How will you plan the Rehabilitation programme in various phases ?

Ans. 1. Acute phase : When the resting ST segment has returned to normal, inflammatory signs have disappeared and symptoms are no longer present. Rehabilitation programmes should only be undertaken when no cardiac symptoms are there.

Proposal for such a programmes.

2. Surveillance of training during hospitalization. I+ constitutes both treatment and test. Following parameters should be checked carefully and no further increase in effort be allowed if:

(i) the heart rate during exercise increases by more than 30beats/minute or decreases more than 10 beats/minute;

(ii) disturbance of rhythm and of conduction appear during or immediately after exercise;

(iii) dysponoea, angina or fatingue appears during or at the end of the test;

(iv) pallor hypotension with bradycardia, or faintness appears.

3. Test for establishing intensity of rehabilitation programme during convalescence : After three or four weeks, if the evolution of disease seems favourable, the patient may undergo a more strenuous rehabilitation programme, either individually at home or collectively in a specialized centre. Most of the programmes involve rhythmic exercises (marching, cycling, etc.) of about 30 minutes duration.

Q.134. What is the W.H.O. proposal for rehabilitation for cardiacs ?

Ans. W.H.O proposal : (between 3rd week and the return to work) Heart rate is the most important and simplest guide in establishing the intensity of exercise programme. For a constant load exercise of 30 minutes duration training, heart rate should not increase beyond the resting heart rate by more than 60% of the difference between the heart rate during maximum exercise and the resting heart rate.

This criterion may be criticized on the grounds that the heavier load is thus imposed on elderly people. It will be better to take it as the upper limit of the training heart rate.

Alternatively, the following limits could be imposed:

I. Heart rate should not increase by more than 50% of the resting value.

II. Heart rate should not increase beyond 120 beats per minute or if no severe subjective symptoms appear, beyond 150 beats/minute;

III. Heart rate should not be more than 70% of the difference between maximum heart rate and resting heart rate.

Above mentioned details have been used and since the average coronary population is relatively homogeneous in respect of age, the usually yield fairly comparable results. In general, the limits proposed seem to be safe. However, no centre has yet experienced with more than 500 patients and there is need for further study.

Appearance of subjective symptoms during exercise should also be watched.

Q.135. Explain once again in one complete answer as "How training or exercise help in prevention of specific Heart Problems ?"

Ans. Degenerative diseases of cardiovascular system are mainly based on oxygen required its supply to tissue area. It is the endurance type of exercise which help the individual by -

A. In the heart itself by-

1. Reduction of Heart rate at rest & in given submaxmal exercise intensities in connection with the enlarged stroke volume.
2. Prolongation of Diastole.
3. Reduced contractility .
4. Redution of Catacholamine release.
5. Stabilization of electrical stability.

Above mention points explain decrease oxygen requirement to Heart muscle, while phase of intramyocardial blood supply gets prolonged. In this disturbances in heart rhythm is counteracted.

B. Due to above facts there is reduction thrombocyte aggregation & adhesion, with less danger of thrombosis.

C High density lipoprotein (HDL), an important protective factor against arteriosclerosis gets strengthened. If we go in further details, especially HDL2 fraction, which is of special anti-arteriosclerotic importance gets improved.

On the other hand simultaneously Low Density lipoprotien (LDL) and triglycerides may be reduced, again having an anti selerotie effect.

Q.136. How metabolic activity in trained skeletal muscle improved ?

Ans. Increased myoglobin content.

Increase in the number and size of the mitochondria.

Increase activity by some anaerobic, but mainly aerobic enzymes.

Increase combustion of free fatty acids, with a reduced demand on enlarged glycogen stores.

Q.137. What is the Diagnostic value of exercise test ?

Ans. During the past 10 years, it is suggested that exercise E.C.G. obtained with gradually increasing load test may be used (bicycle or treadmill), in the interest of preventive medicine or life insurance or sports participation; to detect the subject in a population who are likely in the future, to show high morbidity and mortality from coronary disease. The results seem to be conclusive, particularly in the middle-age population and provided that the presence of a S.T. ischemic response taken as the only positive criterion. This seems to be the only statistically valuable index. The frequency of S.T. depression shows the expected increase, proportional to age and to the intensity of effort. On the contrary, the frequency of T wave abnormalities does not change with age or intensity of effort.

VALUE OF POSITIVE TEST :

Subjects which show S.T. change ischemic type during and after an exercise test seem to have higher probability of dying from coronary disease than the subjects who show no change. The magnitude of ischemic S.T. depression during and after exercise is directly correlated with the severity of coronary disease. An S.T. depression of less than 0.1 mV on maximum or near maximum effort, corresponds to a coronary group in question. A depression of 0.1-0.2 mV is at the same rate, while a depression of more than 0.2 mV would bear a 20 fold increase.

On the average, the probability of coronary deaths in subjects with S.T. ischemic depression is four times higher than in subjects showing no such change.

Q.138. Mention the symptoms of staleness.

Ans. (1) Occurs in endurance sports, such as cross-country racing, track, crew, swimming, wrestling.

(2) "Nonspecific" symptoms, such as fatigue, tiredness, sore throat.

(3) Physical findings are normal.

(4) Laboratory studies are for endurabce athletes.

(5) Psychological factors dominate; anxiety, depression, fatigue.

Q.139. What is the validity of the exercise test ?

Ans. It should be remembered that 'false negative' cases exist, i.e., subjects with a heart condition in whom exertional anginal pain develops without any specific change occurring in the E.C.G. There are also coronary patients whose resting E.C.G. is highly abnormal but who do not present any additional changes during exercise, or even during an attack of again. Further more, it should be mentioned that there are also a number of 'false positive' cases, i.e. clinical condition that in the absence of any organic pathology coronary changes may bring about or accentuate E.C.G. changes during exercise. The following may be mentioned in particular :

— relative or functional insufficiency of coronary output (e.g. left ventricular hypertrophy, mitral stensis),
— hormone imbalance (e.g. adrenal hyperfunction),
— haemoghlobindeficit or blocking (e.g. severe anaemia, increased level of carboxy-haemoglobin),
— impairment of oxygen transport (e.g. hypoxia),
— various drugs (e.g. epinephriue, digitalis, quinine, nicotine),
— meals (post-prandial, hypokalaemia, probably caused by insulin action),
— hyperventilation (changes of intercellular potassium concentration as aresult of respiratory alkalosis).

On the other hand, this may sometimes prevent or improve S.T. change due to neurocirculatory asthemia, left ventricular hypertrophy; pericarditis, or saturation with digitalis.

Many of these conditions, probably as a result of the hypokalaemia that they bring abou, may accentuate E.C.G. anomalies accompanying mild exercise even in the absence of coronary insufficiency. It is applied particularly to digitalis which because of the permeability of the cell-membrane, renders the interpretation of E.C.G. anomalies during exercise subject to considerable difficulty.

Q.140. Justify the relation of Physical Activity, Fat Balance and energy Balance, Keeping in mind the latest research in view.

Ans. For getting fat balance it is necessary to have a stable weight body composition. For this we must examine why fat balance is achieved at such widely differing levels of body fatness. Change in body fat mass itself help, fat balance. Any attempt to promote the healthy body weights should focus on reasons why a particular person can achieve fat balance at low level of fat mass while another person cannot.

Physical exercise can have major effects on both intake and oxidation of total energy and in particular on intake and oxidation of fat. Research data reveal a consistent relationship (negative) between level of physical activity and indices of obesity but do not provide clear evidence of a cause and effect relationship. So, increase in physical activity also increase the proportion of total oxzidation from fat and may decrease the proportion of ingested energy from fat. Due to this reason maintaining an active lifestyle should allow achievement of fat balance at a lower level of body fat mass than would occur with a sedentary life style.

CHAPTER SEVEN
NUTRITION

Q.1. **What do you understand by the word 'FAD' ?**

Ans. A fad is identified by a food or combination of foods that a declared to be beneficial or to serve as a cure. All fads are generally short-lived. They remain very popular for a period of time until replaced by another fad. The originate with individuals who are untutored in nutrition.

Q.2. **What do you understand by word nutrition charlatan ?**

Ans. Athletes have become prime targets for the profit, motivated surveyors of an almost limitless variety of so-called nutrition supplements, vit., proteins, and energy supplements so called health food, body building mixtures and other items. Even though they may know that a diet is optional in meeting the needs of an athlete, the trainer, the coach and the athletes themselves should know how to recognise the nutrition charlatan who is out to exploit the performance motivation of the sport participant.

Q.3. **How will you explain 'Fallacies regarding food' ?**

Ans. Fallacies in regard to food are based on misrepresentation misinterpretation and misinformation. Some folks, for example, believe that the only kind of sugar to be used is honey. Most of the athletes also consider honey as a better replacement of sugar. Many people are thus misinformed about the true nutritive value of food and are ignorant of the fact that the specific qualities cannot be attributed to foods.

A desire for a quick cure will lead many persons to eat a quantity of a certain food. An adolescent with a poor complexion, a man with arthritis, or a young woman who is over weight are potentials for believing that certain food or combination of foods will do miracles.

Q.4. **What is food quackery i.e. Silajeet for strength in weigh lifters. ?**

Ans. Food quackery : usually such people have a product to sell. Such products are offered as important dietary supplements, based on 'secret formulas'. They are sold at high prices and are urged upon the public with half truths and outright misinformation. I have seen many National weight lifters consuming 'Silajeet' for attaining more miraculous strength.

Q.5. Can you quote some examples of Fallacies related to the caloric value of food ?

Ans. Yes, here are a few examples :

1. Honey is not fattening. (The fact is that 1 table spoon gives calories.)
2. Vegetable fats or oils can be used in any amount and are not fattening. (Fact : It contains same caloric value as animal fats and are definitely fattening).

Fallacies related to combination of food :

1. Milk and fish together are poisonous or harmful.
2. Milk and orange juice will explode in the stomach.

Q.6. Can you suggest a few cheap food preparations, which are tasty and provide good quality nutrients ?

Ans. Spinach Soyabean Cutlets (A)

Ingredients :

Spinach	....	100 gms
Soyabean	....	30 gms
Potatoes	....	100 gms
Green Chillies	....	2-4
Bread crumbs	....	20 gms
Salt	....	to taste
Chilli powder	....	1/2 tea spoon
Mango powder	....	a pinch
Oil	....	25 gms

Nutritive Value :

Calories	....	478 Kcal
Protein	....	16.5 gms
Iron	....	15.1 mg
Carotene	....	5720 mg

Bengal Gram Leaf Roti (B)

Ingredients :

Wheat floor	....	200 gms
Bengal gram leaves	....	100 gms
Salt	....	a pinch

Fat	....	15 gms
Nutritive Value :		
Calories	....	914
Protein	....	31.2gms
Iron	....	46.8 mg
Carotene	....	1480 mg

Source : ICMR, Hyderabad.

Q.7. What are the common points to be remembered regarding food ?

Ans. Points to be remembered : Points to be remembered are :

— Leafy vegetables are a rich store-house of many nutrients.

— Leafy vegetables protect our eyes.

— Leafy vegetables supply roughage useful for good digestion and maintain healthy skin and beautiful complexion.

— Leafy vegetables help children to grow and develop.

— Leafy vegetables help in building strong bones, healthy teeth and gums.

— Cook leafy vegetables carefully to preserve all the nutrients.

— Wash leafy vegetables before chopping.

— Avoid excess of water for cooking-because excess of water will leak out the nutrients.

— Do not throw away the water in which the vegetables have been cooked since it is rich in nutrients.

— Use it in dals, soups or making dough if left.

— Cook leafy vegetables for a short time. Too much cooking destroys nutrients.

— Cook them when covered by lid.

— Avoid deep frying of leafy vegetables.

— Consume food immediately after cooking.

— Use leafy vegetables throughout the year by dehydrating them when available in plenty.

— Grow as much leafy vegetables as you can throughout the year.

— Eat at least one leafy vegetable every day.

Q.8. Why do most of the housewives feel weak and tired though they have sufficient amount of weight ?

Ans. It has been found among many athletes that they have fair amount of Haemoglobin in their blood but still they feel weak. It is because during the course of blood loss, stored iron has ben used to generate new haemoglobin and so the tonic iron which is also required for many other metabolic reactions falls short, and so if proper bio-chemical investigations are not performed for the estimation of iron, the cause of weakness remains unknown.

Probably the above mentioned mechanism is responsible for the feeling of generalized weakness among a housewife.

Q.9. Give your comments on young female athletes (Gymnasts) and food intake i.e. Nutrition.

Ans. In my opinion some gymnasts face difficulties associated with the female athlete triad; eating disorders poor bone development and amenorrhora. To help guarantee successful communication with the athlete, her coach, parents and the nutritionist should use an approach that emphasises athletic performance. Example, significant energy deficit during training or sports are likely to impact negatively on performance. It may further reduce metabolic rate, may encourage the gymnast to eat still less food so creating a cycle of even greater deficits and enhancing the likelyhood that the athlete will eventually fall into a serious disordered eating pattern. Increase frequency of meals will diminish the likelyhood of significant energy deficit so she can improve her performance also. It will also help intake of greater nutrient that are important of normal bone development and normal menstruation function. So it seems necessary to take care of diet of ellite athlete in the mentioned contest.

Q.10. Explain in brief how obesity develops and also mention its harmful effects.

Ans. It shortens the life span, restricts joyful movements and exposes one to heart diseases, diabetes etc.

Once obesity has developed, treatment is much more difficult because its nature is to perpetuate itself.

The number of calories spent each day in addition to those spent to keep the body functioning depends on the kind of work a person does and the kind of activities he is engaged in leisure time.

Q.11. What are the causes of obesity ? Why do certain people even take exercise but are not able to control their weight ?

Ans. The earliest contributory factor, i.e., parental nutrition may activate a genetic tendency towards overweight. When on parent is over weight there are 50% chances that the child will be obese. The probability is increased to 80% when both the partners are fat. Studies of adolescent girls reveal a familiar and probably genetic predisposition to the development of obesity with normal food intake. Actually speaking, many middle aged obese do not eat more than a person with normal weight, yet they are obese.

A pattern of obesity can be established in infancy. Over feeding an infant produces a fat baby who tends successively to become a plump child, an obese adolescent and an overweight adult. Yet many parents for sociological and psychological reasons, find a prime source of satisfaction and pride in their body showing a more rapid growth and weight gain than other children. Similarly maturation will occur at an early age.

Q.12. Mention the point for loosing body fat ?

Ans.

1. Remember it require an excess expenditure of 3500 kcal in order to lose 1 pound of pure fat.
2. It is recommended that the caloric deficit not exceed 2000 to 2500 Kcal/day or 4 pounds of fat per week. An ideal loss is 2 to 3 pounds per week. An attempt to estimate daily or weekly caloric intake and expenditure should be made.
3. The caloric deficit should represent both an increased expenditure and a reduced caloric intake. A caloric deficit that is solely the result of diet restriction will also cause fat-free weight loss.
4. For most active athletes, the lower limits of a restricted diet is a 2000-kcal intake per day. Coloric reduction below this level should be medically supervised.

Q.13. Why do the players, after reducing weight start gaining weight quickly if they reduce the activity ?

Ans. Recent investigations have established that in the very obese person, chiefly the number and also the size of adipose cells are greater at a time than normal. The cells of non-obese adults contain 0.605540439 mg of lipid and the cell number (26.83 +1.77) x 107. For obese subjects the lipid cell content is 0.9088 + 0.0828 mg and there are three times as many cells as (77.02 +13.47) x 10. Weight loss in the obese adult following calorie restrictions can only reduce the size of fat cells but does not influence their number which remain fairly constant. This decrease in cell size is not permanent, and it is rapidly restored when restrictions are lifted. As a result, the individual may be morphologically more abnormal after weight loss than before. Therefore, prevention in early life, in childhood, through control of the factors which influence number of size of adipose cells may be the only effective treatment.

Q.14. How moderate exercise helps better than passive procedures in recovery amount of athletes ?

Ans. Moderate exercise performed during recovery appears to facilitate recovery process compared to passive procedures. In most situations, this is reflected in a faster removal of lactic acid.

Q.15. Does obesity have something to do with Metabolic defects ?

Ans. It can be discussed in the following manner :

(a) Metabolic defects :

There is no defect in basal metabolism that can account for obesity outside the known metabolic laws. Investigations have shown nothing which makes it possible for obese people to perform work on less energy than normal or under weight. On the contrary, they spend more energy in performing the same measured amount of work than do normal or underweight subjects (averaging about four calories for each pound of excess of weight)

(b) Specific dynamic action :

Food itself causes an increase in metabolism, which is called dynamic action. This extra or waste heat can neither be converted into muscular exercise nor can be stored as fat. If this dynamic action of food is absent in some persons they would have a tendency to put on fat as compared to others with a normal specific dynamic action. But all investigations under properly controlled conditions have failed to demonstrate any defect in obese.

Q.16. Does weight gain among weight category of athletes have some relation with appetite ?

Ans. Obesity is invariably caused by a greater intake of calories in food than the expenditure of calories as energy. This disproportion results from an appetite for food that is greater than required to maintain normal weight.

Mostly we enjoy such an appetite and regulation mechanism which balances the intake of calories with the expenditure automatically and perfectly. When activity is greater than usual or when tissue is being added as in growth in recuperation from an acute illness, such people automatically eat more. When their expenditure of calories is less, they eat less. If they occasionally eat more one day or at one meal than is needed because of instant hostess they consciously eat less at the next meal. The automatic weight regulating mechanism which operates through appetite is amazingly efficient. Many people go throughout the life without over consciously restricting their food intake or consciously increasing their exercise. The appestat is located in hypothalamus. Atrophy of pituary gland is seen in Simmond's disease which causes the appestat to be set for a low level of food consumption and subsequently emaciation follows.

Q.17. What do you mean by economic and uneconomic food ?

Ans. The hypothesis is expounded that food calorie estimated in a calorimeter is not equal to one nutritional calorie since the body is not a calorimeter and metabolism may higher produce a positive energy balance called economic eating or a negative balance called under economic eating because more energy may have to be expended on breaking down the food than was contained in the food itself. The production of digestive juice consumes a lot of energy. Examples of economic food are soft boiled egg, warm fat in clear soup, orange juice etc., while examples of uneconomic food are hard boiled egg, salad etc.

Q.18. Some young players are labelled as habitual over-eaters. What does it mean ?

Ans. Repeated over-feeding beyond satiety eventually results in the setting of the appestat at a level so high that satisfaction can no longer be obtained by normal food intake. When the appestat is conditioned or set at a higher level the person is not conscious of overeating. This is the physiological explanation of why most of the obese people deny overeating and in their own mind do so truthfully.

Habitual overeating may come solely from environment. In the household where a laden table is regularly set and where the quantity and quality of the food are over-emphasized by constant conversation about it, eating beyond satiety is frequent.

Frequent or habitual use of alcohol is another common cause of an elevated appestat.

Purposeful overeating also occurs through ignorance. It is a popular misconception that eating beyond energy or growth requirement will give added strength. No popular belief is more fallacious than this Excessive calorie consumption whether in children or adults leads to fatness.

Q.19. What is Broca's Index ?

Ans. Standard weight in Kg =Height in centimetres minus 100. This does not take body build into consideration. Anyone weighing more than 10% of their standard weight is considered overweight and over 20% is considered to be obese.

Q.20. Mention basic paints for weight control of a team ?

Ans.
1. Identify the level of fatness associated with elite performances in the specific sport.
2. Project a desired competing weight per each individual. Athlete and on body weight and an estimated level of body fatness.
3. Project a rate of reduction of body fat for each individual to achieve "competing weight" based on existing level of fatness.
4. Initiate the fatness reduction programme prior to the season so that a desired level of fatness will be achieved with weight reduction of no more than 2 or 3 pounds each week.

5. Create the necessary negative energy balance with a controlled modest reduction in food energy intake combined with a significant increase in energy expenditure as preseason conditioners activities.
6. Monitor the progress of fatness reduction with periodic skin-fat fold measures and weight determinations.

Q.21. What are the common approaches to weight reduction?

Ans. The most common methods of reducing obesity are :-

Reduced food intake.

Regulated physical exercise.

It takes about 3500 extra calories to produce a pound of stored fat. For each pound to be gained or lost there must be 3500 calories more or less in the diet than the body uses. For example to lose 2 pounds a week, a person would have to consume 7000 calories less per week or 1000 calories less per day. A person, whose calorie-need is 2400 a day, will have to cut down to 1400/ day.

Reducing diet :

It can be said that the quantity of food what one is taking should be halved to start with. Appetite is better controlled by taking small quantities of food frequently. Fat, ghee, butter, eggs, fried foods, gravies, alcohol, sweets and potatoes should be avoided as far as possible. Leafy vegetables such as cabbage, spinach, lettuce etc. are useful being high residue low calorie diet. Milk is better if taken in skimmed form.

Initially this is due to loss of excess of water content of the obese person as evidenced by frequency of micturition and polyuria. There after the weight remains somewhat stationary for about a couple of months when the system adopts itself to the new weight and then one starts to lose weight again, In this way, when desired weight is reached, one should try to maintain it.

Obesity is never resistant to a low calorie diet but the patient himself is resistent to dieting.

Heavy exercise in reducing weight defeats its purpose, because it increases the appetite. It is said to lose a pound of body weight by exercise one has to walk 36 miles. This is not possible but moderate exercise with controlled appetite is always advocated. Walking one mile a day is sufficient to reduce the load of one pound of fat in about a month if one does not over eat.

Q.22. What other suggestions can be given to weight reducers ?

Ans. Suggestions for weight reducers :

1. Persons who are considerably overweight should reduce it. Those who are only a little overweight may need not reduce it. They should only watch their diet so that they do not put on more weight.
2. If you intend to start a reducing programme, it is wise to consult doctor and check whether you are in good physical condition for reducing it.
3. Take it easy. A loss of pound or two per week is enough.
4. Plan meals around familiar foods. The only effective diet is the one which has been followed faithfully. Hence select foods that give satisfaction and are part of family way of eating.
5. When you have achieved the desired weight, simple additions can be made to the diet so that you can maintain weight at a desirable level. It is important to establish patterns of eating that can be followed when desirable weight is attained. Undersirable foods and attractive combinations may seem to be an alarmous solution to the dieters' problems but they are nearly unacceptable as regular affairs. As a result the dieter may soon be discouraged and go back to the old food habits that will result in weight gain. It is important not to skip meals as this may lead to indiscriminate snacking.
6. Many reducing diets which includes only a few foods are inadequate in essential nutrients. Such diets should not be followed for any length of time.
7. Choose lower calorie foods, avoid such items as sugar added gravies, sauces, fried foods, fatty meats, sweets, pasteries, cookies, cakes, alcohol, soft drinks and creams, Learn to like cereals of fruits with little or no added sugar and cream.
8. Budget your calories to take care of your special occasions such as holiday meals or parties. Save

calories from other meals to allow extra calories for such occasions. Keep busy so that you may not be tempted to eat foods which are not included in your planned meals.

9. Take advantage of daily opportunities to increase the physical activities.

SMOKING

I. Smoking is used as a custom, loathsome to the eyes, hateful to nose, harmful to brain and dangerous lungs.

II. What is smoke ? When a cigarette is lighted, the smoke that is produced contains various vaporized chemicals and millions of minute particles of ash and other solids. During smoking, when the smoke is inhaled, these are drawn into nose, throat and lungs.

III. Nicotine is the most important constituent of tobacco and its content varies from 0.5 to 8.0%. Cigarette tobacco on an average contains about 1.5% of nicotine and the smoke of the average cigarette may yield several therapeutic doses of nicotine (6 to 8 mg.) The smoke of a 10 gm. cigar may contain from 15 to 40 mg. of nicotine.

IV. Most commercial denicotinized tobacco still contains significantly large amounts of alkaloid.*

V. Approximately 90% of the nicotine in inhaled smoke is absorbed. Cigarette smokers who inhale 60 mg. of nicotine after smoking a package of 20 cigarettes while non-inhalers inhale only 7mg.

* Ref: Three enermies by Dr. L.C. Gupta

VI. Another poison is carbon monoxide which is a deadly gas in exhaust fumes. It is the product of incomplete combustion. On an average carbon monoxide comprises from 1% to 2.5% of the volume of cigarettes smoke.

BAD EFFECTS OF SMOKING

Smoker's Throat :

There are number of constituents in tobacco smoke in sufficient concentration to set up an irritation in the throat, the delicate mucous membrane becomes inflammed which induces cough, often of a very persistent character. There is no medical treatment for this condition and as long as the victim smokes, so long his cough persists.

Chronic Bronchitis :

Cigarette smoke paralyses the tiny hair which line the bronchial tubes that sweep foreign particles out of lung. Without this protective action, healthy lung tissue can be injured. Hence cigarette smcke is the most important predisposing cause of chronic bronchitis of cough and expectoration is closely related to the number of cigarettes smoked. These symptoms usually abate rapidly in those who stopped smoking. Smoking may cause and aggravate existing emphysema and flares up tuberculosis.

Effect on Vocal Cords and Larynx :

Specific changes in cells in the epithelium of the larynx were not often observed in the area below vocal cords. The histologic changes including cells with a typical nuclei, carcinoma in situ and early invasive carcinoma are highly related to smoking habit. These conditions are much higher in cigarette smokers than in those who never smoked. They increase in proportion to the number of cigarettes smoked per day and are seen to a greater degree in cigarette smokers than in cigar and pipe smokers. Cells with disintegrated nuclei are found in ex-smokers.

Pre-cancerous :

Chewing and smoking habits are correlated with the presence of lichen planus found among tobacco chewers than among those with no such habits. Lichen planus is located in the buccal mucous, more posteriorly than usual. Histologically an unusual atrophic epithelium, lichen planus and submucous fibrosis are precancerous in nature.

Lung Cancer :

The relationship of cigarette smoking to lung cancer is so overwhelmingly documented that the epidemiological approaches and laboratory data need not prove it. Chemical carcinogens and pulmonary irritants have been identified. Tobacco tars have induced cancer in animal models. Irritants present in tobacco smoke have been shown to significantly interfering with the function of the mucociliary apparatus in the respiratory tract as well as after the functional capability of pulmonary macrophages.

Cancer has been shown to increase with the increase of smoking. Even more important is the repeated observations that cessation of smoking is associated with a reduction in the risk of this disease. Compared to the non-smokers, average smokers have about 20 folds risk of developing the disease. The risk for pipe and cigar smokers are less and that for hookah smokers is still less.

Each cigarette contains a minimum of 19 different poisons which get into blood stream making heart's action difficult. Just one puff of cigarette contracts even tiniest capillary. Pulse increases upto 20 beats per minute and this increase lasts for 10 to 20 minutes after cessation of smoking. Blood pressure rises from 1 to 20 points.

While doing Electrocardiogram (E.C.G.) the most striking change is the configuration of the 'T' waves. These were lowered and sometimes inverted in leads II and III.

The nicotine entering the body by smoking of just one cigarette is sufficient to reduce the skin temperature of the hands and feet by three or four degrees as it reduces the blood flow through blood vessels of reduced size. If one smokes and drinks alcohol at the same time, the effect of 6 pegs of whisky as vasodilatory will be balanced by the vasoconstricting effect of two cigarettes.

Smokers die more often fro coronary heart disease. Myocardial infarcts may be associated with severe symptoms in heavy smokers. It depends, to some extent, on alteration in blood flow due to various mechanisms and not entirely on the degree of sclerosis. In other words, cigarette smokers may be more vulnerable than non-smokers with an equal degree of arterial narrowing. The use of tobacco apparently aggravates or precipitates attacks of angina. Some patients develop thromboangitis when they use tobacco and it remains active as long as they continue its use in any form. The habit is difficult for some people to break. It is on record that patients warned repeatedly to abstain from using tobacco continued to smoke even though they suffered agonising pain from gangrene and multiple amputations until in the most extreme cases they were left without either leg. Relapses in thrombo-angitis obiliterans may occur when patients smoke the filtered cigarettes.

Heavy smoking can cause an accelerated coagulative tendency with deposition of fibrin on arterial walls with incorporation of this fibrin to develop atherosclerotic plaques in larger arteries and thrombotic occlusion of small arteries.

Blood Sugar :

Smoking is being blamed for transitory rise of blood sugar level. An example of the magnitude of this rise has been shown by Heggard & Greenberg. The control blood sugar value was 95 mg% whereas following the smoking of a single cigarettes the blood sugar level rose steadily to 160 mg per cent.

Effect on Gastro Intestinal System :

Carlson was the first to observe that the gastric hunger contraction may be inhibited as long as 15 to 16 minutes following a few puffs of a cigarette. Under basal condition, when one cigarette is smoked there may be three different responses. In one third of the subjects there is immediate cessation of stomach motility, while some may have no effect. Last 1/2 may show hypermotility of stomach contraction. Augmentation of bowel function is noted in the last group.

A rise in total gastric acidity is noted in 60% smokers. The percentage is reduced to 23 only if they smoke fittered cigarette.

In about 90% of peptic ulcer cases, there is an increase in free hydrochloric acid and total acidity. Hence in peptic ulcer smoking will result in increased motility and concomitant epigastric pain.

Heart burn is the most common complaint amongst smokers. Eructation, anorexia, nausea, flatulance and epigastric distress also occurs but to a lesser degree.

Effect on Central Nervous System :

It may be said that the effect of a single cigarette on Central Nervous System is equivalent to that of two ounces of whisky.

Effect on Mucous Gland.

Smoking is associated with increase in size of the mucous glands as measured by the ratio of the thickness of bronchial wall and depth of the gland. Smoking causes hypersecretion of mucous and hypertrophy of the mucous glands which in turn leads to the damage of mucous membrane. Even one to six years after leaving smoking, smoke spirals are seen in sputum.

Smokers need more Red Blood Cells.

Normally oxygen is taken into the lungs and carried by the haemoglobin in the blood to the cells of the body. When carbon-monoxide, which is present in the exhaust fumes of the cigarette, is breathed in it unites with the haemoglobin preventing it from picking up oxygen and thereby depriving the body of oxygen. Smoking 20 cigarettes a day results in upto 10% carbon-monoxide saturation of the blood and blood is now able to carry only nine-tenth of its normal amount of oxygen resulting in severe headache. In order to compensate the needed oxygen, the body has to manufacture extra red cells which in turn may lead to thicker blood. This blood will clot more easily explaining why smokers suffer from a higher rate of heart attack than non-smokers.

Longevity :

Smoking one cigarette reduce life by at least 11 minutes. A man who smokes an average of 40 cigarettes per day will live on an average eleven years less than the one who does not smoke.

Cost of Smoke ;

On 20 cigarettes a day, a man would spend over about Rs. 750/- a year, i.e.,1500 in twenty years and later on is likely to develop cancer of the lung.

Mental Efficiency :

Cigarette smoking impedes simple reaction time for a short period. Smoking immediately before performing a motor skill, requiring quick reactions, probably reduces the performance level.

Effect on Pregnancy :

It is known that some of the toxic substances in the tobacco smoked by the mother actually reach the blood and tissues of her unborn child. It has been reported that the heart beat of an unborn child responds to the mother's smoking in very much the same way as the heart of an adult by significantly increased heart rate.

Babies born to women who smoke during pregnancy are on an average 150 gm lighter than those of non-smokers. There may be still born babies or they die soon after birth or there may be an abortion. One in five babies may be saved if mothers had not smoked.

Prevention :

Please prcctice :

(i) Smoke fewer cigarettes.
(ii) Inhale less frequently and less deeply.
(iii) Take fewer puffs from each cigarette.
(iv) Remove the cigarette from the mouth between putts.
(v) Smoke cigarette of low tar and nicotine content.

Think again, still you are not late and even now if you decide not to smoke, you would not have that pungent smell which makes your breath offensive to others, shortness of breath and choking cough every morning, premature wrinkling over the face and the nicotine straining which colour your fingers' skin.

ALCOHOLISM

Alcohol destroys the total man physically, socio-economically, mentally and spiritually. It involves him in his social, cultural professional and religious life.

Dangers of Alcohol :

Social life :

Alcoholism is prone to people whose socialisation was disturbed in childhood because of the loss of a parent, or lack of affection etc. However, it is the micro-culture of the parental, familial and later reference group which offer restrained drinking as a solution to life problems.

Social drinking ends and problem drinking begins when man wants to drink alone and develop aptitude for it. An alcoholic invariably acts out of character in a variety of areas, for example, a punctual person becomes careless, the neat becomes untidy, the truthful person starts fabricating fantastic stories. A kind and compassionate parent may become vicious and brutal towards his loved ones. It is responsible for divorces and separations, in black mailing, in family quarrels and plays a decisive role in producing emotional ill-health.

Alcoholics are social isolates, more depressed and less active

Crime :

The exists a direct and indirect relation between crime and alcohol. Alcohol can predispose the individual to become a victim as well as make him to commit criminal offences, e.g. homicide, murders, crime against property and sex. 16% cases of chronic alcoholics at one time or the other are likely to develop suicidal tendencies.

Mental Disease :

Six percent alcoholics may suffer from schizophrenia. Old men suffer more often from brain syndrome and alcoholism than old women who show a higher incidence of affective psychosis and neurosis. From the psychodynamics view point, depressive elements predominate among female alcoholics while those of a homosexual nature are less evident in females than in male alcoholics.

Memory :

After an acute prolonged alcohol intake, an amnesia (Loss of memory) of several hours occurs. It involves a short term memory defect while immediate and remote memory remains intact. Hence patient can carry on conversation and even drive a car but cannot remember what was said a minute ago. Short term memory is significantly and progressively impaired with increasing levels of intoxication.

Appetite :

It ruins appetite although in low concentration before dinner. It may increase the hunger contractions. The loss of appetite gradually grows and progresses to the stage of semi-starvation. The energy the drinker collects from alcohol leaves little appetite for food. As a result, the essential elements of nutrition are crowded out and the boy suffers nutritional deficiency. Outwardly, the person may show an appreciable fatty layer under the skin.

Obesity :

Alcohol is a ready source of energy and its utilization does not involve as much biochemical processing as does the utilization of the other substances. That is why some individuals, who over a period of years, are able to substitute alcohol for food to a surprising degree and yet remain well. But the persons who maintain food intake as usual, become fat due to the consumption of extra calories derived from drinks. Each ounce of whisky yield about 64 calories.

Sex :

As regards sexual performance, alcohol gives a desire but takes away its performance. As per statistics more than 30% alcoholics are involved in sex crimes unknowingly and knowingly.

Liver :

Alcohol seriously injuries the liver, the organ without which a man cannot live. Within the body, the liver breaks down fats and proteins into elements from which the body derives its energy. It is associated with the process of blood coagulation, protection against infection and many others. Damaged by alcohol leads to liver cirrohosis, a grave condition where an organ is loaded with fat and is disabled.

Brain damage :

The scientists determined that alcohol affects the brain by depriving it of oxygen. A drinker who consumes enough alcohol to become stuporous suffers a number of small brain haemorrhages and larger number of plugged capillaries. Around each of these plugs some of the brain cells die and infarcts are formed.

That social drinker may knock out brain cells every time he drinks was the most shocking part of the information given by Dr. Kingsley. Also shocking is the fact the occasional drinker incurs some loss of brain cells every time he drinks. Worst of all, these cells are lost for ever.

Vision :

Blue and yellow colour vision disturbances are more in alcoholics. Eighty per cent of the patients with chronic alcoholism and alcoholic psychosis acquire deficient colour vision. Anomalous colour vision was principally red/ green deficiency due to lesions of the visual pathway. Colour vision is disturbed more markedly than visual acuity. Direct toxic effects of alcohol are responsible for the pathogenesis of alcoholic myelopathy.

Optokinetic reactions (movements of eye balls) :

Alcohol inhibits optokinetic reactions in comparison to control group. The observed post-alcoholic changes in vestibular and optokinetic reactions are objective evidence of diminished fitness of individuals under the influence of even small dose of alcohol for work requiring perfect and integrated function of sense of equilibrium and sight.

Cholesterol/serum proteins :

Consumption of 3ml. of 30% aqueous ethyl alcohol daily for 2 months causes 74-80% increase in blood cholesterol in adults. On withdrawing alcohol, cholesterol level comes down to normal in four weeks. Increased serum cholesterol level has been blamed for atherosclerosis and subsequent heart diseases.

There is also a decrease in the serum albumin and an increase in free amino-acids of serum in alcohol fed rats indicating an impairment of protein metabolism.

Q.23. Is there any difference among Male and Female Players regarding Carbohydrate Loadings ?

Ans. Yes, A recent research study shows it :

The study show that female may not have the same magnitude of response to CHO loading as males.

A standard CHO loading protocol (4 days of diet at 75% of energy from CHO VS 4 days of habitual CHO intake (57%) upon muscle glycogen stores, time to cycling fatigue at 85% VO_2 ma, and the metabolic response to running for 60 minutes at 75% of VO_2 in 7 males and 8 female athletes. CHO loading increased muscle glycogen stores for male by 41% but not for females (0%), and time to exhaustion shows parallel changes for males (45% increase in males, $P<.05$, and a 5% increase in females $P>.05$). In addition females oxidired more lipid and less CHO and protein than did males in response to the 60 minute exercise trial. So, metabolic response to endurance exercise is different for males and females.

Q.24. What and why there is need of extra care of water and Electrolyte Replenishment in exercising child ?

Ans. Following points may be kept in mind :

1. In comparison to adults children's sweat has lower concentration Na^+ & Cl^- and somewhat higher concentration of K^+ and lactate.
2. From child to adult pattern should be kept in mind at Midschool level competitions.
3. Dehydration is accomplanied by a faster core temperature increase among children.
4. The volume of voluntary rehydration in a thermo neutral environment, following mild dehydration

(exercise in hot whether), is higher with grape and orange flavoured beverages than with apple flavoured beverage or water.

5. Addition of grape flavour to water, when compared with plane water, increases ad libitum drinking volume by 44.5% in children who exercise intermittently i.e. three hours total exposure time in a hot climate.
6. There opinion may or may not be time or valid for children with acute infections leading to vomitting and or diarrhora.

CHAPTER EIGHT
NUTRIENTS AND DRUGS

Q.1. What are the signs and symptoms of Ageing ?

Ans. Following changes indicate that ageing process has set in :

1. Muscle power starts decreasing. Grip of hand in the aged people will be less than the younger age grip.
2. Greying of hair and their loss. This is more common in men than women. Though heredity is also a factor, this is not a sure and certain sign but when compared for the same individual, it indicates ageing process.
3. Reading becomes difficult. One has to adjust the distance between the eyes and the book or newspaper. It is popularly known as presbiopia.
4. Difficulty in hearing low pitch sounds.
5. Changes take place in heart and blood vessels. Total functional efficiency of all organs shows gradual deterioration.
6. Reduction in height may be observed due to flattening in the cartilaginous discs of vertebrae.
7. Digestion and absorption also show the decline.
8. Loss of fat from underneath the skin-causing wrinkles on face and other places.
9. Power to remember becomes poor although old people are quoted to remember past events better than recent happenings.

Q.2. What do you understand by "energy" ?

Ans. Energy is defined as the ability to perform work and therefore is revealed only when change takes place. Energy exits in either a potential or kinetic form. Potential energy is the energy associated with substances because of structure or position, whereas kinetic energy is the energy of motion. Potential energy is measured when it is transformed into kinetic energy. There are six forms of energy: chemical, mechanical, heat, light, electric and nuclear. Each form of energy can be formed into another form.

Q.3. Suggest basic points which makes a champion ?

Ans.
1. Condition.
2. Will to win.
3. Physically tougher than opponent.
4. Execution of fundamentals.
5. Fewer errors.

Q.4. Mention the opinions about use of drugs in sports ?

Ans.
(1) There are no drugs that improve performance definitely.
(2) Some drugs improve performance and thus provide an unfair advantage for the user.
(3) Such drugs are dangerous to health.

Q.5. How ATP-CP provides energy in different types of exercise ?

Ans. The major means of ATP production differ depending on the intensity and duration of exercise. In intense exercise of short duration (100 yd. dash) (weight lifting), the energy is derrived from already present stores of intramuscular ATP and CP (immediate energy system). For intense exercise of longer duration (1-2 min.), energy is generated mainly from the anarobic reactions of glycosis is (short term energy system). As exercise progresses beyond several minutes, the aerobic system predominates and oxygen consumption becomes an important factor (Long-term energy system).

Q.6. What are the important factors responsible for Ageing?

Ans. These changes depend on the following factors :
1. Heredity : It is an important factor. Like greying of hair, certain diseases like hypertension, coronary heart disease and diabetes may have hereditary linkage.
2. Nutrition : Balanced food habits also play an important role in ageing, as many of the atophic changes, in old age are attributed to nutrition.
3. State of physical activity : Whether over or under-activity both has been found to hasten the process of ageing.
4. Environment : It is as important as the above three. Calm and quiet place with plenty of fresh air to

breathe will reduce tension of modern hectic life, whereas polluted air, noise and heavy fatty food will create problems.

5. Mental make-up : It is another factor influencing ageing. If one is always tense at his home, office or other places, it is going to affect his body. One's attitude towards, these day to day problems should be easy and relaxed, no matter how many and how big these problems are.

Q.7. Explain some common exercises which help in prevention of ageing.

Ans. To help the process of slowing down gaining, certain exercises were tried on people who were between 35-40 years. Ageing cannot be stopped but can be slowed down or delayed. Exercises could not change the colour of hair but they certainly brought some shining on the face. Stamina, physical functions and ability showing better performance have been noticed.

Exercise 1 : Take a slant board which raises the foot end about 2 feet higher than the head. Lie down on the board and relax completely. Lick fingers of one hand into fingers of the other. Pull arms out away from each other as hard as possible, simultaneously press small of the back into the board while lifting the head up and breath count up to 20. Return to the starting position and relax. Remember this exercise is the greatest antidote to the ageing pull of gravity.

Exercise 2 : Stretching is best prevention. A caged animal does not bother about exercise, still he stays limber and supply. Lie down on the floor and stretch slowly in every direction at least 10 times and relax. Repeat it once or twice a day.

Exercise 3 : Walking - It is another miracle. Walking every day and in every weather is the best exercise for aged people. Idea is to walk at least two miles a day but fast walk.

Exercise 4 : Breathing exercises - Preferably in the morning and in open place, if available, like a lawn or roof top. Keep both hands on the sides of the chest. Take a long deep breath through the nose, hold count upto five and breathe out through the mouth, simultaneously pressing the walls of chest with hands. Repeat it 10 times in one sitting every day.

Exercise 5 : Expand the cheeks - Fill air in between the cheeks, try to hold as long as possible. This is the best way to deny the forming of wrinkles from corner of nose to corner of lips.

Exercise 6 : Crows Feet - Small lines due to loosening of the skin emerge around the eyes. Move gently middle or index finger or the hand below the eyes from inner side of the eyes towards the ears for about 5 minutes. Do it every day.

Q.8. How to organise the right sports diet ?

Ans. The energy requirement of an athlete depends on the following factors.

The right sports diet should have adequate provision for the following:

(a) Quantity : Calories according to sports.
(b) Quality : Carbohydrates, protein, Fat. Vitamins, Mineral and Fluids.
(c) Variety : Different types of foods.
(d) Palatability : Proper cooking.
(e) Acceptability : To suit different customs, habits and tastes.

Following table shows approximate percentage of calories which may derived from different components of nutrients:

	Carbohydrates	Protein	Fat
(a) Light Sports	60%	15%	25%
(b) Moderate Sports	60%	14%	26%
(c) Heavy Sports	60%	13%	27%
(d) Endurance Sports	60%	12%	28%

Q.9. What factors should be kept in mind while organising or planning a diet schedule for a particular group ?

Ans. (a) Age : The energy requirement of adolescents and adults are greater than that of children and old people. Most of the active sportsmen belong to the growing age group of adolescents and adults. A recent study of Olympians has shown that 81% of Olympic champions are below 30 years of age, 15% between 30-42 years of age and the rest 4% are above 42 years of age.

(b) Sex : All other factors remaining constant, the energy requirement of women is relatively less than that of men.

(c) Body weight : Energy requirement is directly proportional to the body weight. It increases or decreases according to type of activity and muscles involved during exercise period.

(d) Climate and Environment : In hot and humid environment the energy requirement is less. Higher the altitude and colder the climate, greater the energy requirement. Athletes, who undertake regular motivated physical exercises, develop the capacity to lose heat efficiently. The physical performance of athletic supremacy depends on the ability of the athlete to get rid of excess heat generated during exercise from his body efficiently.

(e) Physical Activities (Sports & Games) : The energy requirement of an athlete depends on the intensity, duration and type of his activities. Based on these factors, sports could be grouped under four categories:

(i) Group I: Light Sports, Sedentary Sports or Skill Games :

These involve high skill, minimum strength and low endurance. The muscie effort of this group is equivalent to the effort involved in walking 2 miles/hr. e.g., Archery, Shooting, Billiards, Bridge, Chess, Carroms.

The energy requirement. The energy requirement of athletes doing these sports would be 50 calories/kgm body weight/day.

(ii) Group II : Moderate Sports : These sports involve skill, moderate strength and moderate endurance. The muscular effort of this group is equivalent to walking 4 miles/hr. e.g., Badminton, Cricket, Golf, Gymnastics, Kabaddi, Kho-Kho, Table Tennis, Tennis, Short Distance Swimming and tract and field events like Spring, Hurding, Jumping and Throwing.

Energy requirement : 6 calories/kgm body weight/ day.

(iii) Group III : Heavy Sports : They involve skill, high strength and high endurance. The muscular effort is equivalent to waling 6 miles/hr., e.g., Boxing, Wresting,

Football, Hockey, Handball, Cycling, Squash, Waterpool Fast bowling in Cricket, Weight lifting, Middle distance running, Middle distance Swimming. Decathlon and Pentathlon.

Energy requirement : 70 calories/kgm body weight/ day.

(iv) Group IV : Endurance Sports : They involve skill, moderate strength and extreme endurance. The muscular effort is equivalent to walking milles/hr. e.g., Marathon, Cross country running, Long distance walking Channel swimming, Mountaineering and Rowing.

Energy requirement : 90 calories/kgm body weight/ day.

The energy requirement of different groups above are calculated based on the athlete's actual physical training hours (4 hrs/day). During of season, when he is not doing active training, his energy requirement considerably less and is calculated as for sedentary sports of moderate sports depending on what types of activities he is doing to maintain his fitness during that period.

For women athletes, the energy requirement would be 2-3 calories per kgm body weight less than that of men.

Note : The above mentioned recommendations are the recent ones and made by the top level committee on sports nutrition in India.

Q.10. What do you know about quality of sports diet ?

Ans. Here the basic principle remains the same with slight variation. The quality of a sports diet depends on the correct proportion of carbohydrates, proteins, fats, mineral salts and vitamins which constitute the main nutrients of the diet.

Proteins : Proteins are the main body building foods and they form the main constituents of muscles, tissues and blood. They supply the building material for the body during the growth process and also repair the wear and tear of the muscles, ligaments and tendons. Hence they are most essential for an active athlete. The ideal sports diet should have both animal and vegetable proteins in adequate quantities. 1gm of protein yields 4 calories of energy.

Carbohydrates : Carbohydrates form the main bulk of the sportsman's diet and are the main sources of energy for physical activities Carbohydrates could be easily oxidised for energy production and as such are the sources of 'instant energy' for athletic activities. This is the reason why athletes are advised to take glucose during physical activities. 1gm of carbohydrate yields 4 calories of energy. Here glucose should be taken a specific dilution in water. Eating large amount of glucose powder during an event may be harmful also.

Fat : Fat is the most concentrated source of energy and 1gm of yields 9 calories which is more than double the energy yielded carbohydrates or proteins.

Physical activity and vigorous exercise appear to help the fat in the diet without much increase in the blood cholesterol which could be the reason why active sportsmen are less prone to high blood pressure and heart attacks.

This explains the recent craze amongst people all over the world towards jogging, Swimming, Tennis etc. Here one thing may be advised. As far as possible consume unsaturated fats like saffola oil, groundnut oil etc.

Q.11. Give Comments about protien intake in the diet ?

Ans. Precise recommendations for fat and carbohydrate intake have not been established. A prudent recommendation is that 30% of the daily calories be obtained from fats, of this half should be in the form of unsaturated fatly acids because excessive intake of saturated fats is related to various disease, especially coronary heart disease. For people who are physically active, atleast 50% to 60% of calories should come from carbohydrates, particularly polysaccatiarides.

Q.12. Give your comments regarding fat and carbohydrate %age in the diet ?

Ans. The recommended protein intake about 0.9 gm. of protein per kg body weight. For the average man and woman, this is liberal requirement and represents about 15% of daily total caloric intake.

Q.13. What is the ideal ratio of proximate principles of diet?

Ans. Ideal ratio of carbohydrates, Proteins, Fats in the Sports Diet, may be in the form of following formula.

While calculating this ratio, the following points should be looked into:

(a) The main source of energy should come from carbohydrates.

(b) The percentage of fat should not exceed more than 30% of the calories requirement.

(c) Protein should be adequate and it should be proportionate to the body weight and physical activities of the athlete. The normal requirement is 1-2.5 gm of protein/kgm body weight/day. Excessive protein quantities are also disadvantageous.

Q.14. Why is more iron needed by Indian athletes ?

Ans. Iron requirements of Indian athletes are comparatively higher (due to increased sweating, chances of worm infestation etc. and hence there should be a minimum provision for 30mgms. of iron per day in the sportsman's diet. Excessive sweating during exercise, especially in hot climate, causes, loss of optimum amount of sodium and more potassium from the body. Hence fruit juice should be added to the fluids taken during and after exercise.

Q.15. Mention what you know about vitamins ?

Ans. During sports activities, the requirement of various vitamins increases, particularly vit. A, vit. B complex and vit. C. Vitamin E, which is present in vegetable oils, plays an important role in the breakdown of energy and as such lot of studies are being carried out on vit. E by sports scientist, which may revolutionise the science of physical training in future. The sports diet, when it is well balanced, is sufficient to cater to the extra demand of vitamins do not carry and advantage for the body. Thus, there is no scientific justification for providing extra vitamin pills to an athlete who is fed on the right balanced sports diet.

Q.16. Suggest diet to provide 5000 K. calories ?

Ans. The following foodstuff consumed per day provides 5000

Kcal to an athlete :

Cereals	600 gm
Butter	15 gm
Jam	15 gm
Eggs	2
Pulses	60 gm
Sugar/Glucose	150 gm
Milk	500 gm
Oil	200 gm
Mutton	200 gm
Chicken/Fish	150-300 gm
Green leafy vegetables	125 gm
Fresh vegetables	100 gm
Roots and Tubers	150 gm
Fruits	150 gm
Tea/Coffee	8/20 gm
Salt	40 gm
Condiments	15 gm

For vegetarians in lieu of mutton and chicken given extra four eggs and 150 ml. of milk. Remember the concept of eggs as non-vegetarian food is to be removed from the minds of athletes. Another substitute is panner or soyabeans.

Q.17. Write the guide lines for pre-game meal ?

Ans. (i) Food intake should be sufficient so that the athlete will not be hungry or feel "weak" during the upcoming event.

(ii) The menu items and the time of eating should be selected so that the upper gastrointestinal tract will be empty at gave time.

(iii) The menu should contain foods that are generally well tolerated by most individuals. The meal for the individual athelete obviously avoids food idiosyncrasies meal or imagined. In all instances atheletes are provided any food that they know "makes them win".

(iv) Food and fluid intakes should contribute to good hydration and carbohydrate strores.

Q.18. What is the common mistake made in pre-game meal?

Ans. Athletes generally consume two to three times the recommended protein intake. This is because the proportionately greater caloric intake of physically active people usually provides proportionately more protein.

Q.19. What is Pre-game meal and carbohydrate leading ?

Ans. This was popularised recently by Western sports scientists to meet the extra demand for energy required by the athlete during actual competition. The athlete who is fed on a sell balanced sports diet is deprived of carbohydrate in his diet. 7 days prior to the competition, he is fed mainly on protein and fat rich food for the first 4 days. During the remaining 3 days prior to the competition, this carbohydrate starved athlete is fed on very rich carbohydrate diet, thereby increasing the glycogen (glucose) storage within the body. This enhanced glycogen reserve in utilised by the athlete to meet his extra demand of energy during actual competition. After the competition, he goes back to his normal sports diet.

Pre-game meal is easily digestible carbohydrates, sweet foods or liquids which quickly get digested and leaves the stomach.

Q.20. Name the points for pre-game a diet ?

Ans.

1. Timing of the diet - The diet plan should ensure that the stomach and upper bowel are empty at the time of competition.
2. Fluid contents of the diet-food and fluid intakes prior to and during prolonged competition should guarantee an optimal state of hydration.
3. Blandness of the diet- The pre-competition diet should offer foods that will minimize upset in the gastrointestinal tract.
4. Psychological aspects of the diet- The diet should include food that the athelete is familiar with, and is convinced will "make him win"

Q.21. Give guidelines for pre-event meal ?

Ans.

1. The meal should be high carbohydrate, low fat and protein, either solid food or a liquid formula.
2. Take solid food three to four hours prior to an event.
3. Take liquid meals two to three hours prior to an event. They should be low in fat and high in carbohydrate, with some vitamins and minerals added.

Some examples are Nutrament, Sustacul and Instant Break fast.

4. Foods should be easily digestable. Avoid fried foods and foods known to cause flatulence, which varies with the individual.
5. Do not ingest foods and beverages high in sugar within one hour of the stant of competition. Sugar taken at the start of a game stimulation insulin production and therefore actually cause an accelerated use of glycogen supplies.
6. Take adequate fluids to insure hydration. Unsweetened beverages may be taken within 15 to 30 minutes of competition. Hyperhydrate in hot environments.

Q.22. Mention the importance factor effecting blood glucose level interrelation to exercise ?

Ans. 1. Peripheral glucose uptake (glucose disposal) will be determinal by :

(a) Insulin concentration.

(b) Counter regulatory hormone concentrations : catechola mines, cortizol, and growth hermone.

(c) Changes at the insulin receptor site, both in receptor number and in insulin blinding to the receptor.

(d) Postreceptor changes in muscle : cyclic adenosine monophosphate (AMP) and rate limiting enzymes in the glycolytic path away are altered, including (changes) in hexokinase, glycogen phosphory case, phosphofructokinase, and pyrurate dehydrogenase.

(2) Hepatic glucose output. Regulatory factors are unknown but may be meuronal under steady-state conditions of moderate-intensity exercise, hepatic glucose output is perfectly matched to peripheral glucose output, independent of indulin or the counter regulatory hormones, at least in short term exercise. However, cender most physiologic situations of high intensity, short bursts of exercise result in hypergly cemia where hepentric glucose output exceeds glucose disposal rate.

Q.23. What factors related to nutrition, if kept in mind, will help in increasing the performance of an athlete ?

Ans. The concerned doctor, coach or manager should keep the following points in mind while observing athlete training programme :

1. Check the body weight regularly and adjust the food intake and physical activities. An athletes's body weight serves an index of his nutritional status. It remains constant at the right level of rutrition, increases with overfeeding and falls if the diet is inadequate.
2. Measure the skin fat fold thickness with the help of skin callipers. It will indicate whether the weight gain is due to increase in fat depots (harmful) or due to muscle mass (helpful). Remember skinfold thickness should be assessed by measuring it at 4 to 6 places on body, i.e. biceps, tricps, subscapular, supra iliac etc.
3. Drastic weight reduction or weight gain - both are harmful. The ideal weight gain or loss should be 1 kgm per week. This could be achieved by increasing or decreasing 1000 calories daily in the diet (to reduce 1 kgm) body weight 7000 calories of energy are to be expended).
4. Get the stool examined periodically and deworming done if required.
5. Periodical blood test should be carried out for haemoglobin estimation. Physical exertion can precipitate sports anaemia. If required, iron tablets should be added to the diet, especially in the case of female athletes from the very beginning of their career.
6. Contaminated water and food could cause diarrhoes, jaundice, typhoid etc. Use boiled filtered water for drinking purposes. Do not eat unaccustomed food at parties, which could upset the next day's training or competition.
7. For a sportsman, a glass of beer or a small whisky after heavy exercises is not harmful. But remember during international competition it may be banned.
8. The practice of chewing gums causes wastage of energy as the act of chewing itself is an exercise. It also causes untimely extra secretions.
9. Vitamin pills do not enhance the performance of an athlete who is getting his right sports diet.

10. The more the number of training sessions, the higher the frequency of meals. The Western athletes prefer 5 meals a day (2 breakfasts, lunch, evening snacks, dinner) compared to Indian's meals.
11. The interval between the last meal and competition should be minimum 3 hours preferably in food has sufficient fat in diet- 4 hours.
12. The last meal before competition should be rich in carbohydrates. Soups, steaks, chocolates etc. may be added to this meal.
13. Avoid food which contains too much oil, chillies and spices before the competition.
14. After heavy exercise, take a liquid meal and delay ordinary meal. Electrolyte drinks, lime juice, glucose water, sugarcane juice etc. are ideal refreshments during exercise. Glucose should not be taken more than 20 gms at a time. Salt may be added to fluid taken if needed so.
16. The temperature of drinks taken during the competition should be based on the environmental temperature. The temperature of drinks should not be too high or too low-both are undesirable.
17. Do not fill the stomach just before the competition with milk, lassi, are ated drinks. It will cause bloating of stomach with resultant lethargy and nausea of stich.
18. Do not undertake endurance events after prolonged hours of fasting as happens in morning competitions like marathon, cross country running, long distance walking, bicycle etc. It is better to have a light liquid meal 1/2 hr. before such competitions. Milk, half boiled eggs, chocolate drinks, fruit juices, Kanji water etc. are ideal for this. Once can even have a good pre-competition meal 2-3 hrs. before such event. If rule permits, take encough fluids during the race. But do not take more than 1/2 pint of fluid at a time.
19. Empty the bladder and bowels before physical exertion.
20. Prefer to remain a non-vegetarian rather than a desi ghee vegetarian. That is the best way to get good sports diet anywhere in the world. But it does not mean that vegetarian diet is inferior to non-vegetarian.

Q.24. Give the basic guidelines of liquid replacement for optimum performance.

Ans. 1. Drink small volumes of water frequently rather than large volumes infrequently, eg. 6-8 ounces every 15 minutes.

2. Drink cold beverages to reduce core temperature.
3. Have fluids accessible, since the thirst mechanism doesn't function adequately when large volumes of water are lost. Athletes will not seek out water if is far away. In many cases, they need to be reminded to drink.
4. After work-out replenish fluids at the rate of 1 pint for every pound lost. Weight should be back to normal prior to the next work-out. Minimal body fat is lost during a wock-out, so weight after an event compared to weight immediately prior to an event is a good "indication of total body water lost.
5. Water is the ideal fluid replacement, although commercially prepared glucose, dectrolyte solutions, juices and other beverages may be used. Consider take preferences of athletes, since whether like a substance will govern how much they drink the following are recommended.

(a) Glucose content of less than 2.5 gm 100 ml of H2O, or 25 gm/quart.
This is equal to 1 1/2 rounded table spoon of sugar per quart.

(b) Favour no electiolyes.

(c) Juice diluted with 5 parts H_2O and walas and sweetened sodas with three parts H_2O to reduce glucose con centration to 25%. These could be adjusted to taste.

Q.25. Give your comments on "Drug Misuse by Adolescent Athletes".

Ans. Athletes have used many substances to augment their performance. These substances have been referred to as ergogenic aids, and as the athletes' abilities carry item closer to international competition or professional athletics, the prevalence of their use seems to increase.

Athletes may believe that the benefits to be accrued include an increase in strength and endurance, a delay in the feeling of onset of fatigue, an increased ability to concentrate and a decreased sensibility to pain. Banning the use of ergogenic aids as is done in International Olympic competitions and enforcing this ban by urine testing may be a practical albeit an expensive approach. This method cannot be used in the usual high school or college athletic programmes. Prescriptions against drugs are not usually considered effective on adolescents. So the answer is to educate the athletes not only about their relative ineffectiveness in achieving "the illegal edge."

Q.26. Explain in details the "Anabolic Steroids".

Ans. These drugs, such as nandrolone phenoproprionate (Durabolin) and methandrostenolone (Dianabol), rank with amphetamines as the principal drugs misused in athletics. They also share with the amphetamines the burden of conflicting scientific reports indicating whether they truly do improve athletic performance or not. An example is a 1969 study indicating an increase in weight gain and strength in the half of a group of weight lifters who received androgen therapy. The treatment arm of the study considered of a group of enthusiastic volunteer athletes willing to try the drug; the control arm consisted of a group of volunteers unwilling to take the drug because they thought it might be dangerous. The mental attitude of the former might well have contributed to their improved performance.

A somewhat similar study in 1965 was performed in a double blined fashion, and it demostrated no improvement in strength, motor performance, or physical capacity.

Another well controlled study was that of Hervey and Associates, who administered an androgen in large doses to athletes for six weeks in a double blind crossover study. There was no difference between the two groups in strength or performance, although the treated group did have an increase in body weight, body water, and muscle mass.

The author concludes that the increase in body weight could be largely caused by the increase in body water. Regardless whether the use of anabolic steroids improves performance, their well known toxic side effects should preclude their use for enhancing performance. The list of adverse reactions is formidable : virilization in the female; oligospermia, testicular atrophy, infertility, and gynecomastia in the male; and premature closure of the epiphyses, acne, increased blood cholesterol and hepatocellular carcinoma in both the sexes. These health hazards clearly outweigh any potential gain the drugs might induce and make it ethically impermissible to perform further studies to answer the question of effectiveness. The substances described have little or no ergogenic capacity, and even if they did, the dangers associated with taking many of them far outweigh the advantage of their giving an athlete an "illegal edge". Using these drugs for this purpose is cheating and a violation of the ethics of fairplay in sports. The use of alleged ergogenic aids by the adolescent athlete is a possibility that should be considered by physician whenever he performs either a routine health maintenance examination or a pre-participation physical examination on the adolescent athlete. This subject should be routinely mentioned by the physician, and the risks and alleged benefits fully discussed.

Q.27. Enlist banned drugs for Olympic Games.

Ans. List of Doping classes and methods :

1. **DOPING CLASSES :**

A. Stimulants,
B. Narcotics,
C. Anabolic Steroids,
D. Beta-blockers,
E. Diuretics.

2. DOPING METHODS :

A. Blood doping.

3. CLASSES OF DRUGS SUBJECT TO CERTAIN RESTRICTIONS :

A. Alcohol,
B. Local anaesthetics,
C. Corticosteroids,

Q.28. Why should the care be taken while taking drugs even for cold or flu at the time of International competition ?

Ans. One group of stimulants is the sumpathomimetic amines of which ephedrine is an example. In high doses, this type of compound produces mental stimulation and increased blood flow, Adverse effects include elevated blood pressure and headache, increased and irregular heart beat, anxiety and tremor. In lower doses, they, e.g., ephedrine, pseudoephedrine, phenylpropanolamine, norpseudophedrine, are often present in drug preparations used for cold which can be purchased in pharmacies and sometimes form other retail outlets without the need of a medical prescription.

Thus the product for use in cold, flu etc. purchased by a competitor or given to him should not be used without first verifying from a doctor or pharmacist that the product does not contain a drug of the banned stimulants class.

Q.29. Enlist Narcotic analgesics.

Ans. They are the following :

alphaprodine	levorphanol
anileridine	methadone
purprenorphine	morphine
codeine	nalbuphine
dextromoramide	phentazocine
dextropoxyphen	pethidine
diamorphine(heroin)	pentazocine
dihydrocodeine	pethidine
dipipanone	phenazocine
ethoheptazinc	trimeperidine
ethylomorphine	related compounds.

Q.30. Why are Narcotic Analgesics banned by I.O.C. ?

Ans. It is felt that the treatment of slight to moderate pain can be effective by using drugs-other than the narcotics-which have analgesic, anti-inflammatory and antipyretic actions. Such alternatives, which have been successfully used for the treatment of sports injuries, include Arthranilic acid derivatives (such as Mefenamic acid, Floctafenine, Glafenine, etc.), Phenylalkanoic acid derivatives (such as Diclofenac, Ibuprofen, Ketoprofen, Naproxen, etc.) and compounds such as Indomethacin and Sulindac. The Medical Commission also reminds athletes and team-doctors that Asprin and its newer derivatives (such as Diflunisal) are not banned but cautions against some pharmaceutical preparations where Aspirin is often associated to the banned drugs such as Codeine etc. needs the same precautions which are often taken for drugs of the banned classes.

Q.31. What common Anabolic Steroids are used by players?

Ans. Anabolic Steroids used are :

bolasterone
boldenone
clostebol
dehydro chlormethyl testosterone
fluoxyme sterone
mesterolone
metandienone

Q.32. How can the Anabolic Steroids harm the athletes ?

Ans. Their use in teenagers who have not fully developed can result in stunting growth by affecting growth at the ends of the long bones. Their use can produce psychological changes, liver damage and adversely affect the cardiovascular system. In males, their use can reduce testicular size and sperm production. In females, their use can produce masculinization, acne, development of male pattern hair growth and suppression of ovarian function and menstruation.

Q.33. How heart is effected by drugs and harmones ?

Ans. Myocordial contractility is increased by digitalis, calcium and catecholamines, including norepinephrine epinephrine, isoproterenot and alopainers. Countratility is also increase by corticasteroids, spironolactone, angiotensin, serotonin, glucagon, some prostagrandins and cardioglobulins. The actions of thyronine on myocardial contractive functions are complex but, in general, it may be said to enhance cadiac contraclility. Myocardial contracility is decreased by hypoxia and by many drugs, including barbiturates, quinidine, propranolol, procainamide and lidocaine. Acidosis also depresses myocardial contraclility, particularly, if the sympathoadrenal system function is impaired.

Q.34. Comment on the use of Diuretics.

Ans. Diuretics have important therapeutic indications for the elimination of fluids from the tissues in certain pathological conditions. However, strict medical control is required. Diuretics are sometimes misused by competitors for two main reasons, namely : to reduce weight quickly in sports where weight categories are involved and to reduce the concentration of drugs in urine by producing a more rapid excrediton of urine to attempt to minimise detection of drugs misuse. Rapid reduction of weight in sports cannot be justified medically. Health risks are involved in such misuse because of serious side effects which might occur. Furthermore, deliberate attempts to reduce weight artificially in order to compete in lower weight classes or to dilute urine constitute clear manipulations which are unacceptable on ethical grounds. Therefore, the IOC Medical Commission has decided to include diuretics on its list of banned classes of drugs.

Q.35. Will you enlighten about Blood Doping ?

Ans. Blood transfusion is the intravenous administration offered blood cells or related blood products that contain red blood cells. Such products can be obtained from blood drawn from the same (autologous) or from a different (non-autologus) individual. The most common indications for red blood transfusion in conventional medical practice are acute blood loss and severe anaemia.

Blood doping is the administration of blood or related red blood products to an athlete other than for legitimate medical treatment. This procedure may be preceded by withdrawal of blood from the athlete who continues to train in this blood depleted state.

These procedures contravene the ethics of medicine and of sports. There are also risks involved in the transusion of blood and related blood products. These include the development of allergic reactions (rash, feveretc.) and acute haemolytic reaction with kidney damage if incorrectly typed blood is used, as well asdelayed transfusion reaction resulting in fever and jaundice, transmission of infectious diseases (viral hepatities and AIDS), overload of the circulation and metabolic shock.

Therefore, the practice of blood doping in sports in banned by the IOC Medical Commission.

Q.36. Mention the drugs which are restricted for their use by athletes.

Ans. CLASSES OF DRUGS SUBJECT TO CERTAIN RESTRICTIONS.

A. Alcohol :

Alcohol is nor prohibited but restricted in selected events. However, breath or blood alcohol levels may be determined at the request of an International Federation.

B. Local anaesthetics :

Injectable local anaesthetics are permitted under the following conditions :

(a) the procaine, xylocaine, carbocaine, etc. are used but not cocaine;

(b) only local or intra-articular injections may be administered (intra-vascular injections are not permitted):

(c) only when medically justified (i.e. the details including diagnosis; dose and route of administration must be submitted immediately in writing to the IOC Medical Commission).

C. Corticosteroids :

The naturally occurring anssynthetic corticosteroids are mainly used as anti-inflammatory drugs which also relieve pain. They influence circulating concentrations of natural corticosteroids in the body. They produce euphoria and side-effects such that their medical use, except when used topically, require medical control.

The use of corticosteroids is banned except for topical use (aural, ophthalmological and dematological), inhalational therapy (asthma, allergic rhinitis) and local or intra-articular injections.

Q.37. What do you think about the use of ergogenic aids ?

Ans. For augmentation of performance athletes use many substances. These substances are referred as ergogenic aids. Competitors may believe that the benefits may be in the form of increase in strength and endurance, a delay in onset of fatigue, an increased ability to concentrate and a decreased sensitivity to pain. Banning the use of ergogenic aids as is done in international competition with the help of urine testing is not the only way of solving problem.

Q.38. What is the possible way to avoid consumption of drugs ?

Ans. There is a need for mass health education campaign to educate the athlete not only about the hazards of most of these ergogenic agents but also about their relative ineffectiveness in achieving the illegal edge.

Q.39. Amphetamines are reported to be used by players. Throw some light about the use of this drug.

Ans. Such type of drugs give an individual a sense of increased alertness and relief of fatigue. It may give advantage in certain track events but it is yet to be proved. Increased physiological fatigue level may allow the athlete to exceed his limits especially during marathons in warm season. Footballers may ignore pain and damage their joints. One may become more aggressive, resulting in unnecessary brutality and rough play in contact sports. When high doses are taken they may induce paranoid, prepsychotic state or a paranoid schzophrenic syndrome.

Q.40. Most widely used drug is anabolic steroids. Mention its harmful effects.

Ans. Regardless of whether the use of anabolic steroies improves performance, their well known toxic effects should preclude their use for enhancing performance :

— Virilization in female,
— Acne and hoarseness of voice,
— Oligospermia,
— Testicular atrophy,
— Infertility and Gynaecomastia in the males,
— Decrease in libido,
— Premature closure of epiphysis,
— Increased blood cholesterol and hepatocellular Carcinoma but it is a rare side effect.

Q.41. Mention the use of nutritional aids by athletes.

Ans. Except during the deficiency state, taking heavy doses of vitamin is wastage of money and health. The excessive use of some vitamins (A and D) can lead to toxic effects.

These days vitamin E is getting popularity not only for athletic and sexual performance but also for increase in aerobic capacity. So far there is no clear cut proof that vitamins improve athletic performance.

The new name of pangamic acid (vitamin B15) is only a chemical with its unknown action.

Q.42. Do the Soft sports drinks, salt etc. give any advantage to the players ?

Ans. Although replacement of body water is critical during strenuous exercise especially in hot and humid climate yet there is no evidence that any drink is preferable to plain water. The more expensive drinks contain sugar and if taken in large amount with lot of glucose (as is the general practice), it can delay gastric emptying of fluids. Thus delaying absorption of water in circulation: Owing to CO2 gas formation it may cause stitch. Loss of electrolytes during sweating is usually quite small and can be replaced after exercise with a glass of fruit juice or electrolyte containing water. Salt tablets are useless and dangerous. Since they may exceed excretion of water, exacerbating dehydration.

Q.43. How may the use of 'local anaesthetic' harm the athlete ?

Ans. Owing to their use, a player is tempted to return to game. It is due to absence of pain that serious injury to that part may result. These drugs may produce cardiac arrhythmias, convulsions or even death. Idiosyncratic death may also be there.

Q.44. Can 'Marijuana' be used as ergogenic aid ?

Ans. Studies has suggested that there is no difference between smoking Marijuana and a placebo in measurements of vital capacity expiratory flow rate, and handgrip strength.

Q.45. Ginseng is marketed for sportsmen also. It is really effective for performances. What latest research says ?

Ans. A seven day study of engesting Panaxginseng did not increase endurance times for individuals cycling at 75% of VO_2-max. Further detail long term studies are to be made before reaching on conclusion.

Q.46. Explain multiple drug abuse ?

Ans. Persons who abuse drugs often take more than one drug at a time, creating combined drug reactions. Try to find out as much as possible about what drug or drugs the patient has been taking. Loof for empty bottles, needles, syringes and paper wrappers that may certain powdered drugs, bottles, spoons, alcohol lamps or other evidence of drug paraphernalia. Send all there to these hospital with the patient. These patients are seriously ill. Drug combinations result in effects for greater than those of individual drugs taken separately. The patient or an acquaintance may be able to tell you exactly what drug or drugs have been taken.

Q.47. What is the rationale behind the movement of vegetarianism ?

Ans. The fast growing medical sciences have been the major factor in converting the people to vegetarianism. In United States of America, United Kingdom, and Scandinavia countries, vegetarianism is being advocated by the medical people. The fibre content of diet, low cholesterol contents, prevention of zoonotic disorders have been the major reasons which have appealed the medical people to propagate vegetarianism. The discovery of human onchogene (mutation of gene by eating) by Prof. Weinberg from Massachussettee Institute has revolutionised the programme of cancer prevention. Bowel cancer per cent is very well known to be due to low fibre content in the animal diet. However, the association of breast cancer and other organ cancers appear to be due to mutant cancer gene.

Prevention of haemorrhoids. Varicosity, constipation, hiatus hernia, ulcerative colitis and peptic ulcer by the fibre rich diet is known to medical scientists since four decades.

Q.48. Are chances of heart attack and stroke more with nonvegetarian food ? Does lack of sports or exercise further contribute to it ?

Ans. Yes, recently the relationship of animal food and the myocardial infraction stroke have gained much attention. In United Kingdom and United State of America, the trend is no animal food and less of eggs in the diet. The cholesterol contents of animal food makes the atherogenesis faster. 1985 Nobel Prize awarded to Prof. Goldstein and Brown for their outstanding work on the cholesterol receptor deprivation with high animal food consumption. Most of the rich and elite people have this fatal illness. Such people are also used to do minimum activity.

Q.49. Is the Immunological state affected by animal food ?

Ans. The foreign body antigenic repose sets up the antigenic response to the antigen antibody reaction. It lowers the immune status and increases the chance of graft rejection in the organ transplants. Animal food increases the chance of bacterial and viral antigens to grow further. Thus the immune system is impaired.

Q.50. In a country like India can people have non-vegetarian food ? What is your opinion ?

Ans. Growing requirement for food energy resources has made the scientists to work as it. The commercial production of meat is very costly. The conversion rate of plant prctein to animal protein is too low. It is, therefore, better to utilise vegetable food directly in human food rather than for animal protein. Not only the conversion of plant protein to animal protein is lower, the calories conversion is much lower. It has been estimated that 7 vegetable calories are required for production of one animal calorie. It is, therefore, evident that the plant animal food conversion is not too costly but too wasteful a proposition in the present day world when all efforts have to be directed to remove the calorie malnutrition throughout the world. At a time when millions are dying of starvation, it is morally indefensible that over half the world's grain is fed to animals, which in turn, would be fed to people.

Q.51. Does Longevity of life and diet have direct relation ?

Ans. Yes, the human survival rate of India may be related to the fat decreasing diet. We have still people who are octogenarian. Attention has been focused on the Soviet Republic of Abkhasia. They live well over one hundred years and are largely vegetarian. They are healthy, vigorous, slim and smart people. A study conducted by the Enthnographic Institute in Sukhumi revealed that arterie-sclerosis is rare there except in extreme old age-after on hundred years. A nine year study of 123 people over one hundred years old revealed no reported cases of mental illness related to type of food we eat.

Q.52. Can physical strength - Strength and endurance also develop with vegetarian diet ?

Ans. Johnny Wwismuller, Pravo Nurmi, Chris Everett-Lloyd and many other marathon runners, body-builders, weight lifters have preferred to be vegetarian. The endurance, stamina have been extraordinary among them. In fact, in scientific tests during a stationary bicycle athletes on vegetable and grans diet averaged three times as long as when eating on animal based diet.

There is a myth among people that meat would make them very strong. They believe that muscles of animals directly incorporate into their muscles. The fact is that whatever you eat, is broken down by digestive system. You must know that elephant, cow, buffalo, bulls, oxen and gorillas are vegetarians. How could they develop so strong without eating other animals.

Q.53. How do the high and low density lipoproteins affect the cholesterol action ?

Ans. Now it is a well know fact that blood vascular diseases are not only due to one factor, i.e. cholesterol but, there are lipoprotein-cholesterols (LDC-C). The elevated level of it may lead to increased risk of coronary heart disease. Contrary to this high density lipoprotein cholesterol in elevated concentrations lead to the reduced risk for CHD. Research workers have proved that exercise causes raised level of HDL-C. There is very low density lipoprotein cholesterol which is neutral in action as far as CHD risk is concerned.

It can also be said that high density lopoproteins can play an important role in CHD. The estimation of only cholesterol and suggesting treatment is not justified.

Q.54. Does screening of individuals by cholesterol estimation help in reducing CHD cases ?

Ans. Definitely, as it has happened in cases of frequent blood pressure measurements and stroke cases, in the same line of total cholesterol estimation done periodically and due steps taken, the chances of coronary heart diseases can be minimized.

Q.55. After total cholesterol estimation, what steps should be taken to help the individual ?

Ans. (i) If total cholesterol is at a low desired level, there is no need to check it again for the next five years;

(ii) In cases of high-risk elevation, aggressive diet therapy, exercise and if needed drug treatment may be given.

Q.56. What to do when cholesterol level is above the optimum level ?

Ans. There is another factor "triglycerides" (amount of fat in blood stream) which should also be estimated. So beyond total cholesterol, there is another important aspect, i.e. triglycerides. To make it more clear here an example is quoted.

A lean man who drinks monderately and exercises a lot may have an elevated total cholesterol level and it is due to this that HDL-C level is elevated. In fact, the cholesterol level is alright. It will be most unfortunate to start any type of treatment. In such case without doing more sophisticated test, even the diet control is not justified.

Q.57. Will you explain further details about lipoproteins etc. ?

Ans. Use of total cholesterol/HDL-C, and LDL-C. Since, rise in HDL-C will affect both sides so to get more correct information both LDL-C/HDL-C are to be accurately estimated.

Q.58. For treatment purposes what are the suggested levels of cholesterol ?

Ans. The table given below is self explanatory :

S.No.	**Age Group** in years	**Moderate Risk** (75th percentile)	**High Risk** (90th percentile)
1.	20-29	Greater than 200 mg/100 ml	Greater than 220 mg/100 ml.
2.	30-39	-do-220 mg/100 ml	Greater than 240 mg/100 ml.
3.	40 & above	-do-240 mg/100 ml	Greater than 260 mg/100 ml.

Source : National Institute of Health Census Development Conference. Statement : "Lowering Blood Pressure to prevent heart disease".

Q.59. "Amount of Cholesterol manufactured by the body may be more of a problem that what an individual eats." Throw some light on the mentioned comment."

Ans. Human body gets cholesterol from two sources, i.e. food and body's own production. In fact, every body's organ can make cholesterol though maximum of it is manufactured in liver and intestine. Generally the body of those who have high cholesterol level, may be making too much. Besides this, food cooking and diet can affect cholesterol production. Foodstuffs having high saturated fats will stimulate the body to make cholesterol.

Actually, diet has two effects :

(a) It provides cholesterol,

(b) It also stimulate the body to make more cholesterol.

Owing to this reason, a person with a family history of high cholesterol needs to modify his diet by reducing cholesterol and saturated fats, and to help the body in making less cholesterol by losing weight and performing regular exercise.

Q.60. Western Press and Media has given lot of popularity to 'SPE'. Actually what is it ?

Ans. If we talk theoretically, S.P.E. is okay for reducing calories; it does not have the effect of raising cholesterol. It has the texture of fat, and it acts like fat in cooking and food preparation. It is an unnatural material like lovastatin. Practical approach to weight control is to increase exercise rather than to too much worry about the number of calories eaten. It is also not wrong that lovastatin and S.P.E. both may be used as substitutes for exercise but remember nothing can replace exercise, neither drug nor S.P.E.

Q.61. Is there optimum level of exercise ? Upto what level should exercises be increased ?

Ans. Though, there is no clear-cut demarcation for it, yet there is a level of exercise below which one cannot get changes in DHL-C levels. That threshold would be due partly to the exercise intensity and partly to its duration. So far researchers have not made authentic longitudinal studies which can show, how much duration and intensity is optimum to get result for an individual.

Q.62. It is said by some people that death rate may start raising after a certain level of vigorous exercise. Explain it briefly.

Ans. There seems to be a plateau effect at exercise level needs 3,500 kcal per week. The apparent increase in CHD at high levels is suspicious because studies are done on limited subjects at those levels. The statistics are weak due to the low number of subjects, so that increase may not be real one.

Q.63. What exercise factors affect most HDL-C levels ?

Ans. There are three separate aspects of exercise that contribute to HDL-C levels.

(a) The amount as measured in calories;

(b) The intensity, i.e., whether the exercise is done all at once and quickly or gradually over a period of time;

(c) The duration of exercise.

The probable effect on HDL-C is the result of these factors. For example, those who have been running at a high intensity level over a period of years would have the highest HDL-C levels. The people who walk great distances over a long period of time, such people may be kept at intermediate level since they have long duration and good intensity. The least effect would be seen in people who participate in a low level activity that is not done often or for an extended period of time.

Q.64. In relation to HDL-C level, how quickly is the exercise effect lost, after total discontinuity ?

Ans. The HDL-C effect certainly does drop off when we talk in terms of months. In the same way, it takes some months for HDL-C levels to be raised while the other aspect like VO2 max and heart rate, occur faster than increase in HDL-C, so these two aspects of fitness may also decrease long before HDL-C level drop. Probably this is the reason that there is no effect on HDL-C in short term studies.

Q.66. Does power lifting affect HDL-C levels ?

Ans. Most of the athletes who go for power exercise also use anabolic steroids. These substances have profound affect on HDL-C; they lower it. Power exercise does not have much effect on C.V. status. Athlete may have terrible

HDL-C levels due to the androgens in their body. Weight lifters who do not take drugs do show increased HDL-C levels, but the effect is not much especially when compared with aerobic athletes. Most probably weight lifting and other power sports probably do not produce high levels of HDL-C.

Q.67. What is blood doping ? Explain it.

Ans. The transfusion of R.B.Cos. to improve oxygen delivery and, thereby, edurance - is widely recognised as an illegal and unethical procedure in competitive sports. Though the ergogenic effect of blood doping is proved in laboratory yet there is disagreement on whether it works in competitive situations in the real field events. It is also true, that blood doping is a very useful tool for examining some physiological questions, such as what limits aerobic exercise. Is it the metabolic capacity of muscle or it is the transport of oxygen to muscle ?

Q.68. What will happen if 100% oxygen is provided to athlete ?

Ans. If we increase an individual's oxygen transport by blood or by providing 100% oxygen, then immediately that individual is able to use more oxygen. This shows that individual's muscle already had metabolic capacity in excess of what was previously thought to be VO2 max. The limiting factor, therefore, is the transport system and not the metabolic capacity of muscle. However, the basic issue still needs clarification; blood doping studies can help resolve this and other physiological questions. There is risk in using 100 percent oxygen.

Q.69. Should hypertensive individuals get special type of diet ?

Ans. Yes, there is an need to modified the diet for such cases. For chronic cases protein may be restricted because without it salt restriction is not possible. Saturated fats as Ghee, hydrogenated oil should be totally avoided. They cause atherosclerosis and then also further raise the blood pressure.

— By low caloric diet weight should be reduced. Restricted sodium but fruits may be given to prevent hypokalemia.

- In case of high blood pressure, fluid restriction may help to some extent only
- Fried food with chillies should not be taken.
- Aspirin and corticosteroids may not be taken as they cause retention of sodium and rise in blood pressure.

Q.69. What points should be kept in mind while planning the diet for Diabetics ?

Ans. Fundamental rule is-Consume which grows above the ground. Sweet things, fruit like ripe banana should be avoided. Soyabean preparations are the best as they are nutritive and contain vary little amount of carbohydrates. Hunger should be satisfied with large amount of green vegetables. Thus total caloric intake becomes low.

Q.70. How to advise the diet for Infective Hepatitis (Jaundice) case ?

Ans. Food rich is protein (2gm/Kg body weight) is good as cystine and methionine amino-acid prevents damage to liver.

Sweet food articles, glucose and sugarcane juice are of great help as due to nausea the patient cannot eat fatty foods. At recovery stage, fats may be included in the diet. Use of alcohol should be forbidden for a few months. It is a hepatotoxic substance.

Q.71. How to increase the weight of an individual ?

Ans. Remember following points :-Regular sleep, exercise and meals is the base for better health. Frequent snacks will reduce the lipogenesis. Alongwith fatty diet, banana, potatoes, groundnuts and sweet foods may be consumed. Avoid green vegetables and do not take water between the eating of foodstuffs as it dilutes the digestive juices and digestion and absorption of food is not complete.

Q.72. What you will suggest for overweight people ?

Ans. Reverse the order of food-stuffs mentioned above. Extra water while eating food and low caloric diet alongwith salt restriction is of great help. Alcohol should be avoided.

Q.73. Explain the word non-cardiac syncope.

Ans. Cardiac syncope results in complete collapse, often with a short.seizure and diaphoresis. Adolesceat athletes, in contrast, may explain of "Passing out" that is better described as a sense of weakness and disorientation. Frequently, these episodes are repetitive and happen at the end of a competitive event. The examination findings, including echocardiography and exercise testing, are normal. Careful questioning often reveals a potential psychological factor in these episodes. One atheletes seen in our clinic was afflicted only during poor performance. Treatment consists of a full evaluation, attention to possible psychological factors, and reassurance for the parents and the athelete.

Q.74. What suggestion will you give to a person who has recovered from Myocardial Infarction (Heart Attack) ?

Ans. Avoid : Hurry, worry and curry.
Prohibit the use of alcohol, roots and tubers and smoking.
Rest after meals and gradually increase the exercises from slow walking to jogging (3 months).
Do not allow the pulse to go above 100 beats/min.
Nicotinic acid and supplementary vitamins may be given.

Q.75. When somebody suffers from fever what type of food should he/she consume ?

Ans. Avoid fried fatty foods, but take carbohydrates, vitamins, electrolytes and extra proteins. Most of the people do not take food which is harmful. They must at least get 1800-2000 Kcal/day in their diets.

Q.76. Is cod-liver oil or vitamin 'AD' capsule Fattening ?

Ans. It is a belief that cod-liver oil will add inches to the wasteline. For information one should know that one tablespoonful of it gives 100 kcal. This dose is for once in 6 months. When the oil is taken on an empty stomach most of the oil is used for lubrication and not for producing energy.

Q.77. Can you give your comments on the problem of 'Acne' ?

Ans. Let us discuss the mechanism of its development in a teenager. Too much of oils in food are dispersed uniformly throughout all fat deposits of body. One must know that the areas of skin over forehead, nose, face, chest and trunk has maximum number of oil glands.

— Mostly people consume saturated fats which may be put as insoluble type.
— These insoluble oils present in glands cannot be burned off easily.

This leads to black heads and acne develops.

Q.78. How to avoid or reduce the severity of acne ?

Ans. — Huge amount of salts and saturated oils may be avoided.
— Cosmetics causing allergies; chocolate, pasteries, sweets should be utilised to minimum.
— Rely on warm water and mild soap for keeping the skin clean as well as clear.
— Keep away many type of face powder, lotions. These will clog the pores.
— Remember one cannot wash faulty diet off his skin.

Q.79. It is said that the elimination of waste product is to maintain without constipation or diarrhoea. How to achieve it ?

Ans. In the diet, sufficient amount of vegetables and green products should be added so that peristaltic waves of intestine are stimulated to move the faecal mass to the last part of intestines.

— Regular timings should be kept of toilets and never resist the evacuation.
— If it is delayed due to nervous tension, take warm water with lemon or tea or coffee.
— If it happens to more than 48 hours take enema.
— Remember that if one take a laxative, it should be taken rerely.
— Visit the doctor whenever failure to have a bowel movement is illness. In such conditions, laxatives should be avoided.

Q.80. How to get good sleep ?

Ans. — Try to go to bed at the same time every night.
— Never relax or sleep longer after lunch.
— Remember too much sleep may contribute to certain diseases.

- Exercise by playing with competitive partner will give sound sleep by reducing continuous worry and causing a bit tiredness.
- Do not drink coffee, tea, cocoa or cola drinks before bed time.
- A warm bath and a glass of warm milk at bed time are effective in producing sleep.
- Read adult book or look at the boring programme of TV.

Q.81. What are the points to be kept in mind to be healthy and young and to live a life of more than 100 years ?

Ans. Always remember : Communicable diseases are not caused by old age. Try to build youthful health and vigour physically as well as mentally.

- Any bad habit that causes chronic fatigue or loss of sleep will speed the aging process.
- Healthy but optimum nutrition and exercise to improve circulation, for example yoga etc. are very important for preventing aging. Very heavy exercises are more damaging than light exercises.
- Take care of posture, heart action, breathing, ingestion and elimination.
- Under weight or over-weight puts load on the body.

Q.82. How to get rid off from fatigue and look young ?

Ans. Fatigue from medical causes should be ruled out as it decreases the resistance.

- Emotional problem will not allow fatigue to be relieved by rest and sleep. So do not let fatigue become a mental habit.
- Always take frequent rest breaks during the day by lying down and elevating legs (especially after meals). Deep breaths may help it.
- If it is due to unhappy job that cannot be changed, one should adopt a happy avocation that will satisfy their need to be creative and useful.
- Lack of exercise, improper diet, inadequate sleep, quick eating of food and other violating healthful, natural living are common causes of fatigue.
- Sit tall, stand tall and walk tall. Wrong posture leaves tiredness.

— Sitting in a rocking chair or rocking at brisk rate will prevent fatigue by pumping blood through the body.

Q.83. How to control the low blood sugar level to normal ?

Ans. Remember the following :

— Low blood sugar (Hypoglycemia) can cause fatigue and hunger, alongwith other symptoms.

— Excessive use of refined sugar can lower blood sugar by overstimulating the pancreas. This is only possible in young healthy individuals.

— A deficiency of blood sugar deprives brain and nervous system of adequate oxygen.

— Refined sugar and white flour products should be eliminated altogether.

— Between the meals candy or coffee should not be taken. However to allay hunger, nuts, fruits and skimmed milk may be taken.

— It is said that Caffeine stimulates adrenal glands (which trigger hypoglycemia). So avoid coffee, tea or cola drinks.

— No alcohol. Combat hangovers with orange juice and honey rather than black coffee or tea.

Q.84. How do the natural foods help in maintaining good health ?

Ans. Remember the following :

— Fresh and unprocessed foods are mostly rich in Calcium, Iron and Iodine alongwith other minerals.

— Milk and its products are needed especially for vegetarians.

— Smoking and boiling reduces the amount of vitamin C in blood. Alcohol destroys vitamin B, and alkalizers disturb the absorption of both Calcium and vitamin C.

— There is definite need of vitamin D for the use of Calcium. When one is away from the exposure to sun rays, one must have cod-liver oil. In Indian conditions it is rare to be away from sunlight.

— Just cook the foodstuffs and do not throw water. Use it as soup.

— Try to have balanced diet, i.e., many food stuffs-wheat, Dal, rice and green vegetables alongwith a glass of milk and fruit juice.

Q.85. We hear so much of cholesterol. Actually what is it ?

Ans. Cholesterol produced in the body as well as consumed in foods, is essential to life. It is needed for the manufacture of call membranes and as a building block in the production of certain hormones. It is transported through the blood by particles known as low density lipoproteins, or LDL. LDL is also absorbed by cells of the liver, where cholesterol can be eliminated from the body so that it does not accumulate in the blood stream and collect in the arteries.

Q.86. Will you mention the latest research in this field ?

Ans. Brown and Goldstein discovered that there is a limit on how much cholesterol a cell can take in and that excessive fats and cholesterol in the blood can slowly accumulate to clog human arteries, causing strokes and heart attacks. The researchers also discovered that some people, due to a genetic flaw, are predisposed toward high blood cholesterol. They found that the cells from people with inherited high cholesterol higher lacked or were deficient in LDL receptors.

Brown and Goldstein also reported that normal individuals who consume large amounts of cholesterol, particularly through red meats and dairy products, may reduce the number of LDL receptors on the cell surface. Fewer receptors mean more cholestors-bearing product remain in the bloodstream, with the risk of deposit build-up on the artery walls.

Goldstein told the reporters that their research could lead to development of new drugs that increase the number of receptors and thus lower cholesterol levels in the bloodstream.

Q.87. What is Diapulse ?

Ans. The latest advances have been made in treatment of injuries to soft tissues, bones and nerves by use of high peak, pulsed, electromagnetic energy called the Diapulse Therapy.

Q.88. What is the mechanism of its working ?

Ans. This machine transmits electromangetic energy in short bursts of micro-seconds with a resting interval of 1600 micro-seconds between the pulses. By this principle Diapulse gives ample time for blood stream to carry off any heat, which may have been produced by the energy pulse, thus permitting deep penetration and high intensity with no significant rise in temperature either locally or systematically. The machine is capable of safely and effectively treating an athlete after acute traumatic injury. It can be used safely over any area of the body, on athletes of all ages, with no danger of hyperpyrexia or tissue damage. It can be used safely and effectively through clothing, surgical dressings, P.O.P and over metal implants.

Q.89. What are the indications of its use ?

Ans. Besides most of medical conditions it can be of great use in sports injuries, hematoma, haemarthrosis, sprains and inflammation.

Q.90. Does this therapy affect nervous tissue also ?

Ans. Yes, healing process naturally occurs in almost all the tissues. A note-worthy exception to the regenerative capacity of living tissue is brain and spinal cord. Peripheral nerves regenerate, but this power is not found in nerve cells in the C.N.S. Diapulse Therapy has produced impressive results in promoting true regeneration of spinal cord nerves with consequent restoration of sensation and function.

Q.91. Besides in the Medical Hospitals where in the sports field is this machine being used ?

Ans. We in India, have used two Diapulse machines for the treatment of sports injuries during the 9th Asian Games at Delhi and thereafter at National Institute of Sports, Patiala. The types of injuries treated were haematomas, haemarthrosis, sprains of various joints, muscle strains and contusions. Most of the cases recovered within 2-3 days, who otherwise would have taken part in the competition after injury because of fast recovery due to Diapulse Therapy. Encouraged by the results of treatment on these machines after the Asiad, N.I.S., Patiala has purchased three more Diapulse machines, one each for their centres at New Delhi, Bangalore and Calcutta.

Q.92. Please write its effectiveness in cases of head and brain injuries.

Ans. The improvement in head injuries and brain oedema is seen with Diapulse measure in parsons getting head injuries as a result of accidents. In cases of haematoma of the brain, only treatment is its removal by brain surgery, which is a very specialised surgical procedure. Very few hospitals in India have the necessary facilities for doing such an operative procedure. Diapulse Therapy can serve as a very useful tool for this. Similarly the effective treatment of sport injuries by Diapulse Therapy shows that it would be equally good in other types of acute injuries commonly seen during every day life.

Now it can be said that Diapulse Therapy is a very useful, cheap and non-invasive type of treatment for many acute injures to soft tissues, bones and nerves. It also hastens the recovery process after operative procedures.

Q.93. What are the wrong notions of an average Indian regarding proteins in diet ?

Ans. The people generally have the following wrong impressions about proteins :

— The quantitative aspects of its requirements are often not appreciated.

— It is assumed that poor man's diet supplies enough protein for all age groups.

— People do not make any distinction between proteins of widely different biological values.

— Baking at high temperature causes damage to proteins which people do not know.

— There is wrong impression that protein hydrolysates are better utilized than intact proteins when taken orally.

— A foolish impression that milkfed infants and children need supplement lysine amino acids.

— Only rich protein food (with very little carbohydrates and fats in diet) makes the balanced diet.

Q.94. What points should be kept in mind while selecting a protein rich food as a dietary supplement ?

Ans. Following scientific aspects may be kept in mind :

— Selection of product : It should be palatable enough

to enable easy administration of the required quantity of protein.

— Of the total protein requirement at least 10-20 grams extra should be taken every day.

— The nutritive value of protein should be high, equivalent to a Net protein Utilization of at least 65.

— It should preferably be in the intact condition and not predigested, i.e., not in the form of protein hydrolysate or mixture of amino-acids.

Q.95. Is there any relation between caloric intake and protein utilization ?

Ans. The main source of energy are fats and carbohydrates. The main work of protein is formation and regeneration of tissues. During starvation or malnutrition proteins may supply the energy as well. This happens when the caloric needs of the body are not adequately met from the intake of carbohydrates and fats, part of protein may be diverted towards energy production. To prevent such wastage of proteins, therefore, care should be taken to raise the intake of carbohydrates and fats to the required levels when protein supplements to cover a dietary protein gap.

Q.96. Will you discuss the protein gap in relation to the common diets of India ?

Ans. Mostly the Indian diet consists of cereals, pulses and rice but the actual quantity consumed by most of Indians is not sufficient. An increased consumption of normal diets would serve to make up the caloric deficit and also ensure a satisfactory level of protein intake. But, for the vulnerable groups the average diet cannot satisfy the needs, as the person findsit inconvenient or physically difficult to eat more of such diets. Therefore the international level athletes, pregnant mothers and little children need more concentrated sources of proteins as dietary supplements.

Q.97. What is your opinion, "Are all dietary proteins equally good ?"

Ans. The answer is,"No." All dietary proteins are not equally good. The proteins differ widely in their nutritive value.

These variations are due to differences in the amino-acids composition and digestibility. The nutritive value of a protein is largely determined by the relative concentrations of the "essential amino-acids" it contains.

Q.98. So far, we have talked about so much of protein, but what exactly protein is ?

Ans. The word protein means which is of first importance. Proteins are complex organic nitrogenous substances made up of carbon, hydrogen, nitrogen, oxygen and sulphur in varying amounts.

Some proteins also contain phosphorus and iron, and occasionally other elements. Proteins differ from fats and carbohydrates as they contain nitrogen.

Q.99. What are "Amino-acids" ?

Ans. Amino-acids are simpler substances which make the proteins. Human body needs 22 amino-acids. Out of these, eight are called essential. Because human body cannot synthesize them in sufficient quantity, therefore, the proteins of food must contain them.

Q.100. Will you enlist these eight essential amino-acids ?

Ans. They are the leucine, isoleucine, lysine, methonine, phynylaline, theonine, tryptophane and valine.

Q.101. What happens to the other 14 amino-acids ?

Ans. As a continuous process body proteins are constantly being broken down into their constituent amino-acids and then resynthesized, but one fifth of the total requirements of body proteins (amino-acids) are to be derived from the diet, and the rest from the amino-acids released by the breakdown of proteins in the body.

Q.102. What do you understand by word "Bioligically Complete Proteins"?

Ans. The protein which contains all the essential amino-acids in adequate amounts to meet human requirements is called Bioligically complete protein. Owing to this fact non-vegetarian food stuffs (including milk) are considered as proteins of high biological value.

Q.103. What is "Poor man's meat" ?

Ans. Soyabean is considered as poor man's meat as it contains most of the amino-acids, oils and minerals in large amount. It is the best vegetarian protein for poor Indian community.

Q.104. What are "bioligically incomplete proteins" ?

Ans. Though pulses contain enough proteins yet they are deficient in one or more amino-acids. The same is applicable to cereals and millets as they have still lower values.

Q.105. What you will suggest for vegetarians ?

Ans. They should take wheat, rice and pulses together in various food preparations. Owing to the "supplementation of amino-acid", the total proteins taken in become proteins of high bioligical value (The poor man's meat).

Q.106. How is the nutritional evaluation of protein done ?

Ans. It is done by two methods :

1. Chemical score calculated from the content of essential amino-acids, and
2. Net protein utilization.

Q.107. What do you mean by Net Protein Utilization ?

Ans. It is the percentage of ingested protein nitrogen that is digested, absorbed and retained in the body for tissue synthesis.

$$NPU = \frac{DxBV}{100}$$

Where, Digestibility (D) represents the percentage of the ingested food in nitrogen that is digested and absorbed. Bioligical Value (BV) represents the percentage of absorbed nitrogen that is retained in the body (the absorbed nitrogen minus that excreted in the urine).

Q.108. How to suggest daily protein requirements for the people ?

Ans. Though there are factors which influence the protein requirements of an individual, i.e. age, height, weight, sex, musculature, type of work, stress etc.; but the mixed proteins of the diets of children and adults are of lower quality, and, therefore, correspondingly higher values should be used in calculating the protein requirements. Example : Suppose the requirement of an adult in terms of ideal reference protein is 0.65 gm/kg body weight, it will be 1 gm/kg in terms of dietary protein with an N.P.U. of 65.

Q.109. How does the heating affect protein quality ?

Ans. During normal process of cooking the foodstuff the quality of proteins improves. Certain beans contain trypsin inhibitor which is destroyed while cooking and thereby digestibility increases. But, there is serious damage to nutritive value as happens in baking stage of biscuits. Sugar or carbohydrates are already there and when formation of an indigestible linkage between the essential amino-acids lysine and a reducing sugar is formed. The ultimate result is fall in nutritive value of careal based products. So, for protein rich food baking or toasting of food-stuffs may be avoided.

Q.110. Does lysine supplement valuable ?

Ans. No, being in free amino-acids from, it is rapidly absorbed and is largely wasted as other essential amino-acids in proportionate concentrations are not supplied simultaneously. It is observed that supplementation of lysine to the wheat based diets did not confer any benefit. It was concluded that a wheat based diet providing adequate amounts of protein and calories would also provide sufficient amounts of lysine to meet the requirements.

Q.111. What do you think about "The Protein needs of diabetics and the elderly higher" ?

Ans. Yes they need extra proteins to offset losses from the excessive gluconeogenesis and ketogenesis that is associated with impaired glucose utilization. If hepatic and renal status permits half of the total amount of daily consumption of proteins may be added. The metabolic condition of diabetic patient alongwith renal status should be assessed.

Q.112. What do you understand by the word "Invisible fats" ?

Ans. Each food stuff may contain fat, proteins or carbohydrates. The amount fat cannot be seen like butter, oil or ghee. Therefore, the fat of milk, soyabean, pulse, nuts etc. is called invisible fats. During the diet survey on average Indian, it is found out that the average diet contains at least 15-20 grams of invisible fats.

Q.113. What are the essential fatty acids and their function ?

Ans. They promote growth as well as dermal integrity. The linoleic and arachindonic acids are two important essential fatty acids. The essential fatty acid content of kardi seed oil, corn oil; cotton seed oil; generally oil; groundnut and mustard oil is very high.

Q.114. Is there any relation between fat and atherosclerosis?

Ans. Food rich in fat (usually animal fat) raises serum cholesterol. If the diet contains more than 30% calories from fats of diet the chances of hypercholesterolemia and coronary heart disease are widely prevalent.

It is also said that in the diet where unsaturated fats (having above the two fatty acids) are used, it exerts preventive action against atherosclerosis.

Q.115. What are Carbohydrates ?

Ans. They are cheapest sources of energy and are made up of carbon, hydrogen and oxygen. They can be divided in three groups : starches sugars and cellulose.

Q.116. What are vitamins ?

Ans. These are complex chemical substances required by the body in very small amounts. Vitamins do not supply energy, but act as catalysts in various body processes. They cannot be manufactured in the body (in sufficient quantity), so the diet should contain these vitamins.

Q.117. What are fat soluble vitamins ?

Ans. A,D,E and K are fat soluble vitamins while vitamin C and B complex group are known as water soluble.

Q.118. What are 'body mineral' ?

Ans. From foodstuffs body needs 19 minerals. Many of these minerals are widely distributed in foodstuffs. Some of these minerals are called trace elements, as they are required in micro-quantities.

Q.119. Enlist important functions of minerals.

Ans. They are :

(a) Calcium, phosphorus and magnesium are required for formation of teeth and bones;

(b) Some minerals are present in body fluids and play a physiological role maintaining osmotic pressure, i.e., sodium, potassium and chlorine.

(c) Few minerals like iron, iodine etc. Serve a special function such as the formation of blood, thyroid secretions etc.

Q.120. How psychology can effect the poor performance of on athlete ? Write only four points.

Ans. (1) The athelete's level of arousal is too low, resulting on slowed reaction times, or in a lack of motivation.

(2) The athelete's level of arousal is too high, resulting in excessive muscle tensim, tying up, or impairment in fine motor coordination.

(3) The athelete is distracted by his own internal thoughts. These may be negative ideas, self-doubts, or fears, or they may result from anger and frustration felt when performance fails to meet the athelete's expectations.

(4) The athelete is distracted by relevant external events at critical times (e.g. movement in the crowd).

Q.121. Define "balanced diet" ?

Ans. Balance diet is defined as a diet which contains different types of food in such quantities and proportions that the need for calories, amino-acids, vitamins, minerals, fats, carbohydrates and other nutrients is adequately met for maintaining health, vitality and general well-being and also makes a small provision for extra nutrients to withstand short duration of leanness.

Q.122. Explain the word stitch ?

Ans. Many atheletes complain about a sharp colicky pain in the left or right upper quadrant during strenuous exercise.

The cause of this condition is not always evident, and may in fact be due to varying factors. The most likely explanation is a traping of intestinal air ('gas') in the hepatic or splenic flexure. Physical activity has been shown to increase propulsive movements in the human colon, an occurrence that would cause intestinal air to move to the hepatic or splenic flexures where intraluminal pressure could cause symptoms. Another possible cause of this synetrome is intestinal is chemia brought on by a shift of blood from the abdominal cavity to the large muscles during strenuous activity.

The symptoms of cranp, abdominal pain often disappear spontaneously during exercise. When the pain persist, a rest period is usually sufficient to relieve the discomfort. Persistent pain, even at rest, would require medical evaluation.

CHAPTER NINE
HEALTH

Q.1. How can Health be defined ?

Ans. According to W.H.O., it can be defined as a state of complete mental, physical and social well-being and not merely absence of disease or infirmity.

Q.2. What is Health ?

Ans. A condition of being hale, safe and sound or it can be said that it is the state in which the individual is mobilized at his resource-intellectual, emotional and physical resources for optimum daily living. According to Lester Breslow*, "The daily habits of people have a great deal more to do with what makes them sick and when they die than all the influences of medicine."

Q.3. Suggest some basic habits for maintaining health and longevity.

Ans. By following 7 golden rules, males can add 11 years to their lives while females are found to be benefited by 7 years.

— Get adequate comfortable sleep (7 to 8 hrs). Out of it, first 3-4 hrs. should be of sound deep sleep.

— Eat fairly heavy breakfast, since after dinner there is a 12 hrs. gap, so stomach is ready for food and gall bladder has fully concentrated bile juice to digest the fatty food stuffs.

— If you are lean and thin, eat regular meals and avoid snacks.

— If overweight, control the weight by avoiding fatty and starchy food -consume enough of green vegetables and fruits.

— Do not smoke cigarettes or bidis. Hukka is less harmful.

— Drink moderately or not at all.

— Do not miss your regular exercise schedule.

Q.4. Is heavy exercise good for getting sound sleep ?

Ans. No, moderate physical activity seems to enhance the ability to fall into deep sleep without altering the time spent in rapid eye movement stage of sleep. Because this REM sleep constitutes about 20% of the nights total, while deeper or quieter periods provide the rest necessary for recovery from fatigue. Always remember : Too little or too much exercise appears to result in sleep disturbance.

What do you understand by emotional headache ?
Headaches may be associated with various types of sporting activities. In most instances they are benign and may be referred to collectively as benign exertional headaches. It is important however, for the sports medicine physician to be aware that headaches associated with exertion may occasionally be a sign of underlying organic disease.

Does the body fat have any relation with aging of an individual ?
Always remember "Waits line increases, life line reduces." It is also proved by many researchers that the major that the major reason for the decline in fitness with age is a rise in per cent body fat. The decline in fitness and performance associated with ageing is largely accounted for by increasing body fat.

What do you understand by moderation in life ?
Moderation is a commondenominator in all phases of life, vices, work, and physical activity. Long term survival in a foot race or the human race depends on pacing.

Explain emotional stress GI Track.
Individuals who have organic disorders of the digestive tract may, with few exceptions, participate in competitive and recreational sports. However, consideration must be given, to possible effects of emotional stress upon the affected and normal organs. Emotions can cause hyper function (Spasm or hyperperistalsis), hypofunction (stasis, hypomotility) and combinations of each of these manifestations of impaired function. It has been estimated that 60 to 70 per cent of gastro in testinal complaints are ultimately found to arise from psychophysiologic factors.

Q.9. How can one achieve and maintain better health ?

Ans. Each and everything in the world is uncertain but Death is certain. So do not worry. Take the things easy. Remember, low calorie diet combined with regular physical activity and sleep, a productive and moderately respected role in society contribute to good health.

By the above mentioned approach, the life expectancy can be increased dramatically. Postponement of chronic illness has extended the period of adult vigour, so life remains physically, emotionally, and intellectually vigorous until shortly before it closes.

Q.10. List the various areas which affect the health of an individual.

Ans. It may be grouped in the following manner :

- Endomorph is likely to put on weight. Imitating family eating habits can contribute to inherited tendency of disease.
- Too much or too less use of water may be harmful.
- Properly cooked and natural foods are always better than tinned, fried food and having lot of chillies.
- Proper chewing and having meals at fixed interval are always helpful.
- Relationship of liquids with solids is important. More liquids may dilute the foodstuff and lead to improper digestion.
- Too hot and too cold foodstuffs harm the eaters.
- Emotional and nervous tension play a very important role.
- Hygienic standards, i.e., virus and bacteriological infection should be avoided and needed inoculation and vaccination should be carried out.

Q.11. What do you understand by posture ?

Ans. It is the position or attitude of the body in space. The antigravity muscles work with maximum efficiency and with minimum effort when posture is correct. Poor posture whether standing or sitting produces unnecessary work for muscles and viscera and may also produce aches.

Q.12. How to find out the good normal posture ? Explain.

Ans. The simplest method is to stand in front of a mirror.

— Keep feet spaced four to five inches apart and toes facing forward.
— Weight should be distributed evenly, and slightly in from of ankles. See that ankle joint has 90 angle.
— Knee should not be locked but they should be kept firm.
— Slight normal curve of spine should be maintained at low, upper back and neck level.
— Head should be well set on spine, so eyes look forward.
— Shoulder and hips should come at a level.

Q.13. List the causes of poor posture.

Ans. It may be congenital or acquired. Acquired may be sub-divided into-Heavy bags carried by school children, from disease, accident and malnutrition, fatigue, wrong furniture, lack of correct exercise, more metal work, poor-health knowledge, obesity and poor muscular development.

Q.14. How can postural defects be avoided ?

Ans. From the very childhood, the following points should be kept in mind :
— Practice of remedial exercises for correction of defects.
— Developing postural sense.
— Investigation and correction of fatigued and strained attention, i.e. eye defects (Myopia).
— Health education and nutritional education.
— Avoiding long sitting and standing.
— Avoiding too much exercise for a particular part of body.

Q.15. Can you suggest simplest exercise for Kyphosis and other back defects ?

Ans. Swimming.

Q.16. What are the common causes of knock knee ?

Ans. They are due to rickets, calcium and vitamin deficiency, prolonged standing, flat foot, obesity, heavy body weight and long illness.

Q.17. How to avoid and correct the knock knee ?

Ans. Remove the cause. Horse riding, massage and at an

early age and especially the use of muscle stimulants may help the patient.

Q.18. What is Club foot ? How to correct it ?

Ans. It may be congenital or acquired defect due to poliomylitis in which one or both feet are affected. There is twisting and sole of the food faces inward. Walking is mostly on upper surface of foot. The gait is defective and the patient develops cellosities. The only treatment is surgery.

Q.19. What is forefoot postural strain ?

Ans. There is an ache in the front of the foot (mostly under 2nd and 3rd metatarsal heads). The tenderness may be found in this area.

Q.20. How to treat this condition ?

Ans. Intrinsic exercises should be given.

Q.21. What is "March fractures" or Stress fracture ?

Ans. The stress fracture of metatarsal is known as Marck Fracture. It is generally developed in soldiers or marathon runners. It may be due to hard sole or hard running surface or marching ground. The symptoms may be gradual or rapid. Tenderness is localized and the callus may be palpable.

Q.22. How to manage this condition ?

Ans. Rest from concerned activity. Support with a felt undersole. Stapping is the treatment of choice.

Q.23. What is Morton's metatarsalgia ?

Ans. It is an inter-digital neuroma. There is pain like a knife which can be relieved by removal of footwear. Tenderness is licalized between the metatarsal heads and the neuroma may be palpable, operative removal is the answer.

Q.24. What is Callus ?

Ans. Thickening of the skin due to pressure is known as callus. High heel shoes, narrow pointed shoes are the cause. It can only be treated when the type of shoe is changed.

Q.25. What do you understand by Ingrown Nail ?

Ans. In toes or mostly on large toe, the sides of the nail may curve downward into the flesh, inflaming it. The commonest cause is the pressure of the toe against either the shoe or the next toe. It is often caused by shoes that are too short, too narrow or too pointed. The nail is painful, may become infected, or may require operation.

Q.26. How to prevent it ?

Ans. Use proper shoes. Nails should never be cut too short at the corners. They should be cut straight across. If a nail begins to grow inward, a V may be cut in the margin and little amount of cotton may be placed under the corner of the nail.

Q.27. What do you understand by the world "Athlete's Foot ?

Ans. If skin of the feet is pale and moist or red and sealy, the cause may be a fungus infection. Since swimmers or athletes acquire this infection from each other so the name has been given a athlete's foot, but anybody can suffer from this disease.

Q.28. How to manage it ?

Ans. Since fungus thrives best in moist condition, so feet should be kept dry and between the digits anti-fungal powder may be used. Even drying of interdigital space and use of talcum powder may help. Use of clean dry and washed socks is a necessity. Rerely oral drugs are suggested.

Q.29. What are the basic points to remember for good posture ?

Ans. Stand tall, walk tall and sit tall.

Q.30. What are the harms of poor posture ?

Ans.

1. When the spinal curves are increased, the chest is usually low and abdomen bulges anteriorly (Kypho-lordosis). The joints are out of alignment, not only those of spine, but also those of hips, knees and ankles. The body weight is disturbed unevenly around its central axis.

2 Extreme slumping posture is often mechanically inefficient and reflects an attitude of laziness and lack of self-confidence. When one reaches the middle age, standing and waling for long duration become burdensome and very active exercise virtually becomes impossible. It is because of joint conditions due to long continued postural strain.

3 The internal organs may be hampered in their action as a result of markedly slack posture. Mental work may slow down due to fatigue and diminished circulation. Owing to bad posture, abdomen is relaxed, organs sag downward and forward and this may interfere with their normal action. Constipation may also be there.

Q.31. What happens in a case of flat foot or weak arches of foot "tripod" ?

Ans. In a weak foot the body weight doe not fall at a desired point but falls on the inner side of the foot where boxes are not there to support the weight. In flat footed person ankle rolls inward and bulges on the inner side. Owing to this reason, the medial side of foot is pressed down to the ground when weight is borne on the foot.

Q.32. How does regular activity contribute to Health ?

Ans. Besides recreation, performance of an athlete, physical activity may contribute to health of an individual in the following ways:

(a) Circulation along with heart is kept in good tone. It gives the ability to individual to respond easily to physical and emotional stresses.

(b) Weight is maintained by burning out the energy.

(c) In place of soft and fleshy skeletal muscles become firm by increase in tone. Person feel more alert, comfortable, free of aches and pains.

(d) Metabolic process of the body in general is geared up. The pituitary-adrenal glandular systems are stimulated, contributing to general sense of well-being.

Q.33. What do you understand by wrinkles ? How to avoid them ?

Ans. It is the ageing process which occurs in the skin. To start with, the oil glands become less active, elastic tissue fibres weaken and underlying fat thinner. The mentioned process makes the skin dry and wrinkled.

It should always be remembered that miracles are not possible with the help of creams. But the development of wrinkles may be retarded by avoiding excessive exposure to sunrays and use of good quality lotions.

Q.34. What do you understand by the word 'birth mark' ? Explain it.

Ans. Discoloration, pogmentation of skin since birth or development shortly after the birth. Misconception is about supernatural influence of forefathers etc. Such type of marks are hardly dangerous and need no treatment. It may be that hemangiom as occurs in a ratio of one out of ten children.

Q.35. What is 'wart' ?

Ans. Cauliflower like overgrowths of horny layer of skin may be caused by specific virus. By direct or indirect contact it may spread from one part to other or from one person to other. Surgical removal is the answer.

Q.36. What do you understand by the world "Boil" ?

Ans. When staphylococus enters the skin near hair follicle, infection develops and as a reaction the boil forms. These are the infections which may spread from one part of the body to the other through direct or indirect contact. People suffering from diabetes should be extra cautious.

Q.37. Explain the disease of poor and unhygienic localities 'Scabies" ?

Ans. It is caused by itch mite which burrows under the skin and lays its eggs. It is transmitted form one person to other by direct contact (shaking hands, use of towels etc). There is itching in the night and due to scraching infection and spread of disease occurs. Usually, three applications of Benzyl Benzoate serve the purpose of treatment.

Q.38. What is impetigo contagious ?

Ans. It is an infectious dermatitis which characteristically develops as small blisters, weaping sores and crusts. Mostly it may be seen on hands and face. It spreads by direct or indirect contact. Scratching is another factor which helps in the spread of the disease.

Q.39. How to treat it ?

Ans. Antibiotics with mild corticosteroids are very effective but as far as possible only antibiotic lotion should be applied. If needed systemic antibiotic may be given.

Q.40. Explain the overgrowth on skin known as "Moles" ?

Ans. The overgrowth of deeper pigment layers of skin is known as moles. Though they are harmless yet may change in skin cancer (melenoma). Risk is involved when the mole at neck or feet gets continuous irritation. If moles are irritated or show a tendency to change in colour or size, the doctor should be consulted immediately.

Q.41. What is Leukoplakia ?

Ans. The white, scaly thickening on the lip or membranes of the mouth is called Leukoplakia. It may predispose to cancer.

Q.42. What basic principles should be kept in mind to avoid skin infections and precancerous conditions ?

Ans.
(i) Ample use of glycerinated soap and water (even the ordinary soap will be better) by people working where cancer producing services are being used.
(ii) Use clean gloves and avoid long use of sooty, tarry or greasy clothing.
(iii) Avoidance of over exposure to the sun. It is more important for light-complexioned people. Indians usually do not have much problem.
(iv) Areas subject to frequent irritation should be examined by the qualified skin expert.

Q.43. How are the face powders made ?

Ans. It usually contains talcum, mangnesium, French chalk, and starch or rice powder. One should be careful from large varieties of cheap powders as they may contain undesirable ingredients.

Q.44. Mention something about Lipstick.

Ans. They are usually harmless consmetics, if used skillfully may contribute much to the attractiveness. The cheap quality products contain certain dyes and may cause allergies.

Q.45. Are addiction and habituation the same ?

Ans. No. Addition indicates a severe physical dependence on a drug while habituation is not exactly dependence. It is severe type of psychological desire for a drug. Addiction has three phases :

(i) Compulsion to take drug or substance, to continue to take; and to obtain it by any means.

(ii) Tolerance to drug, so that larger doses are necessary to obtain the psychic effect.

(iii) Physical and psychological dependence, so that illness follows if the drug or substance is withdrawn.

Habituation : There is intense desire but if one does not get drug or substance one will not fall ill.

Q.46. Can you further explain it by quoting examples ?

Ans. Cigarette smoking is habituation while smoke or alcohol drinking may become addiction.

Q.47. Discuss the beneficial and harmful effects of Caffeine (Tea or coffee).

Ans. It has a stimulating effect on brain; it promotes a sense of well-being and reduces fatigue and drowsiness. Speed to any reaction to given stimuli may increase by caffeine if taken in moderation, but the accuracy of response is reduced.

If taken in large amount, it may lead to nervousness, wakefulness, and other effects such as headaches, and dizziness. Moderate stimulation of respiration and circulation may be there. Urine output also increases.

Q.48. Discuss the role of nicotine on human beings.

Ans. Tobacco contains nicotine, a colourless, oily compound which in concentrated form is one of the most powerful poisons. Seventy milligrams about one drop-will cause the death of a man. In the cigarette, the amount of nicotine varies from 0.5 milligram to 2 milligrams per cigarette.

The amount of nicotine absorbed form tobacco varies with type of tobacco and with the method of use. When it is used in powder form as snuff, the proportion of nicotine absorbed is higher than that in either chewing or smoking. Chewing, in turn, results in more absorption than smoking.

Q.49. "Smoking affects the health." Give your comments.

Ans. Many persons pay a heavy price in terms of health but for fashion and habit and relaxation they pay it. It shortens life expectancy and increases the rate of illness, disability and early death from tuberculosis, cancer or heart-attack.

Q.50. If one is not in a position to leave cigarette smoking, what suggestion can be made to minimise the harmful effects ?

Ans. Pipe or cigar smoking is less harmful. Smoke of cigarette should not be inhaled. filter brand should be used or half of the cigarette should be utilised. Never keep full packet in your pocket.

Q.51. In the light of the above questions, discuss the mental depression.

Ans. It ranges in severity from minor dullness to such deep dejection or melancholia that the person does not wish to live and neglect essential mental and physical activities and functions.

Even the normal individual may experience elation and depression. Elation or optimism usually means a happy disposition and unless completely unrealistic, it is to be desired. The depression is more likely to be troublesome, but such periods should not be considered as abnormal, unless they are severe and prolonged.

Depression, if properly treated, is usually transient and result in no permanent disability or handicap.

Q.52. How to identify a depressed person ?

Ans. Such type of person feels alone, without friends, love, status, or esteem. Nothing excites him, the hobbies are uninteresting, and life has lost its meaning.

Person may feel chronically tired, fatigue frequently worse in the morning. There may be complaints of pain, aches, poor digestion, poor bowel function, diminish or loss of sleep, anorexia or lack of desire to have food, weightloss, menstrual disorders in females, and loss of sexual interest. The individual may be irritable, quarrelsome, negligent for household responsibilities and business. One may start taking alcohol, drug, social withdrawal, or may commit suicide.

Q.53. How to help the depressed person ?

Ans. Friends and relatives have the real responsibilities to help the person especially when he/she is depressed or has tendency to commit suicide. Encouraging talks are of great help. Timely medical help may prove beneficial. Such patients should never be left alone.

Q.54. What type of children can be labelled as emotionally sick ?

Ans. School problems, discipline problems, bed wetting, delinquency, and nervousness are all indicators of disturbance. Such type of problems leads the child to be emotionally sick.

Q.55. Can we help such children ?

Ans. The causes of these symptoms should be investigated and. In selected cases. Corrective action should be taken in order to avoid a life of unhappiness, physical illness or antisocial behaviour.

Q.56. What is schizophrenia ?

Ans. It means split personality, characterised by disorientation, loss of contact with reality, delusions, hallucinations, bizarre actions, strange posture, and sometimes senseless laughter.

Q.57. How to identify that an individual is likely to become schizophrenic ?

Ans. One can easily find out if a personality undergoes the following changes :

A young man or female often bright and attractive, gradually undergoes a personality change.

He or she becomes more listless, eccentric, pre-occupied, and suspicious, stays long for longer times, avoid friends.

Such type of individual may also complain of peculiar physical symptoms and react in a variety of ways. He may give furtive smiles and glances; alongwith secret words and gestures. In the worst stages of the disease, his all contacts with the world seems to have been abandoned.

Q.58. How to manage a case of Schizophrenia ?

Ans. Now the cases are rountinelytreated with electric and insulin shocks; tranquilizers and related drugs.

If Schizophrenic case is recognised early and prompt and proper treatment is instituted, most of the patients may improve and are able to lead relatively normal and useful life. Treatment outside the hospital seems to be more effective.

Q.59. Comment upon psychotic patients.

Ans. Such type of people have great difficulty in making correct interpretations of the world around them. Their behaviour is often peculiar, and occasionally they are dangerous to themselves or to others. Psychotic patients usually require hospital treatment. Suicide attempts are common in this group of people.

Q.60. Some people are grouped as neuro-psychotics, will you throw some light on this aspect ?

Ans. People of this category suffer from unreasonable fears, obsessions, compulsions, depressed feelings and unwarranted exhaustion.

Generally the neurotic is able to carry on his work, but he does so with excessive effort, with reduced efficiency, and with reduced personal satisfaction. Such type of persons are able to interpret their environment correctly, they are usually responsible citizens.

People of this type hardly need hospital care. Every individual has some neurotic trait in him, but it may be of very minor degree.

Q.61. What type of people are grouped in the heading of character disorder ?

Ans. Following groups may fall in this category : Alcoholics, drug addicts, delinquents, criminals, sexual deviants etc.

These people will not be considered as insane or irresponsible for their conduct, yet they often behave as if they were totally usually able to interpret their environment adequately, but they lack a mature conscience and as a result are given to impulsive anti-social behaviour. Most people express it through the religion while others claim to be atheist, speak of the power or of the laws of universe. The recognition and acceptance of this faith can be an important element in maintaining emotional security and a sense of direction in one's life.

Q.62. With reference to the basic emotional needs, discuss the important aspect of 'sex' in life ?

Ans. Sex gives rise to the emotional impulse upon which the perpetuation of human life depends. As such it is a powerful emotion with profound influence on behaviour and feelings. In India healthy satisfaction of this impulse in possible through marriage needs, but it is a tragic mistake to attempt to do so by actions which are morally and socially unacceptable and destructive to the individual involved. Gratification of sexual urges in situations which divorce them from warm, loving feelings in immature behaviour; promiscuity is often the evidence of a psychiatric character disorder.

Q.63. What do you understand by the word 'Companionship' ?

Ans. A basic emotional needs for children and adults too. Prolonged isolation can produce mental abnormality. It is essential therefore that they should recognise the importance of companionship and that they select persons as companions whom they admire and respect, for whom they feel affection, and with whom they can be themselves.

Q.64. What type of reactions may occur if emotional needs are unsatisfied ?

Ans. When people are unable to satisfy emotional needs because of situations or individuals within their family, school, employment, or other associations, such people develop frustration, unhappiness and ill health. Other reactions may be in the form of superiorism, feeling of inferiority; day draming, worry, fear, anxiety, insecurity, hostility, withdrawal, sex conflicts, substitution, rationalization etc.

Q.65. List the seven warning signals of cance ?

Ans. If the following symptoms are there, one must consult the doctor :

— Unusual bleeding or discharge after Menopause.

— A lump or thickening in the breast or elsewhere.

— A sore or ulcer that does not heal.

— Change in bowel or bladder habits.

— Hoarseness or cough.

— Indigestion or difficulty in swallowing.

— Change in the size of wart or mode.

Q.66. What possible treatment can be given for cancer ?

Ans. If detected, early surgical removal of the part is the best but if it is not possible then other treatment includes-radiation, antibiotics, chemicals, hormones and chemotherapy are alternatives. They may be used in conjunction with surgery or separately.

Q.67. Enlist the common emotional needs.

Ans. The basic needs may be-love, independence or individual autonomy (the individual in his own right); security; achievement (recognition, approval, success); faith (belief in God-something greater outside ourselves); sex-creative needs; guidance or examples in living; companionship.

The concept expressed in the above-mentioned list is quite generally accepted, but if someone feels may add to, subtract from; or otherwise modify it.

Q.68. Explain the word faith or God.

Ans. God is nothing but faith in some forces or power outside or and greater than ourselves. For mankind it has always been a basic emotional need. The concept of God means different things for different people but here we are talking in relation to mental health. So the important thing is that people believe in the purposefulness and meaningfulness of their own lives.

Q.69. Describe the syncope among sports world ?

Ans. Syncope cere bral ischemia. It far more likely represents a transient global ischemia with reduced blood flow to brain stem reticular formation, causing a sudden loss of consciousness.

The sport physician may see sudden syncopal episodes following running. In one case, repeated episodes were throught to represent a beta-adrenergic receptor-mediated varsode pressor responses, since it was blocked by a beta blocker. Of course, these episodes can be seen following severe dehydration and we have all seen runners collapse near the end of a long race, such as a marathon, from the combination of dehydration and pooling of blood in the lower extremities.

Another cause of syncope associated with atheletics is an exagge ration of a normal response that most of us have experienced as dizziness or light headedness upon standing after a squat. This results from pooling of blood and a sudden drop in cardiac output upon rising. This response can be highly exaggerated in weight lifters, in whom the squat is often associated with hyperventilation and a volsalvamaneuver. The pooling of blood in the lower extremities upon standing is further accentuated by the sudden release of the intrathorace pressure following the valsalva maneuver. Blood pools in the great viens and splanchnic vessels, further delaying return of normal cardiac output. This has been called "Weight lifter" black-out.

CHAPTER TENTH
FEMALE HEALTH PROBLEMS

Q.1. Give your opinion about Female Participation in Sport ?

Ans. During the last few years it has been observed that a fainly good number of female participate for games and physical activities in a country like India. So far there is very little knowledge about possible type of Injuries and whether these injuries are different thank males or not. More attention is paid towards the brease reproductive organs. It is also an old concept than women should be discouraged from participating "unladylike" active sports. In our country we have also observed an outpouring of women, particularly at the collegiate level competitive sports.

They came from backgrounds in sports in which little was known of conditioning, or pre sport warm-ups. Many schools and colleges had hardly adequate coaching, training or equipments.

Q.2. Comment on common injuries to females ?

Ans. Number of injuries to women in athletics was higher than men. This was attributed to poor conditioning and training. The majority of problems were in the knee and ankles, with women sustaining a higher incidence of shin-pain.

Q.3. What is about chances of getting Breast problems in Athletes?

Ans. Though chances of getting injury to breast are not much but player do suffer from discomfort, resulting primarily from poorly designed brassieres. The primary problems associated with the brassieres are contusions, abrasions from hooks allergies to synthetic materials, the bra-slipping-up over the breast, straps slipping off the shoulders etc: Runners Nipple' occurs when nipple due to friction or movements or get inflamed. When no bra is worn, the breast rub against the shirt and causes the same problem.

Q.4. Please give comments in relation to trauma to the Breast in games & sports ?

Ans. Although we know that serious breast injuries occurring during athletic activities are rare, painful blows to the breast which cause contusions ans haemorrhages into the loose fatty tissue of the breast commonly occur.

Due to the large number of girls participating in Hockey, Kabaddi, Basket ball, Gymnastics etc. has created more interest in minor traumatic breast injuries, especially to school and team physicians. Such injuries can result in fat neurosis which is clinically difficult to differentiate from carcinoma.

Q.5. By research in bra design, can help the athlete - Explain ?

Ans. There have been previous unsuccessful attempt to develop a practical protective bra. There is no doubt that problems such as bulkiness, discomfort and lack of non-toxic material have no developed a standard size, fully protective bra to be worn over the regular bra during athletic games. The material is approved non-porous, non-irritating plastic which will not absorb body perspiration. The bra weights less than 4 ouncess and there is no associated discomfort to the wearer. Each cup will support thirty pounds weight and its designed with a relief-allowing absorption of a direct blow, and will reflect even hard tennis racket or baseball bat blows.

The pro+Tec Bra can also offer protection from external pressure or blows during painful periods of chronic cytic mastitis. The plastic cup can also be used under the regular bra as a protective splint after a breast biopsies. This bra will prove a useful preventive aid in reduction of serious or minor breast injuries in all body-contact activities.

GENITALIA AND REPRODUCTIVE ORGANS ?

Q.6 Among female athletes in there any chance to injure ?

Ans. Yes, there are chances of getting injuries of the vulva occur from falls on the balance beam in gymnastics and during cross country run. There are chances of getting rupture urethera in a fainting attack during certain type of events.

Though the chances of getting pelvic fractures and injuries are there but insipite of severe pelvic fractures so far no worker has reported or seen any injury to the reproductive organs. Off course a lady who is pregnant may go into abortion (Chances of getting injury to reproductive organs are only possible when entire pelvic bones are crushed or when injury is fatal). There may be chances when lady is pregnant for more than 4 months. But again such lady is unlikely to participate in games during pregnancy. Anatomically also if we see it is observed that reproductive organs are very well protected by the bony structure and only a direct blow or penetrating injury is likely to cause damage.

Q.7. What do you think about chances of getting injury to uterus ?

Ans. As far as pregnancy is concern it is once again said that little is known about what can happen to a pregnant player pregnancy. But for information injury is more easily sustained when uterus rises-up out of the pelvis after 4th or 5th months of pregnancy.

Q.8. What are common queries in your mind about female athletes ?

Ans. They are :-

— What are the problems specified to sports?

— Whether these problems are easily avoidable just by changing our life style and the attitudes towards the health and hygienre?

— In what sense do the physical activity help us or harm for our health?

Q.9. Explain the word Monarch ?

Ans. It is the age at puberty when first menstruation starts. This is usually between 12 to 14 years. In many cases it may be delayed. The climate and the physical activity affects the age of Monarchy and it has been found to be delayed among the more physically active girls.

Q.10. What do you understand by word Amenorrohoea in female Athletes ?

Ans. Amenorrhoea may be pathological or physiological are depending upon the age and the causes.

By the term physiological amenorrhoea we mean the absence of menses in normal physiological conditions like pregnancy, lactation, after the menopause or before menarche. The pathological we mean the absence of menses due to some organic or functional defects in the system. It can be primary amenorrhoea if menstruation fails to start upto the age of 18 years. Seasation of menstruation after once it has established in the fertile age is termed as secondary amenorrhoea.

Q.11. Please explain it further for clear picture ?

Ans. The wall of the uterus is made up of connective tissues and the myometrial muscle fibres. Both tissue grew in balance as the child grows. At the time of puberty in some girls the muscle fails to grow as compared to the connective tissue. In such an uterus where there exist the imbalance between connective tissue of the muscle fibres the menses becomes painful. Such a case call be diagnosod on internal examination but, as we know that before marriage female should not be exposed to such examinations, so the cause remain obscure. The physical activity to such a patient helps to develop the muscular part of their urenogenital system and this relieves the pain.

The other important cause of dysmenorrhoea is the congestion and the inflammation of neighbouring organs of the pelvis. The problem of colitis, constipation, urinary tract infection all may lead to such a problem. It happens so because all pelvic organs are supplied by the blood vessels which are the branches of same major vessels, so the conjection of one affects the other.

If the infection is sever than the pain may start a week before onset of the cycle or otherwise it is at the time of usual cycle it create a problem. In case of poor hygiene habits also uterus is affected with infection and gets inflammed and then create more pain during menses. The most important cause of dysmenorrhoea has also been found to be lack of hemoglobin and iron deficiency.

Q.12. Explain the term Menorrhegia for better understanding give details also ?

Ans. Excessive loss of blood during menses is known as Menorrhegia when it is irregulars its cycle then it is known as Meno-metrorrhegia.

The cause can be:-

Gynaecological,

Cardio-vascular,

Hemopoetic, and

overian disfunctional urine bleeding.

When there is the infection and inflammation in the surrounding organs of the ovaries then it leads to the congestion of the overian tissues and affects the ovrial folical, which then fails to shed off its ovum and the follicular phase of the uterus is prolong which leads to the heavy bleeding during normal menstrual cycle. Many players experience heavy blood flow if they play during menses. This happens due to the effect of physical activity on the uterine wall. This is likely to happen among those only who are not perfectly conditioned for their game. Fear to the situation affects through psychological tress and poor conditioning affects through over excitation of cardio-vascular system. Both leads to increase in blood pressure and heavy bleeding. Of course others are the real medical problems and should be consulted with the doctors.

Q.13. Anaemia? It is a big problem among Indian females.

Ans. Anaemia is the another major problem among the female athletes. Though she herself does not know about anaemia and so complains about general weakness and inability to meet the demand of physically active schedule. Such cases are diagnosed only on bio-chemical investigations. The lack of Hemoglobin is known as Anaemia which may be due to several factors. Firstly women are subjected to regular blood loss and it is the iron that always remains deficient because except iron rest of the elements of blood are fulfilled by the diet throughout the month. Element of iron is very less available in vegetarian diet and also its absorption is very specific. Whatsoever iron suppliment you take it is only the certain percentage of it is absorbed and rest is wasted in stool. When the absorption defects are added along with the menstrual loss and dietary deficiency, then the problem of iron deficiency is doubled.

Q.14. What is sports Anaemia? Explain it ?

Ans. It is the another problem with which both group of athletes are affected. It is developed due to distruction of blood cells in the foot steps by the constant running practices. The long distance runners, sprinter and also the players of hockey and foot balls who trained themselves for the development of endurance by running hard everday, are affected with this problem. It has been found among many athletes, that, they have fair amount of Hemoglobin to their blood but still they feel weak. It is because in the course of blood loss the stored iron has been used to generate new hemoglobin and so the tonic iron which is also required for many other metabolic reactions falls short, and so if proper bio-chemical investigations is not perfomed for the estimation of Iron, the cause of weekness remains unknown.

Q.15 What is about problem of Backache among females ?

Ans. It is the another problem which is more often complained by ladies particularly by non active group. Among physically active females this complain is of different origen. The most important cause is weakness of lumbosacral muscles, faulty postures and sometimes the abnormal construction of genital organs, i..e., uterus and cervix. Among sports individual this may be due to strain of lumbosacral muscles when the exercise is performed without proper warming up and conditioning.

Q.16. Do the females have often a trouble which is known as HEADACHE. Give your opinion.

Ans. It is another most common problem and high frequency among ladies.

Common causes may be :-

Organic,

Physiological,

and phychological

The most common one is the psyclogical cause. When no organic and physiological causes are tracable then one should think for the socio-psyclogical problem of the individual. Ofcourse, the organic cause must be ruled out first.

The physiological causes are nothing but the over physical strain with improportionate diet and lack of sleep is very common among people. Gastric upset; over-eating and the premenstrual syndrom are may also lead to headache. So for such a problem proper history, medical check-up and through investigation must be carried out.

It is better for every sports men and women if they maintain their health diary and after filling up the colums may get it signed by Doctor specialist in sports medicine. To remark in close contact with Doctor and off and on discussion on health matter will always help you to understand yourself.

Q.17. Mention some structural difference among male & female ?

Ans. Some structural differences:

a) differential growth at adolescence, hormonally mediated.

b) male adolescent spurt later than female gives both greater absolute size and a longer time for greater lenghtening of limbs relative to trunk.

c) favoured growth of male foremam, relative to whole arm and to leg length.

Q.18. What is the basis of sex difference ?

Ans. Genetic basis of sex :

a) the y-chromosome as the sex determinant
b) embryological differentiation
c) intersexes-Klinefelter's (XX) and Turner's (XY) syndromes.

Q.19. What is average difference in size of two sexes ?

Ans. Human males and females identical until 10 years, then girls are larger until 14, then male growth spurt carries them to approx 10% greater in weight and most external measurements.

Q.20. Mention the basic bony difference among male and & female ?

Ans.

Item	Result
size : Usually smaller, shorter	lower center of gravity Lighter body frame.
Pelvis : Wide	Difference running mechanics
Thighs : Start inward toward knees	Injury may be more likely because of
Lower leg bones:Less "Bowed"	knee instability.
Limbs (relative to body length).	Shorter lever arm for movement important for use of inplements
Shoulder : Narrower, greater sloping	Different mechanics of upper limb motion
upper arms: Do not hang vertically	
Elbows: Marked carrying angle	Important in throwriag pattern.

Q.21. Give the detail account of bony differeneces in both sexes ?

Ans. Here are some important features which show that female skeletion is not actualy the same as that of males.

Main differences - men have broader shoulders, narrower hips, longer legs, and relatively even longer forearms.

Shoulders; male over growth may be a differential response in coracoid, acromial, clavicular and rib cartilages, to produce centres of ossification. Muscles accommodates to skeletal size.

Hips; increased hip width of women is mainly due to pelvic bone structure, but also to fat overlay. Bone growth probably a hormonal response to oestrogen, with Hyperplasia of cartilage at junctions round acetabulam. Female pelvis wider and more spacious; shallower, and with greater diameters. Iliaflare out more to the sides. Sacrum shorter, wider and less curved and coccyx more flexible.

Ischial spines turn outward and are further apart. All contribute to a wider outlet of the true pelvis, to facilitate childbirth.

The pelvic articulations - Sacroiliac joint, public symphysis and sacrococcygeal symphysis - are influenced by hormones during pregnancy. Attributed to 'relaxin' which causes depolymerisation of collagen or of connective tissue ground substance. This, at a basal level, may in part be responsible for much greater general flexibility of women.

Legs; the leg lenght in men is greater than in women, relative to body lenght. In pre-adulescence, legs are growing relatively fastest of all skeletal dimensions.

Q.22. What is the difference between female & male pelvis ?

Ans. Two structural effects are a result of greater female pelvic width :-

i) the femoral shaft is directed downward and medially to approach the femur of the opposite side, the greater female convergence may predispose to an outwara rotation of the lower leg in running;

ii) the femoral neck is incline at a greater angle with the shaft of the femur, than in the male. This results in its being relatively weaker.

Q.23. Is there specifie difference in the arms of two sexes ?

Ans. Yes, there is some specifie difference Arms; the male arm length is greater, relative to body lenght. In part, this is for the same reason as the legs, but even for the same lenght of leg the male arm is longer, due to a sex difference in the develompment of the foream. The difference is already established at two years of age. It is biomecanically important in sports and events involving striking ball with implements and in throwing, in all of which initial velocity of the struck or thrown missile is a ctitical parameter.

The other main difference in arms between the sexes is that when women hold their arms down, with the palms facing forward they have a larger, carrying angle; than men. At puberty, an ossification centre develops for the lateral humeral Epiconyle, and it is probable that a differential growth of cartilage occurs in it in the male, and so acts to stranghten-out the male arm- and which may materially help him to throw better.

A feature of the adult male skeleton in general is that dentsity is greater than that of the adult female. Due to thick cortices of male bones (humerus, femur and cibial, probably occurs at adolescence).

Q.24. As for as composition a fat-content is concern there is some pecuarities explain them with reasons.

Ans. There is a striking difference in body composition between men and women with regard to body fat, in that an 'average' young woman contains twice the amount of fat as a corresponding man, expressed as a percentage of body of body weight. The classification of during and passmore is:-

Men	Women	% Fat
Thin		5
Average		10
Plump	Thin	15
Eat	Average	20
	Plump	25
	Fat	30

Q.25. Mention the difference in relation to body compositio also ?

Ans.

Item	Result
Body fat: Greaterpercentage	contnurs morer ounded, less angular.
Bone and muscle: Less of each	Physique less meso morphic, more ehdomorphic.
Subcutancous adipose tissue: concentration particularly inbuttcks	Less metabrlically active tissue Gretear more bugyant
Muscle: smaller proportion in relation to body fat	Lower ratio of strength 1035 to weight loss.

This implies that there is more fat and less muscle per unit volume of the female body, and imposes a tremendous handicap on her in most aspects of physical activity, relative to her male counterpart. It also tends to distort a variety of physiological measurements such as VO_2 Max. If the female limb contains proportionately less muscle for the same mass, its inertia will be greater than in men, proportionately and its speed of movement will be less.

Q.26. Explain the fluid & blood differences among males & female. If needs give done examples also ?

Ans. Total body fluid in both sexes approximates to 75% of lean body mass. In general terms this amounts to about 60% of male body weight, and 50% of female.

There are wide variations in blood volume, and it varies with the degree of training. A volume of 5 to 6 liters for men and 4 to 4.5 liters for women is considered normal, giving around 75 ml/kg and 65 ml/kg respectively.

Normal haematocrit values are 47% for men and 42% for women with respective haemoglobin levels of 15.8 gms, (+ .0 and + 1.1).

Example :- At submaximal rates of working, 1 litre of oxygen is transported by 8 litres of blood in men, and by 9 litres in women; during maximal exercise, the differences reflect the haemoglobin disparities.

Q.27. Compare male & female in relation to eardio-vascular system?

Ans.

Blood volume : Lower	Total oxygen-carrying capacity of blood lower
Red blood cells : Fewer	
Hemoglobin : Lower	
Heart : smaller	Higher heart rate, smaller stooke volume, and lower oxygen pulse for given cardiac output and maximum oxygen uptake
Maximum cardiac output Lower :	Maximum aerobic capacity lower by 20 to 25%

Q.28. When females are diferently inferior in mentioned questions, then explain the differnces in pulse rate & Blood pressure also ?

Ans. Women operate at a systolic and diastolic pressure about 10% less than men. The maximal heart rate tends to equal in the sexes, e.g., 195 + 10 beats per minute for the 25 years old woman working at 50% of her maximal aerobic power has a rate of 140% min., compared to 130min for comparable male.

Q.29. Is the lung volumes & other respiratory paramaters are also affected in females ?

Ans. Yes, it is true

In women, the lung volumes are about 10% smaller than for men of the same age and weight.

Between 20 and 30 years of age respiratory rates of men and women running at maximal oxygen uptake have been measure at 46/min for men, and 40/min for women, with no overlap at 25D's.

Maximal voluntary ventilation rates have been measured in 25 years old healthy men at 140 litres/ min (100 to 180), and for women 951/min (70 to 120).

Q.30. Females have different size as well as extra fat how it affects is thermal regulation ?

Ans. At beginning of mode rate activity in ambient temperature of 20 Cand 25% humidity, men and women lose heat in following proportions; 40% by convection; 40% by radiation; 20% by avaporation of sweat. As activity proceeds, proportions change, with women tending to loss proportionately more heat by radiation, and men by evaporation. Some workers claim no difference in sweet rates. Lesser ability to dissipate heat does seem to be a barrier in prolonged sessions of very high energy expenditure.

Q.31. Is there any difference in male & female disease & death rate?

Ans. In majority of diseases, morbidity and mortality rates are less for women,e.g., cancer, coronary heart disease, respiratory conditions, ulcers and diabetes. In atheromatous conditions, cestrogans seem definitely protective, and post-menopausal women tend towards the male incidence.

Q.32. Give your views regarding mences & physical training ?

Ans. All over the world Gynacologists are of the view that a sudden strassful event in life of a female with normal menstrual perious can bring about cessation of mences. It is also a fact that certain female athletes during the period of intense training develop either amenorrhoea or irregular periods but once successful training is discontinued the menstraual cycle returns to normal and the women is able to become present. The same type of observations are made for womentraining in ballet dances. It is an expected physiological response and causes no distress.

Q.33. What is mentioned in the literature about psychological aspects, nutrition ets & there relation with mences?

Ans. Lot of literature is being published regarding psychology of the female athlete. Here it will be out of place to mention the details but in nutshell it can be said that women have definate psychological problems which are associated with sports. It is observed that if females have better nutrition, mences starts few months earlier.

Improvement in nutrition has resulted in girls reaching a critical weight. After reaching to optimum weight physiological causes the hypothalamaus to start its regulation of the menstrual cycle.

Q.34. Please comment on mensturation & performance ?

Ans. Several investigetors have compared performance during mences with measures obtained at normal time. Although the physiological variations are more drametic during these times, they certainly are not limited to a binary function. Maximal or near maximal cardiorespiratory efforts has not been investigated in relatioship to potential variations during the intermenstural phase of the cycle. It appeared that if interperformance comparisions were to be made which necessitated measurement at various times during the intermenstrual cycle, that attempts should be made to further determind the periodcity, or lack thereof, of variations in performance.

Q.35. What is DYSMENORRHOEA ? Define it.

Ans. "Lower abdominal pains or cramps during the mentruanal period and is often accompanied by headache, back ache, legache, breast fulness or tenderness, abdominal swelling."

Q.36. Will you further explain it ?

Ans. It occurs most commonly just before the mences or at the beginning of menstrual flow and usually it ceases when the flow is established." The incidence and degree of dysmenorrhoea are difficult to determine because pain is a subjective symptom and tolerance to pain varies among different individuals.

Investigators found the posture of the girls was not generally good. Lack of knowledge and understanding of the meaning of menstruation, lack of regular complete medical examination and proper immediate followup. Hellebrandt also observed that 30% cases develop Dysmenorrhoea from structural, endocrine infections, faulty living habits, lack of exercise, poor posture, fatigue, irritability, and tension resulting from daily activities are considered as more common factors.

Q.37. What education suggestions you will like to give to females regarding mensturation & sports ?

Ans. Athletes may keep following points in the mind.

i) There is no evidence that participation in sports by itself invokes any significant changes in the menstrual cycle, either favourable or unfavourable for the majority of females.

ii) Dysmenorrhoea is apparently neither aggravated nor cured by sports participation. Its appearance and severity appear to depend more on psychological factors and it seldom prevents a high level women athlete from competition.

iii) Physical performance by women seem to be best in the immediate postmenstrual period and upto the 15th day of menstrual cycle. It is also a fact that in sports where endurance is involved, performance during menstruation to be poor; where short bursts, of activity is the only requirment.

iv) Women performing during menstruation have also achieved record breaking-medal winning performances. Top class athlete will almost invariably compete during menstruation although some of them are not psychologically prepared for it.

v) girls or women should not look on mences as sickness. Full participation should be allowed at all times for those who desire to active during menses.

vi) Postponement of mences by the use of hormones is some-time possible but may lead to symptoms which may impair the ability of the athlete to compete.

Q.38. Give Tasular account of percent improvement in selected moscimal & submoscimal performance variables for males & females ?

Ans.

Variable	Male	Female
1. VO2 max (ml/kg/min)	15.0	14.2
2. Heart Volume (me)	11.7	11.0
3. Blood Volume (l)	6.4	4.9
4. Strength (lbs)	20.0	23.0
5. Resting heart rate (Beats/mt)	5.9	7.9
6. Submoscimal Heart rate (Beats/mt)	7.4	10.1

Average for curl- leg press, Bench press.

Q.39. To conclude, about female Athlete, what comments you will like to give?

Ans. Sports activity & females response to acute & chronic excercise by adapting physiologically to the specifie demands of her sport. Due to this fact, her physiological profile closely resembles that of males in the some sport, rather then untrained women or even female athletes in other sports.

The basic difference between the sexes in response to training is related to the differential effects of oestrogen & testosterone on the muscular system. It is well known that male has higher ratio to lean body mass & strength with training, However, females can increase their strenght sufficiently, even without marked muscular hypertrophy, to improve sports performance & to protect them from injury. It also appears that the mechanisms under lying the adaptation to training are more or less the same for male & females.

Few female athletes may experience irregularities in their menstural cycles. There is no long term negative effects on reproductive function. The low aestrogen may affect bone metabolism- decrease mineral density, more stress fractures & ostioporosis.

Q.40. Is there any difference among male & female as far as strenght is concerned ?

Ans. Yes, the absolute strenght of females in our society is about two-thirds that of males. Female are relatively weaker than males in the chest, arms, and shoulders; and there is less difference in leg strenght. Most of this difference is attributed to increased lean body mass secondary to testosterone production puberty. However, some of the general differences may be caused by sociocultural factors. Both women and men are expected to use their lower extrėmities for a certain amount of locomotion, but a minimal use of the upper extremities. This could give men greater baseline upper extremity strenght.

Q.41. Explain the effection that tolerance among athletes ?

Ans. In general, women and men respond similarly to heat at rest. Tolerance to exercises in heat appears to be related to the degree of acclimation and conditioning. Because studies comparing men and women working in heat relate heat tolerance to maximum aerobic capacity, men appear to tolerate heat more effectivaly. With repeated exposure to work in heat, both men and women develop lower mean core and skin temperature, a decreased heart rate, and an increase in the amount of time they can withstand the stress. Thus, physically fit women have a greater tolerance of heat than their untrained ones.

Men have higher sweat rates than women, because women have a higher surface areas to mass ratio and a lower mentabolic rate of heat production, the higher sweat rate may not be essential for the woman athlete.

Q.42. What is about the effect of Altitude on female performance ?

Ans. The performance of women at high altitudes has not been well studied. Hannon, at al. reported that women seem to be at less risk of altitude sickness than men; and, when women do suffer from altitude sickness, it is less severe and of shorter duration. They experience lesser changes in resting heart rate, weight, blood volume, and girls chemistries then men. Nevertheless, women and girls should approach exercise at high altitudes carefully.

Q.43. Please give research openions regarding menarche & mences ?

Ans. Studies of participants in athletic competitions have suggested that, except for swimmers, the age of menarche was 13.7 years. Each group of athletes had an average age of menarche later than that of the general population of their country of origin. Runners and gymnasts had the latest menan ages of menarche, 14.3 years and 14.5 years, respectively; swimmers had the earliest at 13.1 years. An earlier study showed the ages of menarche as 14.2 years in a group of Olympic Volleyball players, 13.0 in high school and college athletes, and 12.2 years in non-athletes. A Swedish study in 1963 showed that swimmers had a mean age of menarche slightly lower than that of the general swedish population. The more rigorous training of swimmers today may delay their menarche as happens with other high-energy consuming sports.

The role of athletic participation in menstrual dysfunction is more difficult to assess because researchers frequently fail to defined or differentiated degrees of of menstrual dysfunction, irregularity, and dysmonorrhea. In addition, the incidence of these problems in control populations frequently is not well established, Estimates of dysmenorrhea have ranged from 36 to 71% in the general population of adolescents. Irregular menstruation has been reported in 6 to 31% of normal girls. In comparison, 8 of 29 champion teen-age swimmers (30%) had "inappreciable menstrual pain," I had moderate menstural pain, and 8 (17%) had irregular menses. Zaharieva reported an incidence of irregular menses of 14.8% in the 1964 Tokyo Olympic athletes less than 16 years old and of 7.6% overall. A study of 557 Hungarian women athletes found no effect of intense athletic participation on the menstrual cycle in 83%, a favourable effect in 5%, and an adverse effect in 12%, disorders were the most common in the 15- to 17- years-old group.

REFERENCES

1a. Allsen, P.E., Harrison, J.M., Vance, B.(1984) : "Fitness for Life, An induvidualised Approach", WMC Brown, Publishers, Dubuque, Iowa.

1b. Arthur E.Ellison, M.D., Arthur L.Boland, Jr.,M.D.Kenneth E.Dettaven, M.D., Paul Grace, A.T., C. George A. Snook, M.D. Heather Cale huff, A.T., C.,P.A.C.(Celetorial Board)- ATHLETIC TRAINING AND SPORTS MEDICINE-1984- (Published by The American Academy of Orthopaedic Surgeons).

1c. A.Dirix, H.G.Knuttgen & K. Tittel-The Oly-MPIC Book of Sports Medicine- 1988.
Published by Balckwell Scientific Publication.

2. Astrand, I. (1960) : "Aerobic Work Capacity in Men and Women with Special Reference to Age", Acta Physiol. Scand. 49 (Suppl.), 169:1-92.

3. Astrand Perolaf and Rhyming Irma(1954) : "A Nomogram for Aerobic Capacity (Physical Fitness) from Pulse Rate during Submaximal Work", Jour. of Appl. Physiol. 7 : 218.

4. Adolph, E.F. Physiology of Man in the Desert : New York, Interscience, 1947.

5. Amold, A. : Korper-Entwicklung and Leibesubungen, pp. 125-157, Leipzig : e Johnn Barth, 1931.

6. Astrand, P.O. and K. Rodhal, Text book of Work Physiology; McGraw Hill, 1970.

7. Adams S.(1980) Ibuprofen : Pharmokinetics. Br. J.Clin, Practice Suppl. 6,3.

8. Adams R.J. and Chandler F.A. (1953) Osteitis pubis of traumatic aetiology. J.Bone Joint Surg. 35A,685.

9. Allemandou A. (1976) A Statistical review of injuries. Injuries in Rugby Football and other Team Sports. Dublin, Irish Rugby Football Union.

10. Alam A., Lamke L.O. and Liljedahl S.O. (1975) Surgical treatment of dislocation of the peroneal tendons. Injury 7, 14.

11. Andersen, N.H. and Ramwell, P.W.(1974) Biological aspects of prostaglandins. Arch. Intern. Med. 133,30.

12. Barber H.M.(1973) Horse play : Survey of accidents with horses. Br. Med. J. 3,532.

13. Bateman J.E. (1969) Shoulder injuries in throwing sports. In

symposium on Sports Medicine, St. Louis, Mosby.
14. Bearden J.M., Hughston, J.C. and Whatley G.S.(1973) Acromioclavicular dislocation rnethods of treatment, J.Sports Med.1,4.
15. Behling F.(1973) Treatment of acromioclavicular separations. Orthop. Clin. North Am. 4,747.
16. Blazina M.E.(1966) Shoulder injuries in athletes. J.Am, Coll. Health Assoc, 15,143.
17. Blazina M.E.(1963) Jumper's knee. Orthop. Clin. North Am. 4,67.
18. Blostein J.L.(1960) Electroencephalography in boxers. J.Sports Med. Phys. Fitness, 1,30.
19. Blonstein J.L. (1966) Medical aspects of amateur boxing. Proc. R.
20. Blonstein J.L. and Schmid L. (1974) Causes of death in ex-boxers. Br. J. Sports Med. 8.205.
21. Blumenkrantz N. and Sondergaard J.(1972) Effects of prostaglandin E.F. on the biosynthesis of collagen. Nature (New Biol.) 1239,246.
22. Bourne M. and Bentley S.(1980) Enhanced recovery from sports 6.72.
23. B.yd.H.B. and Anderson L.D. (1961) A method for reinsertion of the distal biceps brachii lendon. J.Bone Joint Surg. 43A,1041.
24. Buck J.E.(1970) Direct repair of the defect in spond-lolisthesis. J.Bone Joint Surg. 52B,432.
25. Burke Edmond, Keenana Thomus, J.(1984) : "Energy cost, heart rate and perceived exertion during elementary backstroke", The physician and Sports Medicine, Vol. 12, No.2.
26. Borg. G.V. and Linderholm, H. (1967) :"Perceived exertion and pulse rate during graded exercise in various age groups". Acta Med. Scand. (Suppl.): 472-194.
27. Bergstrom,J.,Hultman, E. (1972) : "Nutrition for maximal sports perormance", J.A.M.A.,221:1006.
28. Barrow, H.M. and McGee, R. : "A practical approach to measurements in physical education", Third Edn., 1979, Lea and Febiger, Philadelphia.
29. Barry, L.J. and Nelson, J. (1982): "Practical meaurements for evaluation in physical education", Surjeet Publication, 7-K, Kolhapur Road, Kamala Nagar, New Delhi 110 007, India.
30. Bapat, V.D.(1986) : Jnpublished work, personal communication.

31. Brouha, Lucien (1943) : "The step test - A simple method of measuring physical fitness for muscular work in young men", Research Quarterly, 14:31-36.
32. Balasubramaniam, B. and Pansare, M.S.(1986): "Effect of yoga on cardiovascular efficiency", Unpublished work, paper read in State Conf. of Sports Medicine, Nagpur, Feb.1986.
33. Bhole, M.V., Karambelkar, P.V. and Gharote, M.L. (1970): "Effect of yoga practices on vital capacity" -A preliminary Communication, Ind. Jour. Chest. Dos.,Vol. XII, 1 and 2 : 1-4.
34. Bhole, M.V., Karambelkar, P.V. and Gharote, M.L.K.(1972): "Effect of yoga training on vital capacity"and Breath holding time", Yoga Mimamsa, Vol. XII,3 and 4 : 19-26.
35. Brown, B.S., Payne, T. Kim, C.et al. (1979): "Chronic Response of rat brain norepinephrine and serotonin levels to endurance training",J.Appl. Physiol. 46:19-23.
36. Bennet Collee, L.(1956) : Relative contribution of modern dance, Folk dance, Basketball and swimming to motor abilities of college women:, Research Quarterly, 27 No.3 : 253.
37. Baldwin, K. Klinker, Fuss G., Tejjung R., Mole, P. and Holloszy, J.(1972) : "Respiratory capacity of white, red and intermediate muscles-Adaptative response to exercise", Am. J. Physiol. 222,363.
38a. Bezi, G.,Penceri, P., Debernardi, M.Villa, R.Arcelli, E.,d'Angelo, L.,Arrigoni, E. and Berke, F(1973) : "Mitochondrial Enzymatic adaptation of skeletal muscle to endurance training", J.Appl. Physiol. 34.107.
38b. Bengt O. Eriksson, Tore Mellstrand, Lars Peterson, Per Renstrom, Nils Svedmyr.-SPORTS MEDICINE (Health & Medication)-1990.
(Published in Great Britain by Guinness Publishing Hd, 33 London Road).
39. Bergstorm, J. Hermansen, L., Hultmari, E., and Saltin, B., (1967) :"Diet, muscle glycogen and physical performance" : Acta Physiol. Scand. 71,140
40. Buskirk, E.R. and H.L. Taylor : "Maximal oxygen intake and its relationship to body composition", J. Applied Physiology, 11 : 72-78,1957.
41. Buskirk, E.R. P.F. Lampietro and D.E. Base, " Work performance after dehydration : effects of physical conditioning and heat acclimatization." J.Appl. Physiology. 12:189-194,1958.

42. Buskirk, E.R. and W.C. Graslay, Heat injury and conduct of athletes : Ch. 16 in Science and Medicine of exercise and sports, 2nd edition, W.R. Johnson and E.R. Buskirk, Editors, New York, Harper and Row,1974.
43. Bass, A.L. : Treatment of muscle, tendon and minor joint injuries in sport, Proc. Roy. Soc. Med., 62,925,1969.
44. Costill, D.L., Thomson and E.Roberts : "Fractional utilization on the aerobic capacity during distance running". Med. and science of sports, 5:284-297, Winter, 1973.
45a. Costill, D.L. and B. Saltin. Factors limiting gastric emptying during rest and exercise. J. Appl. Physical 37(5):679-683,1974.
45b. Chandran P.S.M.-outline of Sports Medicine Nutrients and Drugs-1989 (A.P.Publishers, Jhalandur India)
46. Costill, D.L. and B. Saltin. Factors limiting gastric emptying during rest and exercise. J.Appl. Physical 37(5):679-683,1974.
47. Costill, D.L. and E.Fox, : Energetics of marathon running. Med. and Sci. in Sports 1.81-86,169.
48. Costill, D.L.,B. Bowers, and W.F. Kramer : "Skinfold estimates of body fat among Marathon Runners", Med. and Sciences of Sport, 2:93-95,1970.
49. Costill, D.L., W.F. Kammer and A.Fisher, Fluid ingestion during distance running : Arch, Environ. Health 21:520-525, 1970.
50. Cureton, T.K.Jr.: Endurance of young men, (Research monograph of the national society for research in child development, Washington, D.C. : National Research Council, 1945,pp. 293.
51. Cureton, T.K., Jr.: "Interpretation of the oxygen intake test., What is it ?" America corrective therapy journal, 27: 17-23, Jan-Feb., 1973.
52. Cureton, T.K. Jr.: Physical fitness workbook, Compaign Illinois :- Stipes Publication Co., pp. 156, 1944 : (3rd edition, 1947).
53. Curenton, T.K. Jr.and Paul Hunsicker : Physical fitness (Research monograph of Srpingfield College) Supplement to the Research Quarterly, 12.301-330, May 1941.
54. Curreton, T.K. Jr. : Physical fitness of charmpion Athletes, Urbana : University of Illinois Press, 1951, pp.550.
55. Cureton, T.K., Jr. : Proc. of the ACSPFIT and the ICSPET, pp. 139-162, "What does maximum oxygen intake (VO2 max) measure ? How is it interpreted ?" (Lecture 1972 at Colonge, Germany).

56. Cureton, T.K. Jr.: Physical fitness appraisal and guidance, St. Louis : C.V. Mosley Co., 1947,pp. 566.
57. Cureton, T.K.,Jr.: "What does maxinim oxygen intake (VO2 max) measure ? How is it interpreted ? What are its principal limitations ?" Proc. College Physical Education Assn. for men (75th Annual Convention, New Orleans, Jan., 1972.
58. Corrigan, A.B. : Sports injuries, Hosp. Med., 2,1328,1968.
59. Committee on Sports Medicine American Academy on Pediatrics, Sports Medicine. Illinois: American Academy of pediatrics, 1983.
60. Concharov Boris (1986): Sports in USSR, An illustrated Monthly.
61. Clarke, Harrison, H.(1971) : "Basic understanding of physical fitness," Physical Fitness Research Digest Series 1 No.2.
62. Cureton, Thomus, K. (1965): "Improvement of psychological status by means of exercise-fitness programme," Journal of Association for Physical and Mental Rehabilitation.
63. Chopra, R.L.(1983) : "Socio-Econimic aspects of physical fitness," Report and papers on orientation course in scientific aspects of physical fitness.
64. Clarke Harrison, Clarke David (1978): Developmental and adapted physical education, Prentice Hall Inc., Englewood Cliffs, New Jersey 07632.
65. Costill, D.L., Coyle, E.G. Fink, W.F., Lesmese, G.R. and Witzmann, F.A.(1979) : "Adaptations in skeletal muscle following strength training," J. Appl. Physiol. 46-96.
66. Clarke David, H.(1975): Exercise physiology, Prentice Hall Inc., Englewood Cliffs, New Jersey.
67. Clarke Harriet (1943) : "A functional physical fitness test for college women, "Jour. of Health and Physical fitness test for college women," Jour. Of Health and Physical Education, 14, No. 7 : 358.
68. Chigteri, C.V., Melinkeri, R.R. and Pansare M.S. (1986) : "Effect of yoga on serum cholesterol levels," Unpublished work, paper accepted for reading in APPI Conf. in 1986.
69. Cooper Kenneth, H.(1980) : "Aerobics" 31st Printing Bantum Books, Toronto, New York, London, Sydney.
70. Cooper, M.K. "Aerobics for women," Bantum Books, Toronto, New York, London, Sydney.
71. Cooper, K.H. "The new aerobics" 35th printing, Bantum

Books, Toronto, New York, London, Sudney.

72. Costill, DL,Fink, N.J.,Getchell, L.H. et al. (1979) : Lipid Metabolism in skeletal muscle of endurance trained males and females, J.Appl. Physiol. 47 : 782-791.

73. Cave, E.F. and Rowe C.R.(1947) Bankart operation. Surg. Clin. North Am. 27,1289.

74. Cho K.O.(1975) Reconstruction of the anterior cruciate ligament by semitendinous tendon. J.Bone Joint Surg.57A,608.

75. Collins H.R. and Wilde A.H. (1973) Shoulder instability in athletes. Orthop. Clin. North Am. 4,759.

76. Craig R.P.(1975) The quantitative evaluation of the use of oral proteolytic enzymes in the treatment of sprained ankles. injury 6,313.

77. Crane J.,Gibson T.and Busson M. (1980) A comparative study of ibuprofen and indomethacin in ligamentous injuries of the ankle. Br. J. Clin. Practice Suppl. 6.92.

78. Crenshaw, A.H.(1971) Compbell's operative orthopaedics. St. Louis, Mosby.

79. Crenshaw A.H. and Kilgore W.E. (1966) Surgical treatment of bicipital tenosynovitis. J.Bone Joint Surg. 48A,1496.

80. Crompton B.A. and Tubes N. (1977) A survey of sports injuries in Birmingham, Br. J. Sports Med. 11,12.

81. Dandy, D.J. and Jackson, R.W. (1975). The diagnosis of problems after mensectomy. J.Bone Joint Srug. 57B, 349.

82. Devas, M.B. (1969) Stress fractures in athletes. Proc. R.Soc. Med. 62,933.

83. Dexel, M. and Schreiber A. (1979) Diagnois of unstable knee joint. Ital. J. Sp. Traumatology 1,13.

84. Durbin, F.C. (1957) Transcondylar fractures of the humerus in childood. J. Bone Joint Surg. 21,59.

85. Durbin, F.C. (1957) Fracture dislocation of the cervical spine. J. Bone Joint Surg. 39B,23.

86. Duvries, H.J.(1959) Surgery of the Food St. Louis, Mosby.

87. Donoghue, Don H. Treatment of injuries to athletes. Philadelphia : W.B. Saunders Company, 1984.

88a. Devenport, C.B. : "The cural index",the American J., Physical anthropology, 17:333-353, Jan.-Mar. 1973.

88b. Donh. O'Donoughue, M.D.-Treatment of Injuries to Athletes-1984 (Published by W.B. Saunders Company)

89. Devenport, C.B., : Anthropometry, Philadelphia : The Wister Institute of Anatomy and Physiology. pp. 163. Revised, 2nd

ed. 1939, p.246.

90. Derting, R.C. The significance of physical fitness Arch. Phys. Med. 1947, 28,140.
91. Devices, K.J., Packer, L. and Brooks, G.A. (1981) : "Biochemical adaptation of mitochondria, muscle and whole animal respiration to endurance training", Arch. Biocherm, Biophys. 209:539-554.
92. De Vries Herbert (1962) : "Evaluation of static stretching procedures for improvement of flexibility" : Research Quarterly, May, 1962.
93. Dishman Rod, K. (1986) : "Medical psychology in exercise and sport", The Medical Clinics of North America.
94. Dravid, N.G. and Pansare, M.S. (1986): "Effect of yoga on work performance by finger ergography", Unpublished work, paper read in State Conf. of Sports Medicine, Nagpur, Feb. 1985.
95. Ekolom, B., Kilbom, A, and Soltysiak, J. (1973): "Physical Training, Bradycardia and autonomic nervous system," Scan. J. Clin. Lab., Invest. 32:251-256.
96. Essen, B., Hagenfeldt, L.and Kavjser, L. (1977) : "Utilization of blood born and intramuscular substrates during continuous and intermittant exercise in man," J. Appl. Physiol. 265:484-506.
97. Eckert, W.R. and Davies, E.A., Jun. (1976) Acute rupture of the peroneal retinaculum. J. Bone Joint Surg. 58A, 670.
98. Eriksson, E. (1976) Symposium on ski trauma and skiing safety. Orthop. Clin. North Am. 7,3.
99. Fukushima Sho (1980): "Physical conditioning", International Gymnast, May.
100. Fox Edward, L. (1984) : "Sports physiology", 2nd Edn., Holt Saunders International Editions, Japan, Tokyo.
101. Fox E. : Physical training methods and effects, 1971, Orthop. Clin. N. Am. 8(3),545.
102. Fransis, K.T. and Carter, R. (1982) : "Psychological characteristics of joggers." J.Sports Medicine, 22,386-391.
103. Fred Kelly, D.B. (1977) : "Isometric drills for strength and power in athletes", Tarapowala Sons & Co. Pvt. Ltd., Evin Parker, Pub. Co. Inc.
104. Fox, E.L. (1984) : "Sports physiology", 2nd Edn., CBS College Publishing.
105. Fitzgeralad, P.L.(1985) : "Exercise for elderly", Medical Clinics of North America, Vol. 69, No.1.

106. Fox, E.(1981) : "The physiological basis for physical education and athletics", 3rd Edn., Philadelphia, Saunders College Publishing : 620.
107. Fordtran J.A. and B.Saltin. Gastric emptying and intestinalabsorption during prolonged severe exercise; J. Appl. Physical 23: 331-335,1967.
108. Feruguson, R.J.(1974) Low back pain in college football linemmen. J. Bone Joint Surg., 56A, 1300.
109. Flatt, A.E.(1969) Athletic injuries of the hand. In Symposium of Sports Medicine. St. Louis, Mosby.
Flynn, M. and Kelly, J.P. (1976) Local excision of cyst of lateral meniscus of the knee without recurrence. J. Bone Joint Surg. 58B, 88.
111. Garfield, J. (1973) In trauma Surgery (ed. Powley P.) Bristol, Wright.
112a. Gear, M.W.L.(1967) The late results of menisectomy. Br. J. Surg.54,270.
112b. Ghosh Alok: A Book on Sports Medicine 1985 Calcutta.
113. Goldberg B., Wiatman P.A., Gleim G.W. and Nicholas J.A.(1979) Children's sports injuries. Phys. Sportsmen. 7,93.
114. Good C.J., Jones M.A. and Livingstone B.N.(1975) Reconstruction of the lateral ligament of the ankle. Injury 7,63.
115. Ghosh, Aloke. Handbook of Sports medicine and physical fitness. Calcutta : Allied Book Agency, 1980.
116. Grisogono, Virian. Sports injuries. London : John Murray Publishers Ltd., 1984.
117. Gilmore, C.P. and The editors of Time Life Books (1981) : Exercise for fitness library of health/Time Life Books/ Alexandria, Virginia.
118. Gollnick, P.D. Armstrong, R.B. and Saltin et al (1973) : "Effect of training on enzymeactivity and fibre composition of human skeletal muscle", J.Appl. Physiol. 17:107-111.
119. Grimby, G.Haggendal, E. and Saltin, B. (1967) : Local xenon 133 clearness from quadriceps muscle during exercise in Man." J.Appl. Physiol 22:305.
120. Gonyea, W.J., Ericson, G.C. and Bonde Petersen, F. (1977): "Skeletal muscle fibre splitting induced by weight lifting exercise in cats." Acta Physiol. Scan. 99:105.
121. Gonyea, W.J.(1980) : "The role of exercise in inducing skeletal muscle fibre splitting rats", J.Appl. 48:421.
122. Gollnick, P. and King, D. (1969) : "Effect of exercise and

training on mitochondria of rat skeletal muscle", Am. J. Physiol. 216:1502.

123. Geline, R.J.(1978) : "The practical runner", Collier Books, New York.

124. Gharote, M.L. (1973) : "Effect of yogic training on physical fitness, "Yoga Mimamsa, Vol. XV,4:31-55.

125. Gharote, J.L. (1976) : "Effect of short term yogic training programme on the physical fitness of school boys", Vol.1:1:9-15.

126. Gharote. J.L. (1976) : "Physical fitness in relation to the practice of selected yogic exercises", Yoga Mimama, Vol. XVIII :1:14-23.

127. Gharote, M.L. (1979) :"Yogic training and physical fitness", SNIPES Jour., Vol. 2:4:32-38.

128. Ganguly, S.K. (1981) : "Effect of short term yogic training programme on cardio-vascular endurance" ,SNIPES Jour. Vol. 4,2:45-80.

129. Ganguly, S.K. and Gharote, M.L. (1974) : "Cardiovascular efficiency before and after yogic training." Yoga Mimamsa, Vol. XVII, 1:89-97.

130. Gore, M.M. and Gharote, M.L. (1981) : "Effect of yogic training on peak flow rate." Yoga Mimamsa. vol. XX, 1 and 2 :100-104.

131. Gore, M.M. and Bhole, M.V. (1982) : "Respiratory responses to vastra dhauti in asthmetics."

132. Gharote, M.L., Ganguly, S.K. and Moorthy, A.M. (1976) : "Effect of yogic training on minimum muscular fitness". Yoga Mimamsa, Vol. XVIII, 3 and 4:1-20.

133. Gharote, M.L. (1976) : "Effect of yoga exercises on failures on kraus-weber tests, perpetual and motor skills", Vol. 43(2):654.

134. Galbo, H.Christensen, N.J.and Noist, JJ(1977) : "Catecholamines and Pancreatic Hormones during Automonic Blockade in Exercising Man," C. Acta Physiol. Scand. 101:428-437.

135. Ghosh, R.K. and Ahuja, A. (1985): "A modified test for evaluation of physical fitness of sportsmen in endurance games", SNIPES, Vol. 8, No.1.

136. Gitin, E.L., J.E. Olerud and H.W. Carroll : "Maximal oxygen uptake based on lean body mass a meaningful measure of physical fitness ?" J. of applied Physiology, 36:757-760, June, 1974.

137. Gookin. W. Fatigue, dehydration and activity drinks: Running. Fall 1978-21-22.
138. Gradzner, E.N. Athletes of the Ancient World. New Jersey : Oxford University Press, 1930.
139. Guide, W.R. How to keep fit and enjoy it? New York : Harper and Bow,1962.
140. Huduca, O (1928) : "Growth of capillaries in skeletal and cardiac muscle", Circ. Res. 50:451-461.
141. Holloszy J. Boot, F. (1976) : "Biochemical adaptations to endurance exercise in muscle", Ann. Rev. Physiol. 38-276.
142. Hennansen, L.,Hallman E. and Saltin, B.(1967) : "Glycogen during prolonged muscular exercise." Acta Physiol. Scand. 71:129.
143. Hathayoga pradipika with Jyotsna III, 1978.
144. Henry, R.L., Chaiaman, N. Golu, O and Berkman, S. (1960): "Determination of serum lactate dehydrogenase", Ann. J. Clin. Path, 34:381.
145. Hasabnis, G.S. and Sharangpani, R.C. (1985): "A sports syllabus for your child," Sopan Publications, Pune.
146. Health, G.W., Hagberg, J.M., Ehasami, A.A. et al. (1981) : "A physiological comparison of young and older endurance athletes", J. Appl., Physio. 51:634-640.
147. Hanson, P.G. Heat injuries in runners. Phy. and Sports med., 7(6):91-96,1980.
148. Handerson, J. Coping with heated battle. Runners World, 6(4) :39-49, 1971.
149. Hughson, R.L. et.al. Heat injuries in Canadian mass participation runs: CMAJ. 122(10) : 1141-1143, 1980.
150. Harris, N.H. and Murray, R.G. (1974) Lesions of the symphysis pubis in athletes. J. Bone Joint Surg. 56B, 563.
151. Heppenstall R.B. (1975) Fractures and dislocations of the distal clavicle.
152. Hughston J.C., Anderson J.R., Cross M.J. and Moschi A. (1976) Classification of knee ligament instabilities. Part 1 : The medical compartment and cruciate ligaments. J. Bone Joint Surg. 58A, 159.
153. Huskisson E.C., Berry H., Street F.G. and Medhurst H.E. (1973) Indomethacin for soft tissue injuries. Rheum Rehab. 12, 159.
154. Inglis A.E., Scott N.W., Sculo T.T. and Patterson A.H. (1975) Ruputure of the tendo achillis : an objective assessment of non-surgical and surgical treatment. J. Bone Joint Surg.

57A, 1172.
155. Insall J., Flavo K.A. and Wise D.W. (1976) Chondromalacia patellae. J. Bone Joint Surg. 58A, 1.
156. Ismail A.M., Balakrishnana R. and Rajakumar M.K. (1969) Rupture of patellar ligament after steroid injection. J.Bone Joint Surg. 51B, 503.
157. Jackson D.W. (1976) Chronic rotator cuff impingement in the throwing athlete. Am. J. Sports Med. 4,231.
158. Jackson J.P. (1967) Degenerative changes in the knee after menisectomy. J.Bone Joint Surg. 49B, 584.
159. Johansen O. (1955) In Sports injuries, Oslo.
160. Johnson R.J., pope M.H. and Ettlinger C. (1976) Interrelationship between ski accidents, the resultant injury, the skier's characteristics, and the ski boot binding system, Orthop. Clin. North Am. 7,11.
161. James, S.L. Chondromalacia of the patella in the adolescent in Kennedy, J.C.(ed) : The injured adolescent. Knee. Baltimore, Williams and Wilkins, 1978.
162. Johson, W.R. & Black D.K. "Comparison of effects of certain blood alkalinizers and Glucose upon competitive endurance performance.", J. Appl. Physiol, 1953,5,577.
163. Joint Committee of Americn Medical Association and Association for Health, Physical Education and Recreation (1958) : "Exercise and fitness", Jour. of American Medical Association, 16, No.14,1744.
164. Journal of Health, Physical Education and Recreation. 35, No.5, 42, 1964.
165. Jensen and Fischer (1972) : "Scientific basis of athletic condition", Lea Febigner.
166. Joshi, A.R. and Pansare, M.S. (1986) : "Effect of yoga on pulmonary function tests. "Paper for publication in Med. Jour. of West, India.
167. Joshi, L.S. and Pansare, M.S.(1986) : "Effect of yoga on minimum muscular fitness", Unpublished work.
168. Joshi, K.S. (1982) : "Cure yourself with yoga", Indian Yoga Soc., Sagar, M.P.
169. Joshi, A.R., Pansare, M.S.(1983) : "Effect of training on physical fitness and skilled performance", SNIPES Jour., Patiala, Vol.6, No. 3:56-62.
170. Karembelkar, P.V., Ganguly, S.K. and Moorthy, A.M. (1981) : "Effect of yogic practices on cholesterol levels in females," Yoga Mimamsa, Vol. XX, 1and 2:1-8.

171. Kraus, H. and Hirschland, R.P. (1954) : "Minimum muscular fitness tests in school children," Research Quarterly, 25, Nov.2,1978.
172. Kochher, H.C. and Pratap, v. (1971) : "Neurotic trends in yogic practices," Yoga Mimamsa, Vol. XIV, 1 and 2:35-40.
173. Kochher H.C. and Pratap, V (1971) : 'A free association study before and after yogic practices," Yoga Mimamsa, Vol. 1 and 2:41-56.
174. Kochher, H.C. and Pratap, V (1972) : "A Psycho-physioligical study of the effect of short term yogic training on two hand co-ordination," Yoga Mimamsa, Vol. XIV, 3 and 4:45-56.
175. Kochher, H.C. and Patrap, V. (1972) : "Anxiety level and yogic practices-A preliminary communication," Yoga Mimamsa, Vol.SV, 1-11-15.
176. Kochher, H.C. (1973) : "Introverted, extrverted practitioners of yoga and their scores on neuroticism," Anxiety and General Hospitality Yoga Mimamsa, Vol. XV,4,64-73.
177. Kochher, H.C.(1976) : "Influence of yogic practices on mental fatigue," Yoga Mimamsa, Vol SVII, 2.2-13.
178. Kelly, Helen G. : A study of individual differences in breathin capacity in relationship to some physical characteristics, lowa city: University of lowa Press, New Series No. 264, 1033. pp. 59.
179. Khosla. T. : "Grading of sporting events by size", Paper presented at the XVIIth World Congress of sports Medicine, Oxford University, Sept. 11., 1970.
180. Kohirausch, W. : "Zusammenlagne von Korperform and Leisting ergebuise der anthropoimestrischen messungenan athleten der amesterdamer olympiade", Arbeitsphysiologie Berlin : 129,(June 13, 1929).
181. Keen G. (1975) Chest injuries. Bristol, Wright.
182. Kenwright, J.K. and Taylor R.G. (1970) Manor injuries of talus. J.Bone Joint Surg. 52B, 36.
183. Killey H.C.(1976) Cervical spine injuries. In Injuries in Rugby Football and other Team Sports. Bublin, Irish Rugby Football Union,p.116.
185. Longhurst, J.C., Kelly, A.R., Gonyea, W.J. et al (1981) : "Chronic training with static and dynamic exercise-Cardiovascular adaptation and response to exercise." Circ. Resp.48 (Suppl.) 171:178.
186. Lewis, S.G., Nylander, E., Gad, p.et al(1980) : "Non-autonomic component bradycardia of endurance in trained

men at reat and during exercise." Acta Physiol. Scand. 109:297-503.

187. Lorainne Nyelson (1950) : "The effect of swimming on basla metabolism of college women," Master's thesis, University of Illinois.

188. Leger Luc (1982) : "Energy cost of Disco Dancing," Research Quarterly, Vol.5, No.1.46-49.

189. La Cave, G.: A clinical and Statistical investigation of traumatic lesions due to sports, J. Sport Med. (Torino), 1,8(1961).

190. La Cave G. (1960) Indagnie clinico static sulle lesioni traumatische da sport. Turinm Edizioni Mnerva Medica.

191. Lea E.B. and Smith L. (1972) Non-surgical treatment of tendo achillis rupture. J. Bone Joint Surg. 54A, 1398.

192. Leach R.E.O.'Connor P. and Jones R. (1979) Acromionectomy for tendinitis of the shoulder in athletes. Phys. Sportsmen. 7,96. tendinitis of the shoulder in athletes. Phys. Sportsmen.7,96.

193. Leclerc F.P. and Autissier D. (1969) The use of indomethacin in the treatment of limb injuries and their sequalae. Gaz. Hop. Paris 1,31.

194. LINDHOLM A. (1959) A new method of preparation in subcutaneous rupture of the Achilles tendon. Acta Chair. Scand 117,261.

195. LOMBARDO S.T., KERLAN R.K., Jobe F.W. CARTERV.S., BLAZINA M.E. AND SHIELDS V.L., jun. (1976) The modified Bristow procedure for recurrent dislocation of the shoulder. J. Bone joint Surg. 58A, 256.

196. LYNN A.A.(1966) Repair of torn Achilles tendon using the plantaris tendon as reinforcing membrane. J. Bone jointsurg. 48A, 268.

197. Lee. W. In Science and Medicine of Exercise and sports, 2nd Ed. W.R. Honoson and E.R. Buskirk, Editors, New York, Harper and Row, 1974.

198. Luft, U.C.et al., : "Physical performance in relation to body size and composition", Annals of N.Y. Academy of Science, 110 :795-806,1963.

199. Malina, R.M., A.B. Harper, Henrietta H. Avent and D.E. Campbell 'Physique of female track and field athletes'. Med. and Science in Sports, 2:93-95, 1970.

200. Matsui, H.et al.: "Maximal oxygen intake and its relationship to body weight of Japanese Adolescents". Med. and Science in Sports, 4:27-34,1973.

201. Mecloy, C.H.: Appraising physical status (The selection of measurements). lowa city : (University of lowa Press, 1936, New series No. 319,1936, pp.126.
202. McCloy, C.H.: Appraising physical status (Methods and norms), lowa City: University of lowa Press, 1938.
203. Montessori, Meria, : Pedagogical anthropology (Trans. from Italian), New York: A.F.A. Stokes Co., 1913.
204. Mythre, L.G. Shifts in blood volume, during and following acute environmental work stresses in man. Doctoral dissertation: Indian Unversity, Bloomington, Ind.,1969.
205. M.C. Dermott A.G.; Marvle, A.E. ; Yalesley, R.H. ; et al, Monitoring Dynamic Anterior Compartment pressure during exercise AM.J. Sports Med. 10:89,1982.
206. Mangi Richard, Pater Jokl, O'William Dayton; the Runners complete Medical Guide, New York Summit Boo, 1976.
207. Morris, M.A. Sports injury survey of Greater Birmingham, Phys. Edn. 55,41,1963.
208. Maiman, L.A. Wang, VL 1979 Attitudes towards obesity and the obese among professionals. J.Am. Diet, Assoc. 47:331-335.
209. Mayer, J.R. 1068-Overweight : Causes, cost and control. Prentic Hall Inc., Englewood Cliffs N.J.
210. MURPHY, R.J.& Ashe W.F. Prevention of heat illness in football players, J.W.M.A. 1965,194,180.
211. Mcglashan T.P.L.(1976) Current thinking on mouth guards. In Injuries in Rugby football and other team sports. Dublin, Irish Rugby Football Union, p.147.
212. McLatchie G.R.(1979) Surgical and orthopaedic problems in sports karate. Medisport 1,40.
213. McLaughlin H.L. (1947) Repair of major tendon ruptures by buried removable sutures. Am.J.Surg. 74,758.
214. Magnuson P.B. and Stack J.K. (1943) Recurrent dislocation of the shoulder. JAMA 123,889.
215. Miller J.E./(1960) Javelin thrower's elbow. J.Bone Joint Surg.42B, 788.
216. Morrey B.F. and Janes J.M. (1976) Recurrent dislocation of the shoulder. J.Bone Joint Surg. 58A,252.
217. Morris M.(1963) A sports injury survery of Greater Birmingham. Phys. Educ.55,41.
218. Muckle D.S. (1972a) Shoulder injuries in sport. Br. J. Sports Med. 6,77.
219. Muckle D.S.(1972b) Intra-articular ganglion of the knee.

J.Bone Joint Surg. 54B,520.

220. Muckle D.S.(1973) Dislocation of the superior tibio-fibular joint. Br. J.Sports Med. 7,365.

221. Muckle D.S.(1974) Comparative study of ibuprofen and aspirin in soft tissue injuries. Rheum. Rehab. 13,141.

222. Muckle D.S.(1976) First aid in sports. Mod. Med. 21,44.

223. Muckle D.S. (1977) A double mind trial of flubiprofen and aspirin in soft tissue trauma. Rheum. Rehab. 16,58.

224. Muckle D.S.(1980a) Osteoarthrosis of the knee following menisectomy, M.D. Thesis. Univ. Newcastle.

225. Muckle D.S. (1980b) Ipuprofen in soft tissue injuries-a long term clinicl evaluation. Br. J.Clin. Practice Suppl. 6,71.

226. Muckle D.S. and Minns R.J.(1979) The use of flamentous carbon fibre for the repair of osteoarthritic articular cartilarge. J.Bone Joint Surg. 61B,381.

227. Muckle D.S. and Shepherdson H and Injuries. London, Pelham.

228. Muller M.E., Allgower M. and Willengger H.W.(1970) Manual of internal fixation. Berlin, Springer gerlag.

229. MacDougall, J.D.,Ward, G.R.,Sale, D.G., Satton, J.R. (1977) "Biochemical adaptation of human skeletal muscle to heavy resistance training and immobilisation." J.Appl. Physiol. 43:700.

230. Morgan, W.P.(1966) : "The trait psychology controversy", Res. Cl.Exerc. Sports, 50-50.76.

231. Moorthy, A.M., Gnguly, S.K., Gharote, M.L. and Karamblkar, P.V. (1978) : "Cholesterol levels and yogic training programme", Jour Res. Ind. Med. Yoga and Homeopathy XIII,4,1:6,1.

232. Moorthy, A.M.(1982) : "Influence of selected yogic exercises on minimum muscular fitness of the elementary school children", SNIPES Jour. Vol.5,3:21.

233. Manro Robin (1983) : "Towards an epidermiological study of health benefits from yofa, "II Ann. Symp. of Indian Academy of Yoga, Abstract Madras, As quoted by VSSM Rao," Yoga for top performance as well as for heath and physical fitness, reports and papers in orientation course in scientific aspects of physical fitness, Oct. 7to 11, 1983.

234. Mitchel, J., Sproule, B. and Champman, C. (1957) : "The physioligical meaning of the maximum oxygen intake test", J. Clin. Invest, 37.538.

235. Margaria, R., Aghemo, I and Rovelli, E. (1966) :

"Measurement of muscular power (Anaerobic) in man", J.Appl. Physiol. 21:1662.

236. Miller, D.K. and Allen, T. (1982) : "Fitness a lifetime commitment" 2nd Edn. Surjeet Publications, 7-K, Kolhapur and Kamala Nagar, Delhi-110 007.

237. Nowacky Paul (1985) : Lecture delivered on Sports Medicine Certificate Course in Sports Medicine at N.S.N.I.S. Patials, Feb. 1985.

238. Nicholas J.A.(1973a) The five one reconstruction for anteromedical instability of the knee. J. Bone Joint Surg. 55A, 899.

239. Nicholas J.A. (1973b) The five one reconstruction for anteromedical instability of the knee. J. Bone Joint Surg. 55A,899.

240. Nicholas J.A. (1974) Ankle injuries in athletes. Orthlp. Clin. North Am. 5,153.

241. Noble. J. and Hamblen D.L. (1975) The pathology of the degenerate meniscus lesion. J.Bone Joint Surg. 57B,180.

242. Novak, L.P.R.E. Hyatt, and J.F. Alexander. : "Body composition and physioligical function of athletes". J. Am. Med. Assn, 206 :764-770,1986.

243. Norfray, J.F.Schlarchter, L. Kernahan, W.T. et al, early confirmation of stress fractures in Joggers J.Am Med., Assoc. 243:1947-49 1980.

244. Novak, L.P. "Body composition and clinical estimation of desirable body weight", A.M.A. Proceedings of the seventh National Conference on the Medical Aspects of Sports, Chicago, Amer. Medical Ass. 1967 pp.58-64.

245. Orave S. Stress Fracture Br. J. Sports Med. 14:40-44. 1980.

246. O'Donghue D.H. Treatment of injuries to athletes: Philadelphia. W.S. Saunder's Company, 1976.

247. Orave S. and Puranen J. (1979) Athlete's leg pains. Br. J. Sports Med. 13,92.

248. O'Donoghue D.H.(1973) Treatment of acute ligamentous injuries of the knee. Orthop. Clin. North Am. 4,617.

249. Osmono Clarke H.(1948) Habitual dislocation of the shoulder-the Putti Platt operation. J.Bone Joint Surg. 30B,19.

250. Penman, K.(1969) : "Ultrta structural changes in human striated muscle using three medhods of training", Res. Quarterly:40-764.

251. Pattongale, P.K. and Holloszy, J.O.(1967) : "Augmentation of skeletal muscle myoglobin by a programme of treadmill

running", Am.J.of Physiol. 217:783-785.

252. Prentup, Frank, B.(1963): "Skipping the rope for fun and fitness", Boulder Colorade, Pruett Press.

253. Pansare, M.S.(1985) : "Effect of yoga on flexibility:, Unpublished paper read at I.M.A. Conference, Nov. 1985.

254. Paranjape, S.D. and Bhole, M.L.V. (1979) : "Resting neuromuscular activity as influenced by long term yogic training", Youg Mimamsa, Vol.XIX,4:18-26.

255. PANSARE, M.S. and Kulkarni (1986) : "Effect of yoga on plasma LDH levels", Unpublished work, paper read in State Conference of Sports Medicine at Nagpur, Feb. '86.

256. Pratap, V. (1968) : "Steadiness in normals before and after yogic practices", Yoga Mimamsa, Vol. XI,2-1-13.

257. Pansare, M.S., Pradhan, S.G., Kher, J.R., Joshi, A.R., Aundhkar, V.G. (1983) : "Study of physical fitness tests and pulmonary function tests in tribal girls of Maharashtra", SNIPES Journal, Patiala, Vol.4, No.4:39-43.

258. Pansare, M.S., Joshi, A.R., Pradhan, S.G., Aundhkar, V.G.(1985) : "Comparative study of nutritional status, health status and physical fitness in tribal and urban girls of Maharashtra", SNIPES Jour., Patiala, Vol. 8, No.4:44-47.

259. Panssre, M.S., Joshi, L.S., Inamdar, R.S., Joshi, A.R., (1986): "Effect of physical training on minimum muscular fitness in school children", Accepted for publication in Maharashtra Medical Journal.

260. Park, J.E., and Park K. Text book of prevention and social medicine. Jobalpur : Banarsidas Bhanot, 1977.

261. Perbix Joyce A: "Relationship between somatotype and motor fitness in women", The Research Quarterly, 25:85-90, March, 1954.

262. Plagenboet, Stan. : "A biomechemical analysis of Beamon, Williams and an average college long jumper", Track and Field Quarterly Review, 73:221, Dec., 1978.

263. Pugh, L.G.C., J.L. Corbitt and R.H. Johnson, Rectal temperatures, weight losses and sweating rates in marathon running :23: 347-353,1957.

264. Paul, F.Vinger, Eare, F. Hoerner; Sports injuries : The Unthwarted Epidemic, Massachusetts, PSG Publishing Company, 1981.

265. Passmore,R. and Darnin, J.V.G.A. Human energy expenditure, Physiol. Rev. 1955,35,801.

266. Percival L. Vitamin 'E' in athletic efficiency, Ford Foundation

for Medical Research, 1951,3 no.2.
267. Pugh L.G.C. Er and et al; Physiological study of channel swimming 1960,19:257.
268. Ribial, Paul and W.Kachidorian : "Maximal oxygen intake prediction,in young and middle aged males", J. Sports Med. and Physical Fitness, 9:11-10.1968.
269. Ryan Allan J., Fredi All man, Sports Medicine : Academic Press, London, 1974.
270. Ritter M.A. and Gosling C,(1980) The knee : A guide to the examination and diagnosis of ligament injuries. Springfield, 111, Thomas.
271. Roberts R.R. (1963) Triservice medical survey on shoulder dislocation. Dept., Navy. Richard H. Strouss, M.O.,(Editor-SPORTS MEDICINE-1984)
(Published by W.B. Saunders Company)
272. Roles N.C. and Maudsley R.H.(1972) Radial tunnel syndrome: resistant tennis elbow as a nerve entrapment. J. Bone Joint Surg. 54B, 499.
273. Rothman R.H., Marvel J.P. jun and Heppenstall R.B.(1975) Recurrent anterior dislocation of the shoulder. Orthop. Clin. North Am. 6,417.
274. Rowe N.L. and Killey H.C.(1968) Fractures of the facial skeleton. 2nd ed. Edinburgh, Livingstone.
275. Roy, Steven and Irvin Richrd. Sports medicine prevention, evaluation, management, and rehabilitation. New Jersey : Prentice Hall Inc.1983.
276. Reilly, Thomas. Sports fitness and sports injuries. London : Feber and Feber Ltd., 1985.
277. Ryan Allen, J. (1984) : "Sports Injuries-Introduction."
278. Roesko, W.R., 'O'Rourke, R.N. Klein, A.et. al(1976) : "Non-invasive evaluation of ventricular hypertrophy in professional athletes" Circulation, 55:286-292,1975.
279. Rushmer, R.T. (1970) : "Cardiovascular dynamics," Philadelphia, W.B. Saunder Co. 70-112.
280. Roy Shephard, J.(1982) : Physiology and biochemistry of exercise, Preeger Publishers, 521, Fith Avenue, New York, 10175, U.S.A.
281. Roy, Shephard, J.(1982) : Economics of the fitness industries, the Canadian Scene Since 1966, J.Sports Med. 22:245-258.
282. Rodahl, K, Miller, H.J. and Issekutz,B.(1964) : "Plasma free fatty acids in exercise", J.Appl. Physiol. 19.489-492.
282b. Richard H. Strauss, M.D., Edutor - Sports Medicine - 1984

- (Published by W.B. Saunders Company)
283. Strauss, R.H.,(1984) : Sports medicine, W.B. Saunders Co., Philadelphia.
284. Saltin, B. and Grimby, G. (1968) : Physiological analysis of middle aged and old former athletes. Comparison with still active athletes to the same ages." Circulation 38:1104-1115.
285. Saltin, B.Nazark Costil, D.L.et al. (1976) : "The nature of training response, peripheral and central adaptations to one-legged exercise", Acta Physil. Acand. 96:289-305.
286. Sutton, J.R., Cole, A., Gunning. J.et al (1976) : "Control of heart rate in healthy young men", Lancet, 2:1398-1400.
287. Stamford, B.A., Manbacher, W.and Fallica, A.(1974) : "Effects of daily physical exercise on the psychiatric state of institutional geriatric and mental patients", Res. Q.45.34-41.
288. Spirduso (1983) : "Exercise and the Aging Brain", Res. Q. Exerc., Sport, 54,1208,218.
289. Shaver Larry (1981) : "Essentials of exercise physiology", Surjeet Publications 7-K, Kolhapur Road, Kamalanagar, New Delhi-110007.
290. Sidney, K.H. and Shephard, R.J. (1977) : "Maximum and submaximum exercise tests in men and women in Seventh and Ninth Decades Life", J. Appl., Physiol. 43:289-297.
291. Sidney, K.H. and Shephard, R.J., and Harrison, J.E.(1977) : "Endurance training and body composition of the elderly", Am.J. Clin. Nutr. 30:326-333.
292. Strauzsenberg, S.E.(1981) : "Sports in old age : Advantages and risks", The Jour. of Sports Medicine and Physical Fitness, Vol.21, No.4.
293. Saltin, B. Astrand, P.(1967) : "Maximum oxygen intake in athletes", J.Appl. : Hysiol. 23,353.
294. Sheldon, W.H., S.S. Stevens and W.B. Tucker : The varieties of human physique. New York : Harper Bros. 1940,p.347.
295. Sills, Frank D and John D. Mitchem. : "Prediction of performance of physical fitness tests by means of somatotype ratings", Research Quarterly, 28:64-71, Dec.,1957 and also the Research Quarterly, 21:621-437, Dec.1950.
296. Stantiski, C.L. Memaster J.H. and Scranton, P.E. on the nature of stress fractures, Am. J. Sports Med. G. 391:396,1978.
297. Srahms, Mal Fumich, R.M.: and Lappolito, V.D.: A typical stress fracture of the tibia in a professional athlete, Am.J. Sports Med. 8: 131-132,1980.

298. Steinkamp, R.C., "Measures of body fat and related factors in normal adults", Chronic diseases, 1965,18,297.
299. Seltzer, O.C. and Mayer, J.Greater "Reliability of the triceps skinfold over the subscapular skinfold as an index of obesity" Amer, J.Coin, Nutr. Sept 1987, 20,8:950-953.
300. Sunderrajan, G.S. (1983) "Medical aspects of loss and gain of physical fitness," Report and papers on Orientation Course in scientific Aspects of Physical Fitness, October 7 to 11.
301. Salter R.B. and Harris N.R. (1963) Injuries involving the epiphyseal plate. J.Bone Joint Surg. 45A,587.
302. Scott. J.C. and Orr M.M.(1973) Injuries involving the epiphyseal plate. J. Bone Joint Surg. 45A, 587.
303. Shephard R.J. (1974) Sudden death-a significant hazard of exercise. Br. J. Sports Med.,8:101.
304. Slocum D.B. and Larson R.L.(1968) Pes anserinus transplanatation. J. Bone Joint Surg. 50A,226.
305. Solcum D.B. and James S.(1968) Biomechanics of running. J.A. M.A. 205,721.
306. Solcum D.B., Larson R.L. and James S.L. (1973) Late reconstruction procedures used to stabilize the knee. Orthop. Clin. North Am. 4,679.
307. Smillies I.S.(1969) Knee injuries in athletes. Proc. R. Soc. Med. 62. 937.
308. Smillie I.S. (1973) Injuries of the noint, 4th ed. Edinburgh, Churchill Livingstone.
309. Soeur R. and Remy R. (1975) Fractures of the calcaneus with displacement of the thalmic portion. J.Bone Joint Surg. 57B, 413.
310. Sperryn P.N. (1973) Traumatic bursitis in aboxer's hand. Br. J. Sports Med. 7,103.
311. Subotnick S. (1975) Pediatric sports medicine. New York, Furtura Co.
312. Smith, Nothan J. The Pediatric clinics of North America. Philadelphia : W.B. Saunders Company, 1982.
313a. Schneider, Richard C., Kennnedy John C.; and Plant L. Marcus. Sports injuries, mechanism, prevention and treatment. Baltimore: Williams & Williams, 1985.
313b. Sunder Rajan Notes on Sports Medicine 1985 Madras.
314. Thorstenson, A., Hultin, B., Von Dobein, W., Karlsson, J. (1976). "The effects of strength training on enzyme activities and fiber characteristics in human skeletal muscle." Acta Physiol. Scand. 96:392.

315. Tomassoni Teresa, Blanchard, M.S., Gold Farb., A.H. (1985) : "Effects of a rebound exercise training programme on aerobic capacity and body composition", The Physician and Sports Medicine.

316. Tapper E.M. and Hoover N.W. (1969) Late results after. meniscectomy. J.Bone Joint Sssurg. 51A, 517.

317. Troup J.D.G.(1970) The risk of weight training and weight lifting in young people. Br. J.Sports Med.5,27.

318. Tucker W.E. and Armstrong J.R.(1964) Injury in sports. London, Staples Press.

319. Taylor, H.L., Baskirk, E. and Henschol, A(1955) : "Maximal oxygen uptake as an objective measure of cardio-respiratory performance", Jour. of Appl. Physiol. 8,73.

320. Von Itallie, T.B., Yang, M-U 1977. Diet and weight loss N. engl J. Med. 297: 1158-1161.

321. Valtonen E.J. and Busson M. (1978) A comparative study on ibuprofen and indomethacin in non-articular rheumatism. Scand. J.Rheum.7,183.

322. Van Marion W.F.(1973) Indomethacin in the treatment of soft tissue lesions. J.Int. Med. Res. 1,51.

323. Vanderhoof, E.R., Imig, C.J.and Hines, H.M. (1961) : "Effect of muscle strength and endurance development on bloodflow." J.Appl. Physiol. 16,873.

324. Vaidya, S.M. and Pansare, M.S. (1986) : "Effect of yoga on pulse and blood pressure, Unpublished work, paper presented in State Conf. of Assocn. of Sports Medicnie, Nagpur.

325. Vaccaro Paul and Clinton Mary (1981) : "The effects of aerobic dance conditioning on the body composition and maximal oxygen uptake of college women", J.Sports Med. 21:291-294.

326. Von Dobeln W., Astrand, I. and Bergestr'o M.A.(1967) : "An analysis of age and other factors related to maximal oxygen uptake", J.Appl. Physiol. 22:934.

327. Weber B.G. (1966) Die Verletzungen des oberen Sprungglenkes. Aktulle Problems in der Chirugie, Bd.3 Bern and Stuttgart, Huber.

328. Weightamn D. and Browne R.C.(1975) Injuries in eleven selected sports Br. J. Sports Med. 9, 136.

330. Williams J.G.P. (1976) injuries of the lower limbs. In Sports Medicine (Ed.Williams J.G.P. and Sperryn P.) London, Arnold. p.428.

331. Wiltse L.L. and Frantz C.H. (1956) Non-suppurative osteitis

pubis in the female. J.Bone Joint Surg. 38A, 500.
332. Williams J.G.P. Sports Medicine. London : Edward Arnold Publishers Ltd., 1962.
333. Williams, J.G.P. and Sperryn, P.N. Sports Medicine. London: Edward Arnold Publishers Ltd. 1982.
334. Wyndham, C.H. and N.B. Stry lom. The danger of an inadequate water intake during marathon runnings : S.Afr. Med. J., 43 : 893-896,1969.
335. Whyndharm, C.H., et al. : "Physioligical requirements for world class performance in endurance running", S. African Med. J., 41:996-1002., Aig., 1969.
336a. Williams, C.G., et al. : "The capacity for endurance work in highly trained trained man", Int. Z. angew, physiol, einschi. Arbeits physiologic, 26:141-149,1968.
336b. William D. McArle, Franki, Katch, Cictor L. Katch - Exercise Physiology (Energy, Nutrition and human Performance)-1981 (Published in Great Britain by Henry Kimpton Publishers, London).
337. Williams, J.G.P.: Medical aspects of sport and physical fitness. Pergamon, Oxford, 1965.
338. Williams, J.G.P. : Diagnostic pitfalls in the sportsman's knee, Proc. Roy. Soc. Med. 64.640,1971.
339. Williams, J.G.P.;Sperryh, P.N. : Sports Medicine. Edward Arnold. London, 1976.
340. Wilmore, J.H. (1969) : "Oxygen intake and its relationship to endurance capacity on a bicycle ergometer", Research Quarterly: 40-203.
341. Yogeshwar (1980) : "Textbook on yoga," Yoga Centre, 15, Mudhuram Manda, St. Mylapore, Madras 600 004.
342. Yang, M-U, Van Itallie, T.B. 1976. Composition of weight lost during short term weight reduction : metabolic responses of obese subjects to starvation and low-calorie ketogenic and non-ketogenic diets. J. Clin Invest 58:722-730.
343. Zadik F.R.(1950) Obliteration of the nail bed of the great toe without shortening the terminal phalanx. J. Bone Joint Surg. 32B,66.
344. Zuckerman, J.and Stull, G.A. (1969) : "Effect of exercise on knee ligament separation force in rates", Jour. Appl. Physiol. 26,716.